Chronic Intestinal Diseases of Dogs and Cats

Guest Editor

FRÉDÉRIC P. GASCHEN, Dr med vet, Dr habil

VETERINARY CLINICS OF NORTH AMERICA: SMALL ANIMAL PRACTICE

www.vetsmall.theclinics.com

March 2011 • Volume 41 • Number 2

SAUNDERS an imprint of ELSEVIER, Inc.

W.B. SAUNDERS COMPANY
A Division of Elsevier Inc.

1600 John F. Kennedy Blvd. ● Suite 1800 ● Philadelphia, PA 19103-2899
http://www.vetsmall.theclinics.com

**VETERINARY CLINICS OF NORTH AMERICA: SMALL ANIMAL PRACTICE Volume 41, Number 2
March 2011 ISSN 0195-5616, ISBN-13: 978-1-4557-0682-2**

Editor: John Vassallo; j.vassallo@elsevier.com

Veterinary Clinics of North America: Small Animal Practice (ISSN 0195-5616) is published bimonthly (For Post Office use only: volume 41 issue 2 of 6) by Elsevier Inc., 360 Park Avenue South, New York, NY 10010-1710. Months of issue are January, March, May, July, September, and November. Business and Editorial Offices: 1600 John F. Kennedy Blvd., Ste. 1800, Philadelphia, PA 19103-2899. Customer Service Office: 3251 Riverport Lane, Maryland Heights, MO 63043. Periodicals postage paid at New York, NY and additional mailing offices. Subscription prices are $262.00 per year (domestic individuals), $427.00 per year (domestic institutions), $128.00 per year (domestic students/residents), $347.00 per year (Canadian individuals), $525.00 per year (Canadian institutions), $385.00 per year (international individuals), $525.00 per year (international institutions), and $186.00 per year (international and Canadian students/residents). To receive student/resident rate, orders must be accompanied by name of affiliated institution, date of term, and the *signature* of program/residency coordinator on institution letterhead. Orders will be billed at individual rate until proof of status is received. Foreign air speed delivery is included in all *Clinics* subscription prices. All prices are subject to change without notice. **POSTMASTER:** Send address changes to *Veterinary Clinics of North America: Small Animal Practice*, Elsevier Health Sciences Division, Subscription Customer Service, 3251 Riverport Lane, Maryland Heights, MO 63043. Customer Service (orders, claims, online, change of address): Elsevier Periodicals Customer Service, Elsevier Health Sciences Division Subscription Customer Service 3251 Riverport Lane Maryland Heights, MO 63043. Tel: 1-800-654-2452 (U.S. and Canada); 314-447-8871 (outside U.S. and Canada). Fax: 314-447-8029. E-mail: journalscustomerservice-usa@elsevier.com (for print support); journalsonlinesupport-usa@elsevier.com (for online support).

Reprints. For copies of 100 or more of articles in this publication, please contact the Commercial Reprints Department, Elsevier Inc., 360 Park Avenue South, New York, NY 10010-1710. Tel.: 212-633-3812; Fax: 212-462-1935; E-mail: reprints@elsevier.com.

Veterinary Clinics of North America: Small Animal Practice is also published in Japanese by Inter Zoo Publishing Co., Ltd., Aoyama Crystal-Bldg 5F, 3-5-12 Kitaoyama, Minato-ku, Tokyo 107-0061, Japan.

Veterinary Clinics of North America: Small Animal Practice is covered in *Current Contents/Agriculture, Biology and Environmental Sciences, Science Citation Index, ASCA, MEDLINE/PubMed (Index Medicus), Excerpta Medica,* and *BIOSIS.*

Printed in the United States of America.

Contributors

GUEST EDITOR

FRÉDÉRIC P. GASCHEN, Dr med vet, Dr habil
Diplomate, American College of Veterinary Internal Medicine (Small Animal Internal Medicine); Diplomate, European College of Veterinay Internal Medicine–Companion Animals (Internal Medicine); M.L. Martin Professor of Companion Animal Medicine, Department of Veterinary Clinical Sciences, School of Veterinary Medicine, Louisiana State University, Baton Rouge, Louisiana

AUTHORS

KARIN ALLENSPACH, Dr med vet, FVH, PhD, FHEA, MRCVS
Diplomate, European College of Veterinary Internal Medicine–Companion Animals; Senior Lecturer Internal Medicine, Royal Veterinary College, University of London, North Mymms, United Kingdom

NORA BERGHOFF, Dr med vet
Graduate Assistant Research, Gastrointestinal Laboratory, Department of Small Animal Clinical Sciences, College of Veterinary Medicine, Texas A&M University, College Station, Texas

MELANIE CRAVEN, BVetMed, PhD, MRCVS
Diplomate, European College of Veterinary Internal Medicine–Companion Animals; Department of Veterinary Clinical Sciences, Cornell University, Ithaca, New York

OLIVIER DOSSIN, DVM, PhD
Diplomate, European College of Veterinary Internal Medicine–Companion Animals, Internal Medicine; Associate Professor, Department of Clinical Sciences, National Veterinary School, Toulouse, France

FRÉDÉRIC P. GASCHEN, Dr med vet, Dr habil
Diplomate, American College of Veterinary Internal Medicine (Small Animal Internal Medicine); Diplomate, European College of Veterinary Internal Medicine–Companion Animals (Internal Medicine); M.L. Martin Professor of Companion Animal Medicine, Department of Veterinary Clinical Sciences, School of Veterinary Medicine, Louisiana State University, Baton Rouge, Louisiana

LORRIE GASCHEN, PhD, DVM, Dr med vet
Professor of Diagnostic Imaging, Department of Veterinary Clinical Sciences, School of Veterinary Medicine, Louisiana State University, Baton Rouge, Louisiana

TRACY GIEGER, DVM
Diplomate, American College of Veterinary Internal Medicine (Small Animal Internal Medicine and Oncology); Diplomate, American College of Veterinary Radiology (Radiation Oncology); Assistant Professor of Veterinary Medical and Radiation Oncology, Department of Veterinary Clinical Sciences, School of Veterinary Medicine, Louisiana State University, Baton Rouge, Louisiana

EDWARD J. HALL, MA, VetMB, PhD, MRCVS
Diplomate, European College of Veterinary Internal Medicine–Companion Animals;
Professor of Small Animal Internal Medicine, School of Veterinary Sciences,
University of Bristol, Langford, Bristol, England

ALBERT E. JERGENS, DVM, MS, PhD
Diplomate, American College of Veterinary Internal Medicine; Professor,
Veterinary Clinical Sciences, Lloyd Veterinary Medical Center, College of Veterinary
Medicine, Iowa State University, Ames, Iowa

RACHEL LAVOUÉ, DVM, MSc
Assistant Professor, Department of Clinical Sciences, National Veterinary School,
Toulouse, France

PATRICK LECOINDRE, Dr med vet
Diplomate, European College of Veterinary Internal Medicine–Companion Animals,
Clinique Vétérinaire des Cerisioz, St Priest, France

JOANNE MANSELL, DVM, MS
Diplomate, American College of Veterinary Pathologists; Professor of Pathobiology,
Department of Pathobiology, College of Veterinary Medicine, Texas A&M University,
College Station, Texas

CAROLINE S. MANSFIELD, BVMS, MVM
Diplomate, European College of Veterinary Internal Medicine-Companion Animal;
University of Melbourne, Victoria, Australia

SANDRA R. MERCHANT, DVM
Diplomate, American College of Veterinary Dermatology; Professor of Veterinary
Dermatology, Department of Veterinary Clinical Sciences, School of Veterinary Medicine,
Louisiana State University, Baton Rouge, Louisiana

KENNETH W. SIMPSON, BVM&S, PhD
Diplomate, American College of Veterinary Internal Medicine; Diplomate, European
College Veterinary Internal Medicine–Companion Animals; Professor, Veterinary Clinical
Sciences, College of Veterinary Medicine, Cornell University, Ithaca, New York

JÖRG M. STEINER, Dr med vet, PhD
Diplomate, American College of Veterinary Internal Medicine; Diplomate, European
College of Veterinary Internal Medicine–Companion Animals; Director, Gastrointestinal
Laboratory; Associate Professor, Department of Small Animal Clinical Sciences,
College of Veterinary Medicine, Texas A&M University, College Station, Texas

JAN S. SUCHODOLSKI, med vet, Dr med vet, PhD
Department of Small Animal Clinical Sciences, Gastrointestinal Laboratory,
College of Veterinary Medicine, Texas A&M University, College Station, Texas

J. SCOTT WEESE, DVM, DVSc
Diplomate, American College of Veterinary Internal Medicine; Associate Professor,
Department of Pathobiology, Centre for Public Health and Zoonoses, Ontario Veterinary
College, University of Guelph, Guelph, Ontario, Canada

MICHAEL WILLARD, DVM, MS
Diplomate, American College of Veterinary Internal Medicine; Professor of Small Animal
Clinical Sciences, Department of Small Animal Clinical Sciences, College of Veterinary
Medicine, Texas A&M University, College Station, Texas

Contents

Gut microbes play a crucial role in the regulation of host health, but the true complexity of the gastrointestinal microbiota has been underestimated using traditional culture techniques. Recent molecular-phylogenetic and metagenomic studies have revealed a highly diverse microbial community in the canine and feline gastrointestinal tract of healthy animals, consisting of bacteria, archaea, fungi, protozoa, and viruses. Alterations in microbial communities have also been reported in dogs and cats with chronic enteropathies, notably increases in Proteobacteria and depletions of Firmicutes. This review summarizes the current information about the intestinal microbial ecosystem in dogs and cats.

Antibiotic-responsive diarrhea (ARD) is an idiopathic syndrome causing chronic diarrhea in young, large-breed dogs. Why antibiotics are effective in controlling diarrhea is not understood, and whether small intestinal bacterial numbers are truly increased is now doubted, but previous focus on the condition being small intestinal bacterial overgrowth has hampered the understanding of this condition. The name ARD simply defines the condition, and studies are now looking at the interaction of small intestinal bacteria and the mucosa to try to understand why it occurs.

A variety of bacteria are known or suspected of being able to cause enteritis in dogs and cats. *Campylobacter* spp, *Clostridium difficile*, *Clostridium perfringens*, and *Salmonella* spp are most commonly implicated, but many other organisms are likely involved. Poor understanding of the intestinal microflora and the fact that many, if not all, of these microorganisms can also be found in healthy individuals complicates testing, thereby affecting the use of specific treatments and assessment of potential infection control and zoonotic disease risks. An understanding of the strengths and limitations of various diagnostic options is important for the management of canine and feline enteritis.

Chronic enteropathies are commonly encountered in both cats and dogs. Although definitive diagnosis often requires collection of gastrointestinal biopsies for histopathologic evaluation, less invasive laboratory tests can be highly informative and should be performed prior to biopsy collection. Tests for determination of infectious causes comprise those for helminthic, protozoal, bacterial, or fungal organisms. Intestinal function and disease may be assessed by measuring serum concentrations of cobalamin, folate, and C-reactive protein, and fecal concentrations of α_1-proteinase inhibitor. Ongoing research has led to development of tests for serum perinuclear antineutrophilic cytoplasmic antibodies, and fecal inflammatory markers, including S100-proteins and N-methylhistamine.

Ultrasonography, which has become a mainstay of diagnosing intestinal diseases in dogs and cats, is often one of the first diagnostic tools used to differentiate inflammatory from neoplastic infiltration of the small intestine. Although overlap in the sonographic appearances of inflammatory and neoplastic infiltration make a definitive diagnosis difficult, awareness of features of both diseases is important for the accurate interpretation of the sonographic findings. Full-thickness intestinal biopsy remains the gold standard for differentiating inflammatory from neoplastic disease of the small intestine.

The mucosal immune system is at the forefront of defense against invading pathogens, but at the same time, it must maintain tolerance toward commensals and food antigens in the intestinal lumen. The interplay between the innate immune response and commensal microorganisms is essential to maintaining this balance. Great progress has been made in identifying some of the genetic predispositions underlying inflammatory bowel disease in certain breeds, such as the German shepherd dog. Several immunologic markers are discussed with respect to their clinical usefulness in the diagnosis and management of inflammatory bowel disease.

Adverse food reactions (AFR) are a common problem that may cause cutaneous and/or gastrointestinal signs in dogs and cats. They comprise food intolerance, food intoxication, and food allergy. Response to a dietary elimination trial and recurrence of signs during dietary provocation remain the centerpiece of diagnosis and management of dogs and cats with AFR. Response to an elimination trial is frequently observed in dogs and cats with chronic idiopathic enteropathies. However, only a fraction of them relapse after a dietary challenge. These animals may have mild to enteritis and/or colitis and benefit from various additional properties of the elimination diet.

E coli pathotype, "adherent and invasive *E coli*," that are increasingly associated with Crohn's disease in humans. Successful treatment of GC requires antimicrobials that are effective against *E coli* and penetrate intracellularly. Enrofloxacin is widely regarded as the antibiotic of choice.

FORTHCOMING ISSUES

RECENT ISSUES

RELATED INTEREST

THE CLINICS ARE NOW AVAILABLE ONLINE!

Access your subscription at:
www.theclinics.com

Preface

Chronic Intestinal Diseases of Dogs and Cats—Update from the 21ˢᵗ Century

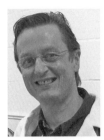

Frédéric P. Gaschen, Dr med vet, Dr habil
Guest Editor

It is very exciting to see this issue of the *Veterinary Clinics of North America: Small Animal Practice* devoted to chronic intestinal disorders in print. Eight long years have gone by since the last issue focusing on small animal gastroenterology was published. Meanwhile, numerous research groups have investigated important issues in the vast field of chronic enteropathies in small animals in many parts of the world, even though it does sometimes feel like we are moving one step forward and then two steps backward in our understanding of these diseases. Despite the fact that each question researchers attempt to answer has the potential to reveal several new questions that need to be investigated, a lot of new data are available that are relevant for small animal veterinarians. It is the goal of this volume to bring the reader up to date.

Some of the best international experts have accepted to write outstanding reviews in their field of research or clinical expertise in this issue, and I am very grateful to all of them who invested a lot of time in this volume's articles. I also want to thank Mr John Vassallo and the staff at Elsevier for their support and flexibility.

The topics include the intestinal flora, a world we cannot ignore any more, as it exerts a major influence on the digestive health of our patients. Other authors will show what hides behind the term "antibiotic-responsive diarrhea," and also what bacteria to consider when infectious enteritis is suspected. Additionally, very practical contributions on laboratory diagnosis and small intestinal ultrasound will be helpful for the diagnostic workup. Our knowledge of gastrointestinal immunology in dogs and cats has exploded and constitutes an essential basis for our understanding of inflammatory bowel disease, protein-losing enteropathies, and adverse reactions to food, which are hot topics for small animal veterinarians. Help is also available in this volume for diagnosis and treatment of alimentary lymphoma, a neoplasia that can be difficult to

Vet Clin Small Anim 41 (2011) xi–xii
doi:10.1016/j.cvsm.2011.02.006
vetsmall.theclinics.com

differentiate from IBD, especially in cats. The article on granulomatous colitis of boxers and English bulldogs is written by the clinicians and researchers who revolutionized our understanding of the disease. The confusing topic of idiopathic large bowel diarrhea in dogs is also revisited. Finally, two experts comment on what correlation can be expected between clinical disease activity and histopathological assessment of gastrointestinal lesion severity and conclude this comprehensive update from the 21st century.

I hope that the reader will come back to this volume regularly and be able to use it to answer important clinical questions.

Frédéric P. Gaschen, Dr med vet, Dr habil
Department of Veterinary Clinical Sciences
School of Veterinary Medicine
Louisiana State University
Baton Rouge, LA 70803, USA

E-mail address:
fgaschen@lsu.edu

Intestinal Microbiota of Dogs and Cats: a Bigger World than We Thought

Jan S. Suchodolski, med vet, Dr med vet, PhD

KEYWORDS

- Feline • Canine • Gastrointestinal • 16S rRNA gene
- Microflora • Microbiota • Gastrointestinal tract
- Metagenomics

Recent molecular studies have revealed that the mammalian gastrointestinal (GI) tract harbors a highly complex microbiota that includes bacteria, archaea, fungi, protozoa, and viruses. The total microbial load in the intestine is estimated to range between 10^{12} to 10^{14} organisms, about 10 times the number of host cells. It is estimated that several thousand bacterial phylotypes reside in the GI tract.[1–3] The gene content of these microbes is defined as the intestinal microbiome. Gut microbes play a crucial role in the regulation of host health, by stimulating the immune system and development of gut structure, aiding in the defense against invading pathogens and providing nutritional benefit to the host (ie, production of short chain fatty acids, vitamin B12). In contrast, a microbial dysbiosis has been identified in dogs and cats with GI disease (**Table 1**).[4–9]

This review summarizes current information about the intestinal microbial ecosystem in dogs and cats.

INTESTINAL BACTERIA
Methods for Characterization of the Intestinal Microbiome

Bacterial culture

Cultivation methods are most useful when targeting a specific pathogen in clinical specimens (eg, *Salmonella*). Culture assesses the viability of organisms and allows antimicrobial susceptibility testing. Isolates can be genotyped for epidemiologic studies. Culture is also valuable for characterizing the metabolic properties of isolates and their virulence factors.

The author has nothing to disclose.

Department of Small Animal Clinical Sciences, Gastrointestinal Laboratory, College of Veterinary Medicine and Biomedical Sciences, Texas A&M University, College Station, TX 77843-4474, USA

E-mail address: jsuchodolski@cvm.tamu.edu

Table 1
Alterations in bacterial groups observed in dogs and cats with GI disease

Refs.	Sample Material	Diagnosis	Method	Microbial Alterations
Dogs				
Suchodolski et al[4]	Duodenal biopsies	IBD	Comparative 16S rRNA gene analysis	↑Proteobacteria ↓Clostridia (class)
Allenspach et al[48]	Duodenal brush samples	GSD with food- or antibiotic-responsive diarrhea	Comparative 16S rRNA gene analysis	↑Streptococcus and Abiotrophia spp
Jergens et al[35]	Duodenal biopsies	IBD	16S rRNA gene 454-pyrosequencing	↑Proteobacteria ↓Clostridium cluster XIVa and IV (ie, Faecalibacterium, Ruminococcus, Dorea spp)
Xenoulis et al[5]	Duodenal brush samples	IBD	Comparative 16S rRNA gene analysis	↑E coli ↓Microbial diversity
Craven et al[49]	Duodenal biopsies	Chronic enteropathies (steroid-, food-, and antibiotic-responsive)	16S rRNA gene 454 pyrosequencing	↓Microbial diversity
Simpson et al[50]	Colonic biopsies	Boxer dogs with granulomatous colitis	Fluorescence in-situ hybridization	Intraepithelial invasion of adherent and invasive E coli
Jia et al[9]	Feces	Chronic diarrhea	Fluorescence in-situ hybridization	↑Bacteroides
Bell et al[7]	Feces	Diarrhea	Terminal restriction fragment polymorphism	↑Clostridium perfringens, Enterococcus spp
Cats				
Janeczko et al[6]	Small intestinal biopsies	IBD	Fluorescence in-situ hybridization	↑Enterobacteriaceae
Inness et al[8]	Feces	Small and large bowel IBD	Fluorescence in-situ hybridization	↓total bacterial load ↓Bifidobacterium spp, Bacteroides ↑Desulfovibrio spp

Abbreviations: GSD, German Shepherd dog; IBD, irritable bowel disease.

It is now well recognized that bacterial cultivation techniques do not yield sufficient information about the microbial diversity in complex biologic ecosystems because of their significant limitations. Firstly, there is currently not enough information available about the optimal growth requirements of most microorganisms, which explains why only a minority of intestinal microbes can be recovered on culture mediums. Secondly, the GI tract harbors predominantly anaerobic bacteria, which may be more prone to damage during sample handling. Thirdly, many microbes live in mutualistic interactions with other microorganisms or the host, and this hinders their growth on culture media. Additionally, many selective culture media lack sufficient specificity and often other organisms than the targets are enumerated.[10] Finally, phenotypic and biochemical identification systems frequently fail to accurately classify many microorganisms residing in the gut. Therefore, DNA sequencing of culture isolates is often required. Because of these limitations, it is estimated that only a small fraction (<5%) of intestinal bacteria can be cultivated, and a much smaller fraction can be correctly identified and classified.

Molecular tools

Because bacterial culture underestimates microbial diversity in the GI tract, molecular tools have now become the standard approach in gut microbial ecology.[1,2,11–14] For molecular analysis, DNA or RNA is extracted from intestinal samples (eg, feces, biopsy specimen, luminal content). For phylogenetic identification or for molecular fingerprinting, a specific gene is amplified using universal primers (either bacterial, fungal, or archaeal) that target conserved regions within these genes. The conserved regions flank variable gene regions, which when sequenced allow the phylogenetic identification of the present organisms. For bacterial and archaeal identification, the 16S ribosomal RNA (16S rRNA) gene is most commonly targeted. Other targets include the 16S-23S internal transcribed spacer (ITS) region and the chaperonin (cpn60) gene.[12]

Molecular fingerprinting Molecular fingerprinting is used to separate a mixture of polymerase chain reaction (PCR) amplicons that were generated by universal primers to yield a fingerprint, which is representative of the bacterial community within the sample. Different techniques include denaturing gradient gel electrophoresis (DGGE), temperature gradient gel electrophoresis (TGGE), and terminal restriction fragment length polymorphism (T-RFLP).[7,15–19] In DGGE and TGGE, differences in nucleotide composition result in unique melting behaviors of the individual PCR amplicons, generating a banding pattern that illustrates the bacterial diversity in the sample. DGGE and TGGE are inexpensive and can be rapidly performed. However, DGGE and TGGE only allow a limited resolution of PCR amplicons because many bacterial phylotypes may have similar melting behaviors. Therefore, these techniques capture only changes in the predominant bacterial groups within the gut community. For identification purposes, bands of interest need to be sequenced. In T-RFLP, amplicons labeled with a fluorescent primer are fragmented in different sizes using sequence specific restriction enzymes, again yielding a characteristic fingerprint of the microbial community.[7]

Identification of bacterial groups For identification of individual bacterial phylotypes, PCR amplicons generated using universal bacterial primers need to be separated and sequenced, which can be achieved by construction of 16S rRNA gene clone libraries,[11,12,20] or more recently by an automated high-throughput sequencing platform (eg, 454-pyrosequencing). This platform allows several thousand sequences to be analyzed within a few hours, yielding deep phylogenetic information about the intestinal microbiome.[1,2,13]

Quantification of bacterial groups Commonly used methods for quantification of bacterial groups are quantitative real-time PCR (qPCR)[12,18] and fluorescent in-situ hybridization (FISH).[6] The use of FISH is currently considered to be the most accurate method for quantification of bacterial groups because it allows direct microscopic counting of fluorescence-labeled bacteria. Furthermore, the location of bacteria with regard to the epithelium (ie, intracellular, adherent, or invasive) can be visualized.

Limitations of molecular methods It is important to realize that molecular methods have some limitations. The use of different DNA extraction methods (eg, bead beating steps, heating in lysis buffer)[1,13] and the use of different PCR primers will yield slightly different results between studies.[12,21] For example, some commonly used PCR primers underestimate the presence of specific bacterial groups, especially those with a high guanine-cytosine content (eg, *Bifidobacterium* spp),[11,21] and some investigators use either a primer mix or group-specific primers for more accurate amplification.[22] Because of the high bacterial diversity in the intestine, groups of low abundance constitute such a low proportion of total bacteria that they escape identification even when high-throughput sequencing techniques using broad-range primers are employed. The additional use of group-specific PCR assays is needed to detect these groups of interest. Furthermore, PCR can exhibit bias in quantification of specific bacterial groups. For example, the bacterial 16S rRNA gene is organized in so-called operons. These operons can vary in number from 1 to 15 within individual bacterial phylotypes. The operon number may also change during the growth phase and changed activity of cells.[23] Therefore, the proportions of bacterial groups with higher operon numbers may be overestimated in 16S rRNA gene libraries or by qPCR, and caution should be used to directly relate molecular results to absolute cell counts. Because of the high diversity of the microbial community, no optimal DNA extraction protocol or PCR-based identification method exists for accurate characterization of all microorganisms, and the various methods available should be used complementarily.

Metagenomics and transcriptomics The amplification of a specific gene (eg, 16S rRNA gene) allows identification of intestinal bacteria and has yielded comprehensive information about which bacterial groups are present in the canine and feline GI tract. However, because only one single gene is evaluated in comparative 16S rRNA gene analysis, these methods yield only phylogenetic information (answering the question: who is there?). They do not provide information about the functional properties of the intestinal microbiome. The microbiota differs substantially at the species and strain level in each individual animal.[2,15,17] Despite these phylogenetic differences, the metabolic end products of the gastrointestinal microbiome are similar between individuals. Also, although some environmental influences (eg, diet, fasting) may lead to changes in bacterial groups, these changes are not immediately associated with any major alterations in gut physiology in healthy animals. For example, antibiotic administration has a profound impact on the composition of gut microbiota but these microbial changes do not correlate with gut function.[1,24] Therefore, for a better understanding of microbial-host interactions in health and disease, the functionality of the intestinal microbiome needs to be explored. New high-throughput sequencing platforms facilitate rapid sequencing of total genomic DNA or mRNA without prior amplification of specific genes. Therefore, in addition to phylogenetic identification of microorganisms, these techniques yield information about the gene content (metagenomics) or the expressed genes (transcriptomics) within the microbiome, and may therefore define the functional potential of the microbiome.[14,25] Metagenomic approaches have revealed the existence of a core microbiome in the mammalian intestine. Despite differences in abundance and prevalence of specific bacterial phylotypes, individuals possess similar microbial genes and metabolic pathways,[14,25] which indicates a functional redundancy of the gastrointestinal microbiota.[24] The various members of the microbial community perform similar functions, and if one group is depressed because of external factors (eg, antibiotic therapy), other members of the community are capable of maintaining the functionality within the ecosystem. These findings emphasize the need for evaluating both phylogenetic relationships and metabolic functions (ie, metagenomics and transcriptomics) of the intestinal microbiome.

Bacteria in the GI tract of dogs and cats

Cultivation results Much of the published data describing the composition of the gastrointestinal microbial ecosystem in dogs and cats has been generated using bacterial cultivation techniques.[26–30] These studies have revealed that total bacterial counts in the stomach range between 10^1 and 10^6 cfu/g or ml.[26] The bacterial load in the duodenum and jejunum of dogs and cats shows pronounced individual variations. Duodenal bacterial counts are low in most dogs (<10^3 cfu/g or ml of duodenal aspirates), but they may reach up 10^9 cfu/g or ml in some dogs.[29,30] The feline duodenum reportedly harbors higher bacterial counts (10^5–10^8 cfu/g or ml), and anaerobic bacteria (*Bacteroides* spp, *Fusobacterium* spp, *Eubacterium* spp) appear to predominate unlike in dogs.[29] The bacterial counts found in the proximal small intestine of some healthy dogs and cats are substantially higher than typically found in humans, where bacterial counts greater than 10^5 cfu/g or ml of small bowel aspirates indicate small intestinal bacterial overgrowth (SIBO). Although initial studies in dogs defined SIBO based on the same numerical criteria as in humans (bacterial counts >10^5 cfu/g or ml for aerobes or >10^4 cfu/g or ml for anaerobes),[31] subsequent investigations showed that healthy dogs can have bacterial counts that by far exceed those proposed cutoffs.[30] Therefore, the use of the term SIBO is now controversial in dogs, and authors prefer the terms antibiotic-responsive diarrhea or small intestinal dysbiosis. SIBO has not been reported in the cat based on the higher physiologic bacterial counts found in that species.[28]

Bacterial concentrations increase aborally along the length of the gastrointestinal tract. The ileum harbors approx. 10^7 cfu/g or ml, whereas bacterial counts in the colon of dogs and cats range between 10^9 and 10^{11} cfu/g or ml of intestinal content. *Bacteroides, Clostridium, Lactobacillus, Bifidobacterium* spp, and *Enterobacteriaceae* are the predominant bacterial groups that have been cultured from canine and feline intestine.

Molecular tools Molecular tools have revealed high numbers of previously unrecognized species in the mammalian GI tract. It is estimated that several thousand bacterial phylotypes inhabit the human colon.[32] Recent high-throughput sequencing studies (based on 454 pyrosequencing of the 16S rRNA gene) have estimated that approximately 200 bacterial species and 900 bacterial strains reside in the canine jejunum[1]; whereas, several thousand phylotypes are thought to be present in fecal samples of dogs and cats.[2] Ten to 12 different bacterial phyla are routinely identified in the mammalian GI tract.[2,12,13,21] Of these, the phyla Firmicutes, Bacteroidetes, and Fusobacteria make the majority of gut microbiota (approximately 95%), followed by Proteobacteria and Actinobacteria, which constitute typically 1% to 5% of total bacteria identified by sequencing.[2,13] The phyla Spirochaetes, Tenericutes, Verrucomicrobia, TM7, Cyanobacteria, Chloroflexi, Planctomycetes, and a few currently unclassified bacterial lineages constitute typically less than 1% of obtained bacterial sequences.

The abundance of these bacterial groups varies along the length of the GI tract as shown by 16S rRNA gene analysis. In the stomach, *Helicobacter* spp represented 99%

of identified sequences in one study; whereas, the remaining 1% consisted of lactic acid bacterial populations and Clostridia spp.[33] Ten and 11 different bacterial phyla were identified in the proximal small intestine of dogs[1] and cats (Suchodolski, unpublished data, 2010), respectively. Firmicutes (mainly Clostridiales and Lactobacillales), Bacteroidetes, Proteobacteria, and Actinobacteria constituted approximately 95% of sequences.

Firmicutes (mainly Clostridiales), Bacteroides, and Fusobacteria have been reported to be the predominant bacterial phyla in the colon and feces of dogs and cats.[2,11,13,14,20,21] However, the observed abundance of these bacterial groups differs between studies. For example, percentages of Firmicutes range between 25% and 95% of obtained 16S rRNA gene sequencing tags.[2,13] These wide ranges are most likely caused by differences in DNA extraction methods and selection of different universal PCR primers. In contrast to results from 16S rRNA gene-based studies, Actinobacteria were documented to be abundant in feline feces in a comparative chaperonin 60 gene analysis.[12] This finding is not surprising because it has been shown that 16S rRNA gene approaches routinely underestimate the abundance of Actinobacteria in intestinal samples when universal bacterial primers are used.[21] In contrast, the use of group-specific primers for Bifidobacterium spp, members of the phylum Actinobacteria, or the use of FISH analysis with Bifidobacterium species-specific probes confirm that this bacterial group is present in the intestinal tract of the majority of dogs and cats.[8,9,21] In a recent metagenomic study, the Bacteroidetes/Chlorobi group and Firmicutes represented each approximately 35% of sequences obtained from canine feces, followed by Proteobacteria (15%) and Fusobacteria (8%). Actinobacteria (including Bifidobacterium spp) represented only 1% of obtained sequences.[14] Similar results were observed in feline fecal samples analyzed by a metagenomic approach.[34]

Firmicutes, which are a highly abundant bacterial phylum in all parts of the canine and feline gastrointestinal tract, are represented mainly by the bacterial order Clostridiales, which in turn is organized into phylogenetically distinct Clostridium clusters. These clusters differ in abundance among the different parts of the intestine.[11,20] Clostridium clusters XIVa and IV make up approximately 60% of all Clostridiales, and encompass many important short-chain fatty acids producing bacteria, such as Ruminococcus spp, Faecalibacterium spp, Dorea spp, and Turicibacter spp. These latter groups are consistently depleted in humans and dogs with acute or chronic enteropathies, emphasizing the importance of these bacterial groups in intestinal health (see **Table 1**).[4,35,36]

Molecular fingerprinting has also demonstrated that every individual dog and cat has a unique and stable microbial ecosystem.[15,17,21] All animals harbor similar bacterial groups when analyzed on a higher phylogenetic level (ie, family or genus level), but the microbiome of each animal differs substantially on a species/strain level, with typically only a 5% to 20% overlap of bacterial species between individual animals. For example, a recent study has shown that only a small percentage (<30%) of dogs and cats harbored the same species of Bifidobacterium spp.[2,21]

OTHER MEMBERS OF THE INTESTINAL ECOSYSTEM

In addition to bacteria, the mammalian gastrointestinal tract harbors a diverse mixture of microorganisms, including fungi, archaea, protozoa, and viruses (mostly bacteriophages). Molecular tools have provided information about the species richness of these microbes, but their role in gastrointestinal health needs to be further elucidated.

Fungal Organisms

Cultivation studies have documented the presence of yeasts and molds in the intestine of approximately 25% of healthy Beagle dogs, with fungal counts ranging from

10^1 cfu/g jejunal content to 10^5 cfu/g of feces, respectively.[26,27,37] Using a PCR assay with universal fungal primers targeting the ITS region, fungal DNA was detected in the small intestine in 39 of 64 (61%) healthy dogs and in 54 of 71 (76%) dogs with chronic enteropathies.[38] Marked differences in the prevalence of different fungi was observed between animals. A total of 51 different fungal phylotypes were identified across all 135 dogs, with the majority harboring only 1.[38] Saccharomycetes were the most commonly identified fungal class, and no significant differences in the prevalence of specific fungal phylotypes were observed between healthy and diseased dogs.[38] Fungi were found to adhere to the intestinal mucosa more frequently than they were detected in the luminal content.[38,39]

Recent high-throughput sequencing data based on 454 pyrosequencing of the 18S rRNA gene revealed 4 fungal phyla in canine and feline fecal samples, with the majority of sequences belonging to the phyla Ascomycota (>90%) and Neocallimastigomycota (>5%).[40] Fungi were present in all 19 evaluated animals, with each animal harboring multiple fungal species, with a median of 40 phylotypes (**Table 2**).[40] Remarkable interanimal differences were observed as each dog harbored a unique profile. Although most dogs harbored similar fungal phyla, each animal had a unique species population.[40]

There is no data describing the precise abundance of fungi in the gastrointestinal tract of healthy dogs and cats. Studies in humans using FISH analysis have estimated fungal abundance as less than 0.3% of the total fecal microbiota.[41] In a recent metagenomic study,[14] the numerical abundance of fungi in canine fecal samples was estimated to be approximately 0.01% of obtained sequences. A similar abundance was observed in a metagenomic analysis of feline feces.[34]

Archaea

Archaea are evolutionarily distinct from bacteria and eukaryotes, and are classified as the third domain of life. Archaea are obligate anaerobes. They are part of the normal

Table 2
Predominant fungal families identified in feces of 12 dogs

Fungal Family	Mean of Total Fungal Sequences (%)	Number of Dogs Positive
Wickerhamomycetaceae	13.78	11
Saccharomycetaceae	12.86	9
Pleosporaceae	12.20	10
Schizothyriaceae	11.68	12
Ophiocordycipitaceae	8.07	11
Taphrinaceae	7.32	11
Trichocomaceae	4.80	12
Papulosaceae	3.71	10
Davidiellaceae	3.28	7
Dothioraceae	2.92	9
Ustilaginaceae	2.84	6
Phaeosphaeriaceae	2.08	6
Hypocreaceae	1.78	6
Sordariaceae	1.49	1
Massarinaceae	1.10	9
Other	10.08	N/A

Data was obtained using high-throughput pyrosequencing of the fungal 18S rRNA gene.
Abbreviation: N/A, not applicable.

intestinal flora in ruminants and have also been characterized in human intestinal samples, with Methanobacteria being the predominant form.[42] The role of archaea in gastrointestinal health is unclear. Hydrogen is an end product generated by other intestinal microbes as a result of microbial fermentation and is metabolized by methanogens and sulfate-reducing bacteria (SRB), which produce methane and hydrogen sulfite, respectively. Hydrogen consumption by methanogens and SRB is an important scavenging pathway. An abnormal accumulation of hydrogen would inhibit further microbial fermentation, resulting in a decreased production of short-chain fatty acids. An imbalance of SRB to methanogens may result in increased production of hydrogen sulfite, which has the potential to damage epithelial cells.[43] Initial studies have revealed a higher abundance of sulfite-producing bacteria in the colon of cats with inflammatory bowel disease (IBD).[8]

In a comparative 16S rRNA gene analysis with universal archaeal primers, 2 archaeal phyla were observed in the intestine of dogs and cats: Crenarchaeota and Euryarchaeota (Suchodolski and colleagues, unpublished data, 2010). Similar to humans, Methanobacteria (ie, *Methanosphaera, Methanobrevibacter*) were the most abundant archaeal class (**Box 1**). Recent metagenomic studies in fecal samples of

---

Box 1
Archaeal genera identified in canine and feline fecal samples by 16S rRNA gene sequencing or metagenomic approaches

Archaeal genera identified in canine and feline fecal samples

Ferroplasma

Haloarcula

Ignisphaera

Methanobrevibacter

Methanocaldococcus

Methanococcoides

Methanococcus

Methanocorpusculum

Methanoculleus

Methanopyrus

Methanoregula

Methanosaeta

Methanosarcina

Methanosphaera

Methanospirillum

Methanothermobacter

Pyrococcus

Thermococcus

Thermoplasma

Thermosphaera

dogs and cats revealed the numerical abundance of archaea as 1.1% of total microbiota.[14] Methanogens were the most abundant and diverse group.

Viruses

Because of the heterogeneity of viruses (ie, DNA viruses, RNA viruses, ssDNA viruses), an approach with universal primers, the preferred method for bacteria, archaea, and fungi, is not possible. Therefore, it remains challenging to characterize the viral communities present in the intestine of dogs and cats. Reported viral phylotypes include rotavirus, coronavirus, parvovirus, norovirus, astrovirus, distemper virus, and paramyxovirus.[44–46] The coinfection rate with multiple viruses is suspected to be low. In a recent study using electron microscopy, only 6.5% of 935 evaluated fecal samples contained more than 1 virus.[44] However, recent metagenomic studies in humans revealed a highly diverse viral community in the gastrointestinal tract, with several hundred different genotypes, with the vast majority of these genotypes representing bacteriophages.[47] New metagenomic studies have described dsDNA viruses in fecal samples of dogs and cats.[14,34] Approx. 0.38% of all obtained sequences represented dsDNA viruses, with the vast majority representing bacteriophages. Future studies will require more detailed characterization of the viral metagenomes for better understanding of their contributions to gastrointestinal health and disease.

SUMMARY

Although molecular-phylogenetic and metagenomic studies have brought insight into the complexity of gut microbes, the medical importance of other members of the intestinal ecosystem, such as fungi, archaea, and viruses, needs to be further evaluated. New technological advances (ie, high-throughput sequencing techniques) will allow not only exploring the presence of microbes in the GI tract but also their metabolic functions. These approaches may yield a better understanding of microbial-host relationships Glossary.

GLOSSARY

Intestinal microbiota	Collection of all microorganisms residing in the GI tract
Intestinal microbiome	The collection of all microbial genes in the GI tract
Phylotype	A phylotype defines a microbe by its phylogenetic relationship to other microbes. In molecular studies, a phylotype is defined as an organism that is different from all other organisms at a specific cutoff (for example: 95%, 97%, or 99% genetic similarity for genus, species or strain, respectively).
Metagenomics	The metagenome is defined as the collection of all host and microbial genes in the GI tract. In metagenomics, DNA extracted from intestinal samples is sequenced randomly (ie, without amplification of specific genes), which provides characterization of all genes (host and microbial) present in the sample, providing a snap shot of the functional property of the metagenome.
Transcriptomics	The meta-transcriptome is defined as the collection of all expressed host and microbial genes in the GI tract. In transcriptomics, mRNA extracted from intestinal samples is sequenced randomly (ie, without amplification of specific genes), which provides characterization of expressed genes present in the sample.

REFERENCES

1. Suchodolski JS, Dowd SE, Westermarck E, et al. The effect of the macrolide antibiotic tylosin on microbial diversity in the canine small intestine as demonstrated by massive parallel 16S rDNA sequencing. BMC Microbiol 2009;10:210.
2. Handl S, Dowd SE, Garcia-Mazcorro JF, et al. Massive parallel 16S rRNA gene pyrosequencing reveals highly diverse fecal bacterial and fungal communities in healthy dogs and cats. FEMS Microbiol Ecol. DOI:10.1111/j.1574-6941.2011.01058.x.
3. Frank DN, Amand ALS, Feldman RA, et al. Molecular-phylogenetic characterization of microbial community imbalances in human inflammatory bowel diseases. Proc Natl Acad Sci U S A 2007;104:13780–5.
4. Suchodolski JS, Xenoulis PG, Paddock CG, et al. Molecular analysis of the bacterial microbiota in duodenal biopsies from dogs with idiopathic inflammatory bowel disease. Vet Microbiol 2010;142:394–400.
5. Xenoulis PG, Palculict B, Allenspach K, et al. Molecular-phylogenetic characterization of microbial communities imbalances in the small intestine of dogs with inflammatory bowel disease. FEMS Microbiol Ecol 2008;66:579–89.
6. Janeczko S, Atwater D, Bogel E, et al. The relationship of mucosal bacteria to duodenal histopathology, cytokine mRNA, and clinical disease activity in cats with inflammatory bowel disease. Vet Microbiol 2008;128:178–93.
7. Bell JA, Kopper JJ, Turnbull JA, et al. Ecological characterization of the colonic microbiota of normal and diarrheic dogs. Interdiscip Perspect Infect Dis 2008; 2008:149694.
8. Inness VL, McCartney AL, Khoo C, et al. Molecular characterisation of the gut microflora of healthy and inflammatory bowel disease cats using fluorescence in situ hybridisation with special reference to Desulfovibrio spp. J Anim Physiol Anim Nutr 2007;91:48–53.
9. Jia J, Frantz N, Khoo C, et al. Investigation of the faecal microbiota associated with canine chronic diarrhoea. FEMS Microbiol Ecol 2010;71:304–12.
10. Greetham HL, Giffard C, Hutson RA, et al. Bacteriology of the Labrador dog gut: a cultural and genotypic approach. J Appl Microbiol 2002;93:640–6.
11. Suchodolski JS, Camacho J, Steiner JM. Analysis of bacterial diversity in the canine duodenum, jejunum, ileum, and colon by comparative 16S rRNA gene analysis. FEMS Microbiol Ecol 2008;66:567–78.
12. Desai AR, Musil KM, Carr AP, et al. Characterization and quantification of feline fecal microbiota using cpn60 sequence-based methods and investigation of animal-to-animal variation in microbial population structure. Vet Microbiol 2008; 137:120–8.
13. Middelbos IS, Boler BMV, Qu A, et al. Phylogenetic characterization of fecal microbial communities of dogs fed diets with or without supplemental dietary fiber using 454 pyrosequencing. PLoS One 2010;5:e9768.
14. Swanson KS, Dowd SE, Suchodolski JS, et al. Phylogenetic and gene-centric metagenomics of the canine intestinal microbiome reveals similarities with humans and mice. ISME J 2010. DOI:10.1038/ismej.2010.162.
15. Suchodolski JS, Ruaux CG, Steiner JM, et al. Assessment of the qualitative variation in bacterial microflora among compartments of the intestinal tract of dogs by use of a molecular fingerprinting technique. Am J Vet Res 2005;66:1556–62.
16. Suchodolski JS, Ruaux CG, Steiner JM, et al. Application of molecular fingerprinting for qualitative assessment of small-intestinal bacterial diversity in dogs. J Clin Microbiol 2004;42:4702–8.

17. Simpson JM, Martineau B, Jones WE, et al. Characterization of fecal bacterial populations in canines: effects of age, breed and dietary fiber. Microb Ecol 2002;44:186–97.
18. Lubbs DC, Vester BM, Fastinger ND, et al. Dietary protein concentration affects intestinal microbiota of adult cats: a study using DGGE and qPCR to evaluate differences in microbial populations in the feline gastrointestinal tract. J Anim Physiol Anim Nutr 2009;93:113–21.
19. Lappin MR, Veir JK, Satyaraj E, et al. Pilot study to evaluate the effect of oral supplementation of *Enterococcus faecium* SF68 on cats with latent feline herpesvirus 1. J Feline Med Surg 2009;11:650–4.
20. Ritchie LE, Steiner JM, Suchodolski JS. Assessment of microbial diversity along the feline intestinal tract using 16S rRNA gene analysis. FEMS Microbiol Ecol 2008;66:590–8.
21. Ritchie LE, Burke KF, Garcia-Mazcorro JF, et al. Characterization of fecal microbiota in cats using universal 16S rRNA gene and group-specific primers for lactobacillus and Bifidobacterium spp. Vet Microbiol 2010;144:140–6.
22. Ramirez-Farias C, Slezak K, Fuller Z, et al. Effect of inulin on the human gut microbiota: stimulation of Bifidobacterium adolescentis and *Faecalibacterium prausnitzii*. Br J Nutr 2009;101:541–50.
23. Rastogi R, Wu M, DasGupta I, et al. Visualization of ribosomal RNA operon copy number distribution. BMC Microbiol 2009;9:208.
24. Dethlefsen L, Huse S, Sogin ML, et al. The pervasive effects of an antibiotic on the human gut microbiota, as revealed by deep 16S rRNA sequencing. PLoS Biol 2008;6:e280.
25. Turnbaugh PJ, Hamady M, Yatsunenko T, et al. A core gut microbiome in obese and lean twins. Nature 2009;457:480–4.
26. Benno Y, Nakao H, Uchida K, et al. Impact of the advances in age on the gastrointestinal microflora of beagle dogs. J Vet Med Sci 1992;54:703–6.
27. Mentula S, Harmoinen J, Heikkila M, et al. Comparison between cultured small-intestinal and fecal microbiotas in beagle dogs. Appl Environ Microbiol 2005; 71:4169–75.
28. Johnston KL, Swift NC, Forster-van Hijfte M, et al. Comparison of the bacterial flora of the duodenum in healthy cats and cats with signs of gastrointestinal tract disease. J Am Vet Med Assoc 2001;218:48–51.
29. Johnston KL, Lamport A, Batt RM. An unexpected bacterial flora in the proximal small intestine of normal cats. Vet Rec 1993;132:362–3.
30. German AJ, Day MJ, Ruaux CG, et al. Comparison of direct and indirect tests for small intestinal bacterial overgrowth and antibiotic-responsive diarrhea in dogs. J Vet Intern Med 2003;17:33–43.
31. Rutgers HC, Batt RM, Elwood CM, et al. Small intestinal bacterial overgrowth in dogs with chronic intestinal disease. J Am Vet Med Assoc 1995;206: 187–93.
32. Frank JD, Reimer SB, Kass PH, et al. Clinical outcomes of 30 cases (1997–2004) of canine gastrointestinal lymphoma. J Am Anim Hosp Assoc 2007;43: 313–21.
33. Dossin O, Jones K, Clark-Price S, et al. Effect of omeprazole treatment on gastric and duodenal bacterial populations in healthy dogs [abstract]. J Vet Intern Med 2010;24:747–8.
34. Barry KA. Indices of gut health and intestinal microbiology in the cat as affected by ingestion of select carbohydrates varying in fermentative capacity [PhD dissertations]. Urbana (IL): University of Illinois; 2010.

35. Jergens AE, Nettleton D, Suchodolski JS, et al. Relationship of mucosal gene expression to microbiota composition in dogs with inflammatory bowel disease. J Vet Intern Med 2010;24:725.

36. Sokol H, Pigneur B, Watterlot L, et al. *Faecalibacterium prausnitzii* is an anti-inflammatory commensal bacterium identified by gut microbiota analysis of Crohn disease patients. Proc Natl Acad Sci U S A 2008;105:16731–6.

37. Davis CP, Cleven D, Balish E, et al. Bacterial association in the gastrointestinal tract of beagle dogs. Appl Environ Microbiol 1977;34:194–206.

38. Suchodolski JS, Morris EK, Allenspach K, et al. Prevalence and identification of fungal DNA in the small intestine of healthy dogs and dogs with chronic enteropathies. Vet Microbiol 2008;132:379–88.

39. Scupham AJ, Presley LL, Wei B, et al. Abundant and diverse fungal microbiota in the murine intestine. Appl Environ Microbiol 2006;72:793–801.

40. Suchodolski JS, Dowd SE, Steiner JM. Pyrosequencing reveals a diverse fungal microbiota in canine and feline fecal samples [abstract]. J Vet Intern Med 2010; 24:748.

41. Ott SJ, Kuhbacher T, Musfeldt M, et al. Fungi and inflammatory bowel diseases: alterations of composition and diversity. Scand J Gastroenterol 2008;43:831–41.

42. Eckburg PB, Bik EM, Bernstein CN, et al. Diversity of the human intestinal microbial flora. Science 2005;308:1635–8.

43. Conway de Macario E, Macario AJ. Methanogenic archaea in health and disease: a novel paradigm of microbial pathogenesis. Int J Med Microbiol 2009;299(2): 99–108.

44. Kempf C, Schulz B, Strauch C, et al. Virusnachweis in Kotproben und klinische sowie labordiagnostische Befunde von Hunden mit akutem haemorrhagischem Durchfall. Tieraerztliche Praxis 2010;38:79–86.

45. Mesquita JR, Barclay L, Nascimento MSJ, et al. Novel norovirus in dogs with diarrhea. Emerg Infect Dis 2010;16:980–2.

46. Mochizuki M, Hashimoto M, Ishida T. Recent epidemiological status of canine viral enteric infections and Giardia infection in Japan. J Vet Med Sci 2001;63: 573–5.

47. Breitbart M, Hewson I, Felts B, et al. Metagenomic analyses of an uncultured viral community from human feces. J Bacteriol 2003;185:6220–3.

48. Allenspach K, House A, Smith K, et al. Evaluation of mucosal bacteria and histopathology, clinical disease activity and expression of Toll-like receptors in German shepherd dogs with chronic enteropathies. Vet Microbiol 2010; 146(3–4):326–35. DOI: 10.1016/j.vetmic.2010.05.025.

49. Craven M, Dowd SE, McDonough SP, et al. High throughput pyrosequencing reveals reduced bacterial diversity in the duodenal mucosa of dogs with IBD [abstract]. J Vet Intern Med 2009;23:731.

50. Simpson KW, Dogan B, Rishniw M, et al. Adherent and invasive *Escherichia coli* is associated with granulomatous colitis in boxer dogs. Infect Immun 2006;74: 4778–92.

Antibiotic-Responsive Diarrhea in Small Animals

Edward J. Hall, MA, VetMB, PhD, MRCVS

KEYWORDS
- Bacterial overgrowth • Diarrhea • Dog • Enteropathy

Chronic diarrhea in dogs for which no underlying cause can be found and which is completely responsive to antibiotic treatment historically was termed *small intestinal bacterial overgrowth* (SIBO).[1–5] This name implied that the pathogenesis of the condition depended on the number of bacteria in the small intestine. However, given subsequent concerns about whether a true overgrowth (ie, increased bacterial numbers) exists in dogs, the preferred alternative name of *antibiotic-responsive diarrhea* (ARD) has been recommended.[6]

Idiopathic SIBO is recognized in humans as a true syndrome, particularly in children.[7] However, studies suggest that the overgrowth develops in pockets of fluid between annular mucosal folds found in the human small intestine, and these anatomic structures are not seen in dogs or cats. Thus, although the existence of SIBO in humans is accepted, the subject remains controversial in small animal gastroenterology, with no clear understanding of why and how the condition develops, or exactly why it is antibiotic-responsive.

Through a series of questions and answers, this article explores the current evidence and the existing areas of controversy concerning ARD.

WHAT ARE THE CLINICAL FEATURES OF ARD?

The syndrome of ARD, originally termed *idiopathic SIBO*, is characteristically a problem of young, large-breed dogs, especially German shepherds.[3,4] Idiopathic ARD does not seem to start de novo in older dogs, and is not recognized in small dogs. It has also never been definitively identified in cats, although mild inflammatory bowel disease (IBD) in cats may be controlled with metronidazole alone. Whether metronidazole's immunomodulatory or antibacterial or antiprotozoal properties are responsible for the positive response is unknown.[8]

The author has nothing to disclose.
School of Veterinary Sciences, University of Bristol, Langford, Bristol, England
E-mail address: dred.hall@bristol.ac.uk

Chronic or recurrent small intestine diarrhea is typical in ARD, but some dogs show colitis-like signs. Most dogs are polyphagic and many are coprophagic, but anorexia is sometimes seen and may be related to acquired cobalamin deficiency. Weight loss or stunting in seen in dogs that are more severely affected.[9]

When examined using conventional microbiologic techniques, the small intestine flora of affected dogs may comprise either predominantly aerobic or predominantly anaerobic bacteria, but tends to consist of a mixed population, with staphylococci, streptococci, coliforms, enterococci, and corynebacteria and anaerobes such as bacteroides, fusobacteria, and clostridia.[4] These bacteria are typically commensals found normally in the oropharynx, small intestine, and large intestine. However, culture of fecal bacteria cannot be correlated with bacterial numbers or species in the small intestine and cannot be used to diagnose ARD.[10] An overgrowth of a single bacterial species is not seen in ARD; instead, a disturbance of the flora, or dysbiosis, is present.

A positive clinical response to the administration of a range of antibacterials is the hallmark of ARD, and is how the condition is defined. Characteristically, affected dogs will be asymptomatic while on antimicrobials and will experience relapse either immediately or some weeks to months after antimicrobial therapy is discontinued. Oxytetracycline, metronidazole, and tylosin are believed to be the most efficacious antibacterials for ARD, although an enteropathy responsive only to tylosin has also been reported.[11-13] The choice of antibiotic is often based on drug availability, the cost of chronic treatment, and the potential impact of the development of antibiotic resistance, rather than on proven efficacy.

WHAT IS SIBO?

Genuine bacterial overgrowth is defined as an increase in the absolute number of bacteria, and therefore increased numbers of bacteria in the upper small intestine during the fasted state is called *SIBO*. Normally, the bacterial population of the small intestine is controlled by several mechanisms (**Box 1**), and SIBO is characterized by an uncontrolled proliferation of these bacteria.

In humans, SIBO occurs secondary to several underlying disorders (**Box 2**) that interfere with the normal control mechanisms, and the presence of SIBO can lead to clinical signs. These causes have subsequently been arbitrarily extrapolated to dogs.

In humans, the upper limit for normal duodenal bacterial numbers (reported as the number of colony-forming units cultured per milliliter [cfu/mL] of duodenal juice) is agreed at $\leq 1 \times 10^5$ total or $\leq 1 \times 10^4$ anaerobic cfu/ml. Unfortunately, that number has been extrapolated to the canine small intestine,[3] and controversy exists regarding its validity.[4,14] The original work used a small number of dogs and questionable bacteriologic techniques, whereas subsequent studies with different collection methods and improved anaerobic culture techniques have shown that much higher counts are commonly found in clinically healthy dogs and cats.[4,9,15,16] Therefore, a genuine bacterial overgrowth may exist in secondary conditions equivalent to those in humans. However, to accept that idiopathic ARD is a true SIBO based on the original numerical limit is incorrect. The term ARD should be used for idiopathic antibiotic-responsive conditions without an obvious underlying cause, whereas secondary SIBO may be diagnosed in cases with a documented underlying cause.

CAN THE NUMBERS OF BACTERIA IN THE SMALL INTESTINE BE COUNTED RELIABLY?

Although culturing and counting the numbers of organisms in the duodenum has been considered the gold standard for diagnosing SIBO, it is actually technically demanding and prone to significant error and natural variability.[9] Collection of duodenal juice

---

Box 1
Mechanisms affecting the normal small intestinal bacterial flora diversity and numbers

- Environmental factors

    Diet

    Hygiene

- Bacterial factors

    Competition for substrate

    Competition for binding sites

    Production of endogenous antibiotics

    Interaction with epithelial cell function

    Immune modulation

- Host factors

    Clearance by peristalsis

    Gastric acid secretion

    Digestive proteases

    Antibacterial pancreatic, biliary, and intestinal secretions

    Innate immune system

    Secretory IgA and other immunoglobulins

---

endoscopically is difficult, because often very little luminal fluid is present in the anesthetized patient. In dogs and cats, the duodenum is a relatively smooth tube in contrast to the human duodenum, in which annular folds trap pockets of fluid. When a large amount of duodenal fluid is found in dogs and cats, it more likely consists of recently secreted gastric, pancreatic, or biliary fluid, and therefore is not truly representative of duodenal juice. It is also not uncommon to contaminate samples by sucking up tissue and blood when trying to collect juice. The alternatives of flushing with sterile saline, trying to culture adherent bacteria from endoscopic biopsy specimens, or collecting fluid through transmural aspiration at laparotomy are also flawed.[16–19]

Even when a representative juice sample is obtained, many organisms, especially anaerobes, will die unless the sample is collected and transported under anaerobic conditions for immediate plating-out. Furthermore, counting is performed manually on serial dilutions of samples and requires excellent microbiologic technique. Finally, recent molecular techniques analyzing 16S bacterial rRNA in duodenal juice have identified a large number of organisms that are unculturable using conventional techniques, and therefore absolute numbers of just the culturable bacteria are probably meaningless (see the article by Jan S. Suchodolski elsewhere in this issue for further exploration of this topic).[20,21]

In summary, the technique of bacterial quantification of duodenal juice is so difficult and prone to error, not to mention labor-intensive and expensive, that it should not be contemplated in practice.

HOW MANY BACTERIA NORMALLY LIVE IN THE SMALL INTESTINE?

Accepting the limitations of current bacteriologic technique, experts generally agree that in all monogastric species, including dogs and cats, bacterial numbers in the intestine gradually increase towards the ileocolic valve, with the colon containing

Box 2
Underlying conditions recognized as potential causes of secondary small intestinal bacterial overgrowth in humans

- Decreased gastric acid
  - Hypochlorhydria or achlorhydria
    - Atrophic gastritis
  - Acid blockers
    - H_2 antagonists
    - Proton pump inhibitors
- Increased substrate
  - Exocrine pancreatic insufficiency
- Small intestinal mucosal disease
  - Chronic giardiasis
  - Dietary sensitivity
  - IBD
- Failure of clearance
  - Partial intestinal obstruction
    - Annular tumor
    - Chronic intussusception
    - Stricture/adhesion
  - Blind loop
    - Afferent loop of Bilroth II partial gastrectomy
    - Duodenal-jejunal diverticulosis
    - Surgical blind loop (end-to-side anastomosis)
  - Motility disorder
    - Absent or disordered migrating motor complex
    - Diabetic autonomic neuropathy
    - Hypothyroidism
    - Idiopathic intestinal pseudo-obstruction
    - Scleroderma
- Recurrent ascending infection
  - Abnormal communication between proximal and distal gut
    - Gastrocolic or jejunocolic fistula
  - Short bowel syndrome
  - Surgical resection of ileocolic valve
- Miscellaneous
  - Immunodeficiency syndromes
  - Pancreatitis

approximately 10^{13} organisms per gram of feces. Besides bacterial concentrations, the composition of the flora also changes along the tract, with a progressively increasing proportion of gram-negative and obligate anaerobic bacteria. However, the assumption that the proximal small intestine in dogs is virtually sterile has been extrapolated from human gastroenterology. The suggested numerical cutoff for normality of 1×10^5 cfu/mL total bacterial numbers or 1×10^4 cfu/mL anaerobes in dogs was based inappropriately on the numbers found in the human small intestine.[3]

Initially these cutoff numbers were considered valid because canine control results matched numbers found in the healthy human small intestine. However, they were obtained by a methodology that was suspect: duodenal juice samples were originally placed in transport medium and mailed to a laboratory for enumeration, and undoubtedly the numbers of viable organisms initially present were underestimated.[3] Other workers then struggled to confirm this cutoff, with numbers up to 1×10^9 cfu/mL being reported in clinically healthy dogs and dogs with other diseases of the small intestine.[4,9,22] However, when bacterial numbers in the duodenum of cats were first reported almost 2 decades later as being up to 1×10^9 cfu/mL, it was assumed that this was because cats were different, and that their strictly carnivorous diet encouraged the growth of anaerobes, especially Clostridia.[16] In fact, the numbers actually reflected the true situation more closely because of better technique.

DOES SIBO EXIST?

Ignoring the problems of bacteriologic methodology, does any evidence show that a true increase in small intestinal luminal bacterial numbers (ie, SIBO) can occur? In humans with intestinal blind loops constructed because of radical bypass surgery, good evidence shows bacterial numbers as high as 10^{12} cfu/mL. Clinical consequences (eg, diarrhea, raised serum folate, low serum cobalamin) are well documented in these patients. Similar overgrowth is seen when strictures (benign or neoplastic) prevent passage of ingesta (see **Box 2**).

Diseases such as abnormal intestinal motility or achlorhydria that might predispose to secondary SIBO are not proven in dogs, and blind loops are very uncommon, but overgrowth could occur when partial obstructions cause luminal contents to stagnate. For example, SIBO could be seen with a focal annular adenocarcinoma when the limited extent of the tumor would not be expected to produce diarrhea directly. Similarly, the profound ileus seen in pseudo-obstruction (eg, visceral myopathy) is associated with both vomiting and diarrhea, and the failure to clear bacteria by peristalsis might permit secondary SIBO. Overgrowth has been described in 100% of dogs with exocrine pancreatic insufficiency, although these results were still based on quantitative duodenal juice culture.[23] However, the lack of antibacterial pancreatic secretions and the presence of undigested food seem logical reasons for SIBO to develop, and the requirement for antibiotics in some patients with exocrine pancreatic insufficiency before an optimal response to enzyme replacement occurs supports the idea of secondary SIBO.[24]

Thus, secondary SIBO likely can exist in dogs and cats, but there is no evidence to suggest that idiopathic SIBO occurs in dogs or cats. The crucial debate focuses on the following question: could the idiopathic condition characterized as ARD in fact represent idiopathic SIBO?

DOES IDIOPATHIC SIBO EXIST?

Controversy still exists regarding the ARD syndrome seen in large-breed dogs and whether it represents idiopathic SIBO. It has become evident that great variation in bacterial numbers exists among individuals, and even within individuals on a daily basis.[25,26] The influence of coprophagia on duodenal bacterial numbers also has largely been ignored.[27] However, even if duodenal juice culture could be relied on for consistent results, the finding of numbers of similar magnitude in clinically healthy dogs and dogs with gastrointestinal disease challenges the relevance of absolute numbers. Use of an inappropriately low cutoff value leads to overdiagnosis of SIBO, which probably explains why it was previously reported in 50% of dogs with chronic intestinal disease.[28]

Established reference ranges for small intestine bacterial numbers in cats are set higher than in dogs, and a similar idiopathic antibiotic-responsive condition has not been documented in cats.[15] This absence may reflect a more realistic reference range for bacterial numbers in the feline small intestine but still does not explain why cats do not experience ARD.[15]

Therefore, experts have suggested that the type of flora or how the host and flora interact is more important than numbers. Dogs treated successfully with antibacterial agents do not necessarily show a decrease in duodenal bacterial numbers.[6,29] Hence, idiopathic SIBO is undoubtedly a misnomer, although clearly some dogs with diarrhea have responded to antibiotics.

WHAT IS ARD?

Even if idiopathic SIBO cannot be confirmed through proving the existence of increased small intestinal luminal bacterial numbers, a characteristic syndrome is recognized in dogs in which no underlying cause for gastrointestinal signs can be found but these signs are controlled by antibiotics. The term ARD is more appropriate than idiopathic SIBO, because bacterial numbers cannot be reliably counted and may not be increased, but a response to antibiotics can be observed.[6,30] Moreover, some cases of ARD may actually have a specific but undiagnosed infection that responds to antimicrobials.

WHAT CAUSES ARD?

Several hypotheses exist as to the cause of ARD. Historically, these were based on the belief that an increase in small intestine bacterial numbers was present and therefore pathogenesis was related to this abnormality. More recent hypotheses focus on host–bacterial interactions. ARD may develop secondary to defects in the mucosal barrier, aberrant mucosal immune responses, qualitative changes in the enteric bacterial flora (dysbiosis), or a combination of these mechanisms.

Defects in the mucosal barrier are supported by studies documenting abnormal permeability and the presence of brush border enzyme defects, but these are likely the effect of the disease rather than the cause.

A relative deficiency in serum IgA is reported in German shepherds, but serum IgA concentrations are not relevant to the amounts of IgA secreted at mucosal surfaces.[31,32] Absolute deficiency of fecal IgA in German shepherds has also been described but has been denied by later studies.[33–35] However, a possible underlying selective IgA deficiency caused by defective IgA secretion at the small intestine mucosal surface has also been postulated in this breed. Decreased IgA production by intestinal biopsies cultured in vitro was found in German shepherds.[36] Affected shepherds may have defective small intestine IgA production, although mucosal IgA+ plasma cell numbers are either normal or increased.[37]

The cause of this IgA secretory deficiency is not clear, but a complex defect is likely and could involve abnormalities either in the production and release of IgA from the plasma cell or in the pathway of translocation of IgA across the epithelium during secretion. However, no abnormalities have been found in the expression of the J-chain that links IgA molecules in secretory IgA (SIgA) or the polymeric immunoglobulin receptor that transports SIgA across the enterocyte to the small intestine lumen.[38] However, a specific allotype of the IgA heavy chain gene has been found in German shepherds.[39] Mutations in the code for the hinge region of the IgA molecule could affect the efficacy of the molecule or its susceptibility to proteolysis, and hence predispose to disease. Unfortunately, all German shepherds tested so far, irrespective of health status and including some claimed to have absent fecal IgA, are the same variant, namely variant C. Therefore, this mutation is probably merely a breed-specific phenomenon.[39,40]

Alternatively, altered IgA secretion may simply be an epiphenomenon related to a more fundamental defect in the mucosal immune system. Enteric bacteria are recognized in the small intestine by the innate immune system through interaction with toll-like receptors (TLRs), and a possible polymorphism in the signaling system shown in German shepherds with perianal fistula could be the basis of abnormal microbial–mucosal interactions.[41] Studies show that German shepherds with ARD have increased lamina propria CD4 T cells and increased expression of certain cytokines, suggesting immune dysregulation and perhaps a loss of tolerance toward endogenous bacterial antigens.[30,42] This hypothesis is supported by the fact that antibacterials lead to resolution of clinical signs and decreased cytokine expression but not necessarily to a decline in bacterial numbers. The fact that the most commonly recommended antimicrobials also have immune-modulating properties (eg, oxytetracycline, metronidazole, tylosin) may also support this hypothesis. Furthermore, anecdotal evidence shows that some German shepherds affected by ARD in younger life develop IBD later.

An alternative hypothesis is that an unidentified pathogen is involved in ARD; candidates include intestinal *Helicobacter* spp or enteropathogenic *Escherichia coli*. The predisposition of German shepherds to this syndrome could therefore be explained by either genetic susceptibility to infection as a result of major histocompatibility complex (MHC) II or TLR polymorphism, or transmission of infection in the perinatal period. This latter mechanism would be similar to the perinatal infection of young Boxers with attaching and invading *E coli*, which seems likely to lead to the development of granulomatous (histiocytic ulcerative) colitis in that breed.[43]

WHY DO ARD AND SIBO CAUSE DIARRHEA?

The development of diarrhea has been related to several mechanisms[5,7,8] that are all largely based on the premise of increased numbers of intestinal bacteria:

- Competition for nutrients
- Damage to brush border enzymes
- Deconjugation of bile salts impairing fat absorption
- Hydroxylation of fatty acids, with these products and deconjugated bile salts stimulating colonic secretion.

In particular, changes in the expression of brush border enzymes have been shown in the absence of light microscopic changes. Furthermore, these changes have been shown to normalize after successful antibiotic treatment. Therefore, if ARD is not truly associated with increased bacterial numbers, the type of bacteria present and the mucosal damage may lead to diarrhea.

IF SIBO EXISTS, CAN IT BE RELIABLY DIAGNOSED?

The definitive diagnosis of SIBO is difficult because quantitative culture of duodenal juice is flawed. A presumptive diagnosis of idiopathic ARD may be made through ruling out other conditions and showing a response to antibiotics, but that still does not prove that an overgrowth exists. Exocrine pancreatic insufficiency produces similar clinical signs and is also seen in German shepherds, and must be ruled out by finding a normal serum trypsin-like immunoreactivity. Intestinal biopsies evaluated through routine histopathologic examination of hematoxylin and eosin–stained sections should also be normal, thus ruling out IBD and other diseases characterized by their morphology.

To facilitate the diagnosis of SIBO without attempting quantitative duodenal juice culture, several indirect tests have been proposed, but all are probably irrelevant if idiopathic SIBO does not exist. None has been shown to be a reliable marker of antibiotic responsiveness.

Serum Folate and Cobalamin

When canine SIBO was first described, it was identified in a subset of dogs with chronic diarrhea that showed increased folate and decreased cobalamin (vitamin B_{12}) serum concentrations.[44] This pattern resembled that seen in humans with intestinal blind loops and diarrhea from secondary SIBO.[7] All of the dogs in this subset were subsequently found to have increased bacterial numbers (compared with human small intestine bacterial numbers), and therefore a specificity of 100% was claimed. The hypotheses for the changes in serum folate and cobalamin concentrations were first that bacteria produce folic acid and therefore SIBO leads to increased production and uptake of folate. Second, bacteria bind cobalamin, making it unavailable for absorption, causing hypocobalaminemia (**Fig. 1**). However, further studies showed that this pattern of folate/cobalamin was only present in 5% of dogs with culture-proven SIBO (**Table 1**).[28] Thus, with such a poor sensitivity, serum folate and cobalamin concentrations cannot be used to diagnose SIBO, although a low serum cobalamin still has value as an indication to treat.

Breath Hydrogen

Intestinal bacteria are the sole source of breath hydrogen. Theoretically SIBO should cause increased breath hydrogen or at least an early peak of hydrogen excretion after ingestion of carbohydrate.[45] Unfortunately, the technique is technically demanding, and other causes of carbohydrate malabsorption and increased intestinal transit rate will cause similar abnormal results.[46]

Unconjugated Bile Salts

Intestinal bacteria can deconjugate bile salts, which are absorbed but then poorly extracted by the liver and are therefore measurable in serum. Theoretically SIBO should cause increased serum unconjugated bile acids (SUCA).[47] Unfortunately, SUCA concentrations fluctuate significantly after a meal. Furthermore, lactobacilli are one of the major organisms able to deconjugate bile acids and are recognized as commensals in the canine small intestine (see the article by Jan S. Suchodolski elsewhere in this issue for further exploration of this topic). Therefore, the relevance of SUCA to disease is questionable. No correlation was found with duodenal bacterial numbers or serum folate and cobalamin concentrations in dogs with ARD.[6]

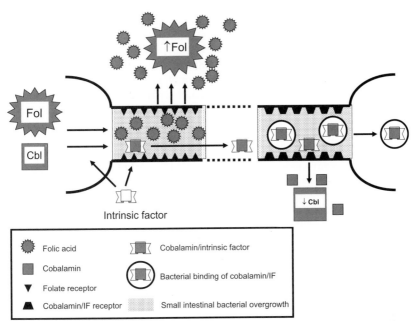

Fig. 1. Cartoon of the small intestine showing the predicted effect of small intestinal bacterial overgrowth (SIBO) on serum folate and cobalamin concentrations. Folic acid and cobalamin (vitamin B_{12}) are dietary vitamins, but their absorption by proximal folate carriers and distal carriers (recognizing cobalamin bound to intrinsic factor secreted by the stomach and pancreas in dogs) can be affected by SIBO. Increased numbers of luminal bacteria may synthesize folate, leading to increased serum folate concentration. Conversely, the bacteria bind cobalamin making it unavailable for absorption and leading to reduced serum cobalamin concentration. Therefore, SIBO is supposedly associated with increased serum folate and decreased serum cobalamin, the pattern seen in humans with SIBO caused by blind loops. However, the sensitivity of raised folate and decreased cobalamin is only 5% for finding greater than 10^5 bacteria per mL duodenal juice in dogs.

Intestinal Permeability

Intestinal permeability, as measured by ^{51}Cr-EDTA or differential sugar absorption, can be abnormal in ARD and can improve after antibiotic treatment.[48,49] However, these findings are not pathognomonic for either secondary SIBO or idiopathic ARD. Moreover, measurement of intestinal permeability is not readily available in practice.

Table 1
Sensitivity and specificity for increased serum folate and/or serum cobalamin concentrations in dogs for the detection of small intestinal bacterial numbers[a]

	Sensitivity (%)	Specificity (%)
↑ folate and ↓ cobalamin	5	100
↑ folate only	50	80
↓ cobalamin only	30	90

[a] Greater than 1×10^5 cfu/mL total or greater than 1×10^4 cfu/mL anaerobic.
   Data from Rutgers HC, Batt RM, Elwood CM, et al. Small intestinal bacterial overgrowth in dogs with chronic intestinal disease. J Am Vet Med Assoc 1995;206:190.

Markers of Bacterial Metabolism

The measurement of increased products of bacterial metabolism, either in blood or excreted in the urine, potentially provides a tool for detecting SIBO, but may not be relevant in ARD if bacterial numbers are not increased. The markers can be normal bacterial metabolites (eg, indican, p-nitrosonaphthol, glycocholic acid).[50,51] Alternatively, they may be produced by breakdown of orally administered substances (eg, bacterial release of sulfapyridine from sulfasalazine or p-amino benzoic acid [PABA] from its bile salt conjugate [PABA-UDCA]).[52,53]

Lack of Histopathologic Changes on Intestinal Biopsy

Histopathologic examination of intestinal biopsies is most often normal or shows only subtle abnormalities in ARD.[9] However, these findings are not pathognomonic, because other conditions such as brush border enzyme deficiencies or type 1 food hypersensitivities may yield similar results but do help rule out small intestine diseases with recognized histopathologic changes.

CAN IDIOPATHIC ARD BE DIAGNOSED?

The definitive test for idiopathic ARD is, logically, response to empiric antibiotic therapy. However, a response to antibacterials is not specific, and antibiotics may be beneficial in IBD, infectious diarrhea, and even a range of nonenteric diseases such as portovascular anomalies. Furthermore, response to antibiotic therapy does not discriminate idiopathic ARD from secondary SIBO.

Although both direct and indirect tests were previously advocated for idiopathic SIBO, recent studies suggest that they have limited value in diagnosing ARD and that neither indirect biochemical markers (folate, cobalamin, unconjugated bile acids) nor quantitative bacterial culture can reliably identify cases of ARD.[6,46] Therefore, the only available diagnostic test for ARD is an antibacterial treatment trial. However, this diagnostic modality is appropriate only after thorough diagnostic investigations have eliminated all other causes of antibacterial responsiveness.

In conclusion, suggested criteria for a diagnosis of idiopathic ARD are as follows:

(1) A positive response to the antibiotic treatment trial judged on resolution of relevant clinical signs
(2) Immediate or delayed relapse of signs on withdrawal of treatment
(3) Remission occurring on reintroduction of antibiotics after relapse
(4) Elimination of other etiologic causes based on the results of other diagnostic tests and histopathologic assessment.

WHAT IS THE BEST CHOICE OF ANTIMICROBIALS FOR ARD?

No cure is available for idiopathic ARD, but signs can be controlled with antibacterials.[29] A broad-spectrum antimicrobial is indicated, and suitable choices include oxytetracycline (10–20 mg/kg given orally every 8 hours), metronidazole (10 mg/kg given orally every 8–12 hours), and tylosin (20 mg/kg given orally every 8–12 hours). Oxytetracycline is cheap, and because systemic absorption is not required, it can be given with food. It cannot be used before permanent tooth eruption because it causes staining of tooth enamel, and it is not universally available. Some authors have criticized the use of oxytetracycline because it is associated with rapid development of plasmid-mediated antibiotic resistance.[54] However, given that long-term efficacy is maintained in most cases, oxytetracycline may not be acting through its antibacterial properties, especially because it does not significantly reduce small intestine bacterial numbers. Rather, it may provide a selective pressure on the intestinal flora, encouraging the establishment of less harmful bacteria, or it may exert immunomodulatory effects. Oxytetracycline has been shown to exert an effect on microvillus membrane (brush border) enzyme activity, although whether this is a direct effect on protein synthesis or if it occurs through inhibition of microbial activity is unknown. Immunomodulatory activity has also been suggested for metronidazole and tylosin.

Whichever antibacterial is chosen, a 4- to 6-week course is recommended initially, although the antibiotic should be changed after 2 weeks if the response has been suboptimal. In some cases, premature cessation of treatment can lead to relapse, and therefore prolonged therapy is usually necessary. In some animals, a delayed relapse occurs several months after cessation of antibiotics, and these cases require either repeated courses or indefinite therapy. Efficacy is often maintained despite a reduction in dosage frequency from three times to even once daily, again calling into question the mode of action of these antimicrobials. Dogs may also outgrow the problem with age, either as a result of a decrease in caloric intake or because of developing maturity of the mucosal immune system. In view of the public health concerns over prolonged use of antibiotics, periodically stopping treatment to determine whether it is still required is appropriate.

ARE OTHER TREATMENTS FOR ARD AVAILABLE OTHER THAN ANTIMICROBIALS?

Adjunctive therapy may be helpful, and mild cases of ARD may be controlled with diet alone. A highly digestible, low-fat diet seems beneficial, but the inclusion of prebiotics such as fructo-oligosaccharides is logical, although not of proven efficacy.[25,55] This syndrome is also a potential target for probiotic therapy. Any acquired cobalamin deficiency should be treated with parenteral vitamin B_{12}.

SUMMARY

ARD is a syndrome causing disease in young large-breed dogs. It was previously believed to represent small intestinal bacterial overgrowth, but initial descriptions of increased bacterial numbers are now recognized as spurious. Instead, the type of flora and its interaction with the host mucosa and immune system is believed to be of paramount importance in the etiopathogenesis. ARD currently can only be diagnosed after excluding other conditions and the response to empiric treatment with antibiotics. Why and how this disease occurs and how antibiotics control signs are currently unknown.

REFERENCES

1. Batt RM, Carter MW, Peters TJ. Sub-cellular biochemical changes in the jejunal mucosa of dogs with naturally occurring bacterial overgrowth. Clin Sci 1982;63:55.
2. Simpson JW. Bacterial overgrowth causing intestinal malabsorption in a dog. Vet Rec 1982;110:335–6.
3. Batt RM, Needham JR, Carter MW. Bacterial overgrowth associated with a naturally-occurring enteropathy in the German shepherd dog. Res Vet Sci 1983;35:42–6.
4. Johnston KL. Small intestinal bacterial overgrowth. Vet Clin North Am Small Anim Pract 1999;29:523–50.

5. Westermarck E, Siltanen R, Maijala R. Small intestinal bacterial overgrowth in 7 dogs with gastrointestinal signs. Acta Vet Scand 1993;34:311–4.

6. German AJ, Day MJ, Ruaux CG, et al. Comparison of direct and indirect tests for small intestinal bacterial overgrowth and antibiotic-responsive diarrhea in dogs. J Vet Intern Med 2003;17:33–43.

7. O'Mahoney S, Shanahan F. Enteric bacterial flora and bacterial overgrowth syndrome. In: Feldman M, Friedman LS, Brandt LJ, editors. Sleisenger & Fordtran's gastrointestinal and liver disease; Pathophysiology/diagnosis/management. 8th edition. Philadelphia: Saunders Elsevier; 2006. p. 2243–56.

8. Johnston KL, Lamport A, Batt RM. Effects of metronidazole on intestinal bacteria and disaccharidase activities in normal cats. Gastroenterology 1994;106:A242.

9. Willard MD, Simpson RB, Fossum TW, et al. Characterization of naturally developing small intestinal bacterial overgrowth in 16 German shepherd dogs. J Am Vet Med Assoc 1994;204:1201–6.

10. Mentula S, Harmoinen J, Heikkila M, et al. Comparison between cultured small-intestinal and fecal microbiotas in beagle dogs. Appl Environ Microbiol 2005; 71:4169–75.

11. Lecoindre P, Chevallier M, Gillard R, et al. Small intestinal bacterial overgrowth and inflammatory bowel diseases in dogs. Evaluation of the therapeutic efficacity of Spiramycine-Metronidazole association. Rev Med Vet (Toulouse) 1998;149:843–52.

12. Westermarck E, Skrzypczak T, Harmoinen J, et al. Tylosin-responsive chronic diarrhea in dogs. J Vet Intern Med 2005;19:177–86.

13. Westermarck E, Frias R, Skrzypczak T. Effect of diet and tylosin on chronic diarrhea in beagles. J Vet Intern Med 2005;19:822–7.

14. Simpson KW. Small intestinal bacterial overgrowth. J Am Vet Med Assoc 1994; 205:405–6.

15. Johnston K, Lamport A, Batt RM. An unexpected bacterial flora in the proximal small intestine of normal cats. Vet Rec 1993;132:362–3.

16. Johnston KL, Lamport A, Ballevre O, et al. A comparison of endoscopic and surgical collection procedures for the analysis of the bacterial flora in duodenal fluid from cats. Vet J 1999;157:85–9.

17. Delles EK, Willard MD, Simpson RB, et al. Comparison of species and numbers of bacteria in concurrently cultured samples of proximal small-intestinal fluid and endoscopically obtained duodenal mucosa in dogs with intestinal bacterial overgrowth. Am J Vet Res 1994;55:957–64.

18. Papasouliotis K, Sparkes AH, Werrett G, et al. Assessment of the bacterial flora of the proximal part of the small intestine in healthy cats, and the effect of sample collection method. Am J Vet Res 1998;59:48–51.

19. Lynch TM, Morris TH, Dix J, et al. Bacterial counts in canine duodenal fluid after exposure to saline, sodium bicarbonate and hypertonic dextrose solutions used to maintain patency of chronically implanted catheters. Lab Anim 1999;33: 143–8.

20. Suchodolski JS, Ruaux CG, Steiner JM, et al. Application of molecular fingerprinting for qualitative assessment of small-intestinal bacterial diversity in dogs. J Clin Microbiol 2004;42:4702–8.

21. Suchodolski JS, Ruaux CG, Steiner JM, et al. Assessment of the qualitative variation in bacterial microflora among compartments of the intestinal tract of dogs by use of a molecular fingerprinting technique. Am J Vet Res 2005;66:1556–62.

22. Kunkle BN, Norrdin RW, Brooks RK, et al. Osteopenia with decreased bone formation in Beagles with malabsorption syndrome. Calcif Tissue Int 1982;34: 396–402.

23. Williams DA, Batt RM, McLean L. Bacterial overgrowth in the duodenum of dogs with exocrine pancreatic insufficiency. J Am Vet Med Assoc 1987;191:201–6.
24. Westermarck E, Myllys V, Aho M. Effect of treatment on the jejunal and colonic bacterial flora of dogs with exocrine pancreatic insufficiency. Pancreas 1993;8: 559–62.
25. Willard MD, Simpson RB, Delles EK, et al. Effects of dietary supplementation of fructo-oligosaccharides on small-intestinal bacterial overgrowth in dogs. Am J Vet Res 1994;55:654–9.
26. Suchodolski JS, Harmoinen JA, Ruaux CG, et al. Dynamics of the jejunal microflora in response to feeding and over time. J Vet Intern Med 2005;19:473.
27. Pierson P. Coprophagy in kennels. Point Veterinaire 2000;31:11–5.
28. Rutgers HC, Batt RM, Elwood CM, et al. Small intestinal bacterial overgrowth in dogs with chronic intestinal disease. J Am Vet Med Assoc 1995;206:187–93.
29. Batt RM, McLean L, Riley JE. Response of the jejunal mucosa of dogs with aerobic and anaerobic bacterial overgrowth to antibiotic therapy. Gut 1988;29: 473–82.
30. German AJ, Helps CR, Hall EJ, et al. Cytokine mRNA expression in mucosal biopsies from German Shepherd dogs with small intestinal enteropathies. Dig Dis Sci 2000;45:7–17.
31. Batt RM, Barnes A, Rutgers HC, et al. Relative IgA deficiency and small intestinal bacterial overgrowth in German shepherd dogs. Res Vet Sci 1991;50:106–11.
32. German AJ, Hall EJ, Day MJ. Measurement of IgG, IgM and IgA concentrations in canine serum, saliva, tears and bile. Vet Immunol Immunopathol 1998;64:107–21.
33. Peters IR, Calvert EL, Hall EJ, et al. Measurement of immunoglobulin concentrations in the feces of healthy dogs. Clin Diagn Lab Immunol 2004;11:841–8.
34. Littler RM, Batt RM, Lloyd DH. Total and relative deficiency of gut mucosal IgA In German shepherd dogs demonstrated by faecal analysis. Vet Rec 2006;158: 334–41.
35. Peters IR, Hall EJ, Day MJ. Faecal IgA concentrations in dogs. Vet Rec 2006;158: 743.
36. German AJ, Hall EJ, Day MJ. Relative deficiency in IgA production by duodenal explants from German shepherd dogs with small intestinal disease. Vet Immunol Immunopathol 2000;76:25–43.
37. German AJ, Hall EJ, Day MJ. Immune cell populations within the duodenal mucosa of dogs with enteropathies. J Vet Intern Med 2001;15:14–25.
38. Peters IR, Helps CR, Calvert EL, et al. Measurement of messenger RNA encoding the alpha-chain, polymeric immunoglobulin receptor, and J-chain in duodenal mucosa from dogs with and without chronic diarrhea by use of quantitative real-time reverse transcription-polymerase chain reaction assays. Am J Vet Res 2005;66:11–6.
39. Peters IR, Helps CR, Calvert EL, et al. Identification of four allelic variants of the dog IGHA gene. Immunogenetics 2004;56:254–60.
40. Peters IR, Helps CR, Lait PL, et al. Detection of allelic variants of the canine IGHA gene by fluorescence resonance energy transfer melting temperature examination. J Immunol Methods 2005;304:60–7.
41. House AK, Gregory SP, Catchpole B. Pattern-recognition receptor mRNA expression and function in canine monocyte/macrophages and relevance to canine anal furunuculosis. Vet Immunol Immunopathol 2008;124:230–40.
42. Peters IR, Helps CR, Calvert EL, et al. Cytokine mRNA quantification in duodenal mucosa from dogs with chronic enteropathies by real-time reverse transcriptase polymerase chain reaction. J Vet Intern Med 2005;19:644–53.

43. Simpson KW, Dogan B, Rishniw M, et al. Adherent and invasive *Escherichia coli* is associated with granulomatous colitis in boxer dogs. Infect Immun 2006;74: 4778–92.

44. Batt RM, Morgan JO. Role of serum folate and vitamin-B12 concentrations in the differentiation of small intestinal abnormalities in the dog. Res Vet Sci 1982;32: 17–22.

45. King CE, Toskes PP. Breath tests in the diagnosis of small intestine bacterial overgrowth. Crit Rev Clin Lab Sci 1984;21:269–81.

46. Neiger R, Simpson JW. Accuracy of folate, cobalamin and the hydrogen breath test to diagnose small intestinal bacterial overgrowth in dogs. J Vet Intern Med 2000;14:376.

47. Melgarejo T, Williams DA, O'Connell NC, et al. Serum unconjugated bile acids as a test for intestinal bacterial overgrowth in dogs. Dig Dis Sci 2000;45:407–14.

48. Batt RM, Hall EJ, McLean L, et al. Small intestinal bacterial overgrowth and enhanced intestinal permeability in healthy Beagles. Am J Vet Res 1992;53: 1935–40.

49. Rutgers HC, Batt RM, Proud FJ, et al. Intestinal permeability and function in dogs with small intestinal bacterial overgrowth. J Small Anim Pract 1996;37:428–34.

50. Burrows CF, Jezyk PF. Nitrosonapthol test for screening of small intestinal diarrheal disease in the dog. J Am Vet Med Assoc 1983;183:318–22.

51. Suchodolski JS, Ruaux CG, Steiner JM, et al. Development of a C-13-glycocholic acid blood test to assess bacterial metabolic activity of the small intestine in canines. Can J Vet Res 2005;69:313–7.

52. Papasouliotis K, Gruffyddjones TJ, Sparkes AH, et al. A comparison of orocecal transit times assessed by the breath hydrogen test and the sulphasalazine/sulphapyridine method in healthy beagle dogs. Res Vet Sci 1995;58:263–7.

53. Takahashi M, Maeda Y, Tashiro H, et al. A new simple test for evaluation of intestinal bacteria. World J Surg 1990;14:628–35.

54. Marks SL. Editorial: small intestinal bacterial overgrowth in dogs—less common than you think? J Vet Intern Med 2003;17:5–7.

55. Ruaux CG, Suchodolski JS, Berghoff N, et al. Alterations in markers assessing the canine small intestinal microflora in response to altered housing and tylosin administration. J Vet Intern Med 2005;19:441.

Bacterial Enteritis in Dogs and Cats: Diagnosis, Therapy, and Zoonotic Potential

J. Scott Weese, DVM, DVSc

KEYWORDS

- Enteritis • Salmonella • Campylobacter • Clostridium
- Zoonotic

Enteritis, most commonly manifested as diarrhea, is a common problem in dogs and cats and can be frustrating for clinicians and owners alike. As described elsewhere in this issue, the intestinal microflora of the dog and cat is a complex and poorly understood population. The poor understanding of what truly constitutes normal versus abnormal, along with the ability to only superficially characterize the gut microbial population, limits understanding of the pathophysiology of enteritis. Diagnostic tests are of variable sensitivity and specificity, and new molecular tests are becoming increasingly available with limited validation. Accordingly, diagnosis of bacterial enteritis can be a challenge, but proper use of available tests can improve diagnosis rates, provide a better understanding of disease patterns, guide specific treatment, and identify potential zoonotic concerns.

CAMPYLOBACTER
Introduction

Campylobacter is a genus of gram-negative microaerophilic curved bacteria that can be found in a wide range of animals. At least 37 species and subspecies have been identified. Most are considered nonpathogenic but some cause of disease in companion animals, humans, and other species. *Campylobacter* spp can be grouped into thermophilic and nonthermophilic species, based on their ability to grow at 42°C.

The author has nothing to disclose.
Department of Pathobiology, Centre for Public Health and Zoonoses, Ontario Veterinary College, University of Guelph, Guelph, ON N1G2W1, Canada
E-mail address: jsweese@uoguelph.ca

Vet Clin Small Anim 41 (2011) 287–309
doi:10.1016/j.cvsm.2010.12.005   **vetsmall.theclinics.com**
0195-5616/11/$ – see front matter © 2011 Elsevier Inc. All rights reserved.

They can also be classified according to their catalase status. In general, most pathogenic *Campylobacter* spp are thermophilic and catalase positive.

Campylobacter spp are commonly found in healthy and diarrheic dogs and cats (**Table 1**). The presence of *Campylobacter* is hardly surprising and can be considered an expected finding, regardless of health status, particularly in young and/or stressed animals. In dogs, the catalase-negative species *Campylobacter upsaliensis* tends to predominate, accounting for up to 96% of isolates.[1–6] The relevance of *Campylobacter upsaliensis* for animal health is unclear, and there is no clear evidence that it is a cause of disease in dogs and cats. *Campylobacter jejuni* is the most common catalase-positive species[1,2,7] and presumably the most common cause of campylobacteriosis (disease caused by *Campylobacter* spp). Despite the known pathogenicity of this species, it can be found in clinically normal individuals. Other species, such as *Campylobacter coli*, *Campylobacter lari*, and *Campylobacter helveticus*, are less commonly identified,[8–11] but the recent use of molecular (nonculture dependent) methods has demonstrated a rather remarkable diversity in *Campylobacter* species in dogs.[5,9,11,12]

Cats are similar, with a variable and potentially high prevalence of *Campylobacter* shedding in both diarrheic and healthy cats. *Campylobacter upsaliensis, Campylobacter helveticus*, and *Campylobacter jejuni* have all been reported as the predominant species in different studies.[2,8,13]

The true role of *Campylobacter* in diarrhea in dogs and cats is difficult to determine, largely because of the high prevalence in healthy animals and frequent reports of a lack of difference in *Campylobacter* shedding by diarrheic and nondiarrheic individuals.[13–17] An association between the presence of *Campylobacter jejuni* or *Campylobacter upsaliensis* and diarrhea in dogs has been reported, but this was

Table 1				
Prevalence of *Campylobacter* spp isolation from dogs and cats				
Species	**Group**	**Prevalence (%)**	**References**
Canine	Healthy dogs	47	2
	Healthy dogs	21	18
	Healthy dogs	38	4
	Healthy dogs	56	9
	Healthy dogs	58	5
	Healthy 5- to 12-month-old dogs	76	9
	Dogs in animal shelter	51	14
	Stray dogs	51	90
	Healthy young pet dogs	76	3
	Healthy puppies	29	10
	Diarrheic dogs	60	2
	Diarrheic dogs	97	5
Feline	Healthy	44	2
	Healthy	42	13
	Healthy cats in quarantine facility	58	91
	Healthy	16 (*Campylobacter jejuni* only)	92
	In animal shelter	75	14
	Diarrheic	31	13
	Diarrheic	16	17

only in animals less than 1 year of age.[18] Experimental infection with *Campylobacter* has yielded variable results, with mild disease reproduced in puppies but no illness in kittens.[19–21] It is likely that some *Campylobacter* species, in particular *Campylobacter jejuni*, are pathogenic in dogs and cats but that colonization occurs much more commonly. Factors that lead to infection versus colonization (shedding of the bacterium in the absence of disease) are not known. *Campylobacter coli* is also likely a potential pathogen, albeit rare. The role of *Campylobacter helveticus* and *Campylobacter upsaliensis* is even less clear.

Diagnosis

Diagnosis of campylobacteriosis is a challenge, largely because of the high prevalence in healthy animals but also because of issues regarding successful isolation and identification of *Campylobacter* spp.

Fecal cytology

Cytologic examination of fecal smears can be used to detect bacteria with the typical curved rod appearance of *Campylobacter*, yet this only identifies *Campylobacter*-like organisms (CLOs), not necessarily *Campylobacter* spp. Other organisms, such as *Helicobacter*, *Arcobacter*, and *Anaerobiospirillum*, have a similar morphology and *Campylobacter* and CLOs are commonly present as part of the normal microflora. Furthermore, appearance does not differentiate between pathogenic and harmless commensal species. At best, detection of CLOs is mildly suggestive of campylobacteriosis, but this test has essentially no clinical utility.

Culture

Fecal culture is currently the standard for diagnosis, although the high prevalence in healthy dogs and cats creates problems with interpretation of results. False-negative results are also a concern, particularly with poorly handled samples or laboratories with limited experience with *Campylobacter*. As microaerophilic bacteria, they require alteration of atmospheric conditions, with 3% to 15% O_2 and 3% to 10% CO_2. Selective media are required for successful isolation, and broth enrichment methods can be used to increase yield. Isolation of *Campylobacter* spp is complicated by the preference of different species for different selective media. Consequently, there can be bias in the species isolated because of media selection. Most methods are optimized for recovery of the species thought to be of greatest clinical relevance: *Campylobacter jejuni* and *Campylobacter coli*.

Incubation is usually performed at 42°C to select for thermophilic *Campylobacter*; however, a temperature of 37°C should be used to ensure isolation of variable or nonthermophilic species.

Determination of the *Campylobacter* species is critical because of the variable pathogenicity of different species. At a minimum, determination of catalase-positive (*Campylobacter jejuni* and *Campylobacter coli*) versus catalase-negative species is important, because catalase-positive species are more likely clinically relevant. Biochemical and thermotolerance testing used to identify *Campylobacter* can be highly variable, resulting in inaccurate identification, and molecular methods are preferred for speciation.

Detection of *Campylobacter jejuni* or *Campylobacter coli* in a diarrheic animal should be taken as a presumptive diagnosis, with the understanding that it could just represent colonization. The relevance of detection of other species is unclear, and care must be taken not to overinterpret the finding of unspeciated *Campylobacter* or species such as *Campylobacter upsaliensis*, that may not be pathogenic.

Molecular Diagnostic Testing

Polymerase chain reaction (PCR) can be used to detect *Campylobacter* from feces but the clinical utility is currently unclear. PCR has the potential to be more sensitive and rapid and able to detect a broader range of species, but validated assays are not available and it is unclear whether or not increased sensitivity will help diagnose this disease.

Treatment

Campylobacteriosis is often self-limiting. In humans, antimicrobials are most commonly recommended in patients with high fever, bloody diarrhea, patients passing more than 8 stools per day, patients whose symptoms have not lessened or are worsening by the time diagnosis is made, or patients in whose symptoms have persisted for more than 1 week.[22] Positive effects of antimicrobial therapy have been reported in children treated early in disease[23] but not in those where treatment was initiated a few days after culture results.[24] Although veterinary data are lacking, these human guidelines should be considered and treatment is perhaps best reserved for moderate to severe cases and early infections. Optimal treatment regimens are not known. Erythromycin, fluoroquinolones, and second-generation cephalosporins are often recommended[25] but the relative efficacy is unclear (**Table 2**). Chloramphenicol has been recommended but considering the questionable need and lack of proved superiority over other options, it is difficult to justify the associated human health risks. Treatment seems more successful at controlling clinical signs than elimination of the bacterium, and treatment decisions should be based on clinical signs, not laboratory results.

Treatment of healthy carriers is not recommended because there is no evidence that it is effective or needed, both from animal health and public health standpoints. Treatment of carriers is most often considered in high-risk environments, such as pet stores or kennels, but the high risk of re-exposure, particularly with suboptimal hygiene and infection control practices, limits the chance of efficacy and could simply increase antimicrobial resistance.

Zoonotic Implications

Campylobacter is an important enteropathogen in humans, and studies of various strengths have implicated pets in human infections. Living with a diarrheic pet has been identified as a risk factor for campylobacteriosis in three different case-control

Table 2 Treatment options for campylobacteriosis		
Drug	**Dose**	**Comment**
Erythromycin	Dog: 10–15 mg/kg PO q8h Cat: 10 mg/kg PO q8h	Drug of choice
Tylosin	11 mg/kg PO q8h	
Enrofloxacin	Dog: 5 mg/kg PO q12h Cat: 2.5 mg/kg PO q12h	Resistance can develop during treatment Avoid in young growing animals
Tetracycline	10–20 mg/kg PO q8h	
Cefoxitin	15–20 mg/kg SC/IV/IM q8h	Rarely indicated

studies.[26–28] Recent acquisition of a new pet dog has also been identified as a risk factor for campylobacteriosis,[29] whereas puppy ownership has been reported as a risk factor for campylobacteriosis in children less than 3 years of age.[30] Identification of indistinguishable isolates of *Campylobacter jejuni* from infected people and their pets[31] provides further evidence of the potential for interspecies transmission; however, the source of infection and direction of transmission cannot be ascertained.

Overall, pet-associated infections certainly play a minor role compared with food-borne infections. The relevance of pets in campylobacteriosis may be higher in certain human populations, particularly in people with close contact with young or diarrheic animals. *Campylobacter jejuni* has historically attracted the greatest attention, but *Campylobacter upsaliensis* should be of concern. The role of this species in human disease has not been well characterized, perhaps in part to the variable ability of diagnostic laboratories to isolate this species.[32] *Campylobacter upsaliensis* was the second-most common species in a study of quinolone-resistant *Campylobacter* in California but only accounted for 4% of isolates.[32] Concurrent isolation of *Campylobacter upsaliensis* from diarrheic individuals and their pet dog or cat has been reported.[33,34] Highly related *Campylobacter upsaliensis* isolates were also recovered from both a pet cat and fetoplacental material of a pregnant woman after spontaneous abortion.[34] Therefore, although *Campylobacter upsaliensis* may be of minimal concern for animal health, it should be regarded as a potential zoonotic pathogen.

CLOSTRIDIUM DIFFICILE

Introduction

C difficile is a gram-positive anaerobic spore-forming bacterium that is a critically important human pathogen but of uncertain relevance in dogs and cats. Some studies have indicated that it may be a leading cause of enteritis in dogs[35,36] and an outbreak has been reported in a veterinary teaching hospital.[37] Limitations in testing (described later), however, hamper clear understanding of the role of this bacterium in enteritis in dogs and cats, and it could range from a leading cause of diarrhea to a minimally pathogenic secondary invader.

As with many other enteropathogens, *C difficile* can be isolated from the feces of a small percentage (0%–10%) of companion animals, typically with higher rates in shelters, breeding kennels, and veterinary hospitals.[38–42] Unlike the situation in humans, canine and feline *C difficile* infection (CDI) seems more commonly a community-associated disease rather than hospital and antimicrobial associated.

CDI is associated with proliferation of toxigenic strains of *C difficile* in the intestinal tract and production of bacterial toxins. Two toxins, toxin A (an enterotoxin) and toxin B (a cytotoxin), are involved in disease, with an additional toxin, CDT (binary toxin), of unknown significance. Some strains of *C difficile* do not possess genes encoding production of any known toxins and these nontoxigenic strains are clinically irrelevant.

Clinical signs attributed to CDI range from mild self-limiting diarrhea to a potentially fatal acute hemorrhagic diarrheal syndrome. Large bowel, small bowel, and mixed signs can be present,[36] as can chronic diarrhea.[43]

Diagnosis

Because there are no clear historical or clinical predictors of CDI, identification of animals with an increased likelihood of *C difficile* is currently impossible. A lack of recent antimicrobial use or hospitalization does not rule out CDI. Testing for *C difficile* should be considered in any diarrheic animal, but objective information regarding optimal methods for diagnosis of CDI in dogs and cats is limited.

Culture

Although *C difficile* is a fastidious organism, culture is relatively easy for laboratories with adequate experience and anaerobic culture facilities. The positive predictive value of culture is limited, because some strains are nontoxigenic and because toxigenic strains can be shed in the absence of CDI. The main potential role of culture in diagnosis is to rule out CDI, because a negative result from a properly collected and handled stool sample processed by an experienced laboratory has an excellent negative predictive value. The time required, particularly if enrichment methods are used for optimal sensitivity, limits the usefulness of this approach. Positive culture results can be useful as an adjunctive test to provide increased confidence in positive fecal toxin assays. Culture is most useful, however, for epidemiologic studies.

Common antigen detection

Commercial enzyme-linked immunosorbent assay (ELISAs) are available to detect common antigen (glutamate dehydrogenase), which is produced constitutively by all *C difficile* strains. These tests are rapid, inexpensive, and highly sensitive (up to 100%).[44] The main limitations are the same as with culture, with the main advantages being ease of testing, short turnaround time, and no need for specialized equipment or personnel. As with culture, common antigen testing cannot be relied on as a sole test for diagnosis of CDI, but its ease and high sensitivity make it a useful screening test. Negative results have an excellent negative predictive value and essentially rule out the possibility of CDI. Positive results should be investigated further (ie, toxin ELISA).

Fecal toxin detection

The clinical standard for diagnosis of CDI in humans has been detection of *C difficile* toxins A and/or B in stool.[45] The gold standard for toxin detection is the cell culture cytotoxicity assay, which detects toxin B activity; however, this test is not readily available because it is expensive, time consuming, and laborious. Many ELISAs are available commercially for detection of toxins A or toxins A and/or B in feces. The latter group is preferred because toxin A-negative, toxin B–positive strains can be encountered.[46]

ELISAs are quick and relatively inexpensive, with good sensitivities and specificities when used with human specimens (88%–97% and up to 100%, respectively)[47,48]; however, the performance characteristics of the human-based assays are poor in dogs with sensitivities ranging from 7% to 60 % and specificities ranging from 65% to 100% in one study.[44] Despite these limitations, ELISAs are commonly used for diagnosis of CDI in dogs and cats, because of their availability, ease, cost, and lack of other options. Positive ELISA results, particularly when combined with a positive common antigen assay or positive culture, are suggestive of CDI; however, the low sensitivity of some assays means the negative predictive value of ELISAs is marginal. Interpreting discrepant (antigen or culture positive but toxin negative results; antigen or culture negative but toxin positive results) is more problematic. Antigen or culture positive but toxin negative results could occur from the presence of nontoxigenic *C difficile* or colonization without the presence of toxins (both of which would not be CDI) or CDI with a false-negative toxin result because of poor specificity or the presence of a toxin A-negative, B-positive strain if the assay only detects toxin A.

Therefore, interpretation of this type of result is difficult and it could be considered weakly suggestive of CDI at best.

Molecular techniques

There are two main potential approaches to using PCR for diagnosis of CDI. One approach is direct PCR on stool to detect toxin B genes, something increasingly used in human hospitals because of the rapid turnaround time and high sensitivity (when used in combination with an appropriate clinical case definition).[49] The main limitation is lack of specificity because of the low but present baseline colonization rate in healthy dogs and cats. There are currently no validated PCR tests for C difficile in animals and no evidence that these tests are useful clinically as sole tests. Although validated human assays are available, specific validation for dogs and cats is required because human diagnostic PCR assays do not necessarily perform the same when used on specimens from animals.[50] The use of direct PCR for diagnosis of CDI in dogs and cats is not currently recommended; however, a validated assay could be a useful adjunctive test in combination with toxin ELISA.

The other potential use for PCR is in conjunction with culture. Testing of C difficile isolates for toxin genes can differentiate toxigenic and nontoxigenic strains, thereby improving the specificity of culture but still having the limitations in specificity associated with the presence of toxigenic strains in the feces of a small percentage of healthy individuals.

Treatment

There is no objective information regarding treatment of CDI in dogs or cats. In general, CDI is treated similarly to any other diarrheic disease, with supportive therapy as required. If antimicrobial-associated diarrhea has developed, cessation of antimicrobial therapy is ideal, if possible.

Specific antimicrobial treatment directed against enteric C difficile is commonly used, although it is unclear whether or not it is needed in all cases and many infections may be self-limiting. Metronidazole (dogs: 10–15 mg/kg orally every 8–12 hours for 5 days; cats: 62.5 mg every 12 hour for 5 days) tends to be the drug of choice. Intravenous metronidazole (15 mg/kg every 12 hours for 5 days) can be used if oral therapy is not an option. In humans, oral vancomycin is often used; however, some individuals consider this drug inappropriate in dogs and cats because a lack of evidence of either need or efficacy in small animals combined with the importance of this drug in humans. Other treatment options used by some clinicians include intestinal adsorbents, probiotics, and dietary changes. Di-tri-octahedral smectite is a type of clay that adsorbs to C difficile toxins in vitro[51] and which is commonly used in the treatment of CDI in horses. It has been used in dogs[37] but its efficacy is unclear. Probiotic therapy has been evaluated in humans with CDI, yet there is currently not a clear answer regarding efficacy.[52] Increasing soluble fiber in the diet is commonly recommended for clostridial diarrhea, but evidence of efficacy is currently lacking.

Treatment of apparently healthy dogs and cats is not indicated. There is no evidence that treatment of healthy animals can successfully eliminate C difficile colonization or that elimination of colonization is needed in healthy pets. Treatment of pets in households where humans have CDI, or even recurrent CDI, is not indicated. If there is any suspicion that pets may be involved in transmission, efforts are better focused on infection control practices. Duration of therapy should depend on clinical response, not laboratory results, and there is no indication to repeat testing as a basis of determining duration of therapy.

Zoonotic Implications

The risk of zoonotic transmission is currently unclear. Transmission of C difficile from animals to humans has not been documented; however, there is circumstantial evidence suggesting that interspecies transmission of the organism can occur. The strains of C difficile recovered from dogs and cats are almost always indistinguishable from those found in people with CDI.[53–55] In a study of therapy dogs, antimicrobial treatment of a human in the household was a risk factor for colonization in the dog, presumably from increased risk of C difficile colonization in the person with subsequent direct or indirect transmission to the pet.[46] Additionally, living with an immunocompromised owner is a reported risk factor for C difficile colonization in dogs,[55] giving further support to the notion that C difficile can be transmitted within households. The clinical implications of this, for both humans and animals, are not clear.

CLOSTRIDIUM PERFRINGENS
Introduction

C perfringens is a highly diverse and essentially ubiquitous, gram-positive, spore-forming anaerobic bacterium. Isolates are divided into 5 major types (A–E) (**Table 3**), based on the presence of one or more major toxin genes, cpa (alpha toxin), cpb (beta toxin), etx (epsilon toxin), and iap (iota toxin). Additionally, at least 11 other toxins have been identified,[56] although information regarding the potential role in disease is limited largely to two of them, C perfringens enterotoxin (CPE) and beta2 (B2) toxin. The presence or absence of these toxins is not dependent on the C perfringens type.

This bacterium can be found in a variable but often high (up to 11%–100%) percentage of healthy dogs and a similar percentage (27%–86%) of diarrheic dogs[16,35,57,58] and is essentially a normal component of the intestinal microflora.

The most common C perfringens strain in dogs and cats is type A. The clinical relevance of this strain is questionable because of its commonness in healthy animals and the apparently low virulence of alpha toxin. The potential for disease from type A strains probably relates more to the presence or absence of CPE and B2 toxin rather than effects of alpha toxin.

Enterotoxin has received the most attention, and an association between the presence of CPE in feces (as detected by ELISA) and diarrhea has been reported in dogs.[16,59] Although not proving a causal relationship, this, combined with the known role of CPE in disease in some other species, supports the potential for CPE-associated diarrhea in dogs. cpe, the gene encoding CPE, has been reported in

Table 3
Clostridium perfringens types and toxins

Type	Alpha/cpa	Beta/cpb	Epsilon/etx	Iota/iap	Beta2/cpb2	Enterotoxin/cpe
A	+	−	−	−	±	±
B	+	+	+	−	±	±
C	+	+	−	−	±	±
D	+	−	+	−	±	±
E	+	−	−	+	±	±

Abbreviations: +, Type produces this toxin; −, type does not produce this toxin; ±, some strains of that type produce this toxin.

15% to 33% of *C perfringens* isolates from diarrheic dogs[16,60] but can also be found in health animals.[16]

The role of B2 toxin is unclear but there is increasing interest in this toxin because it has been implicated as a cause of enteritis in horses and piglets.[61–63] Canine and feline data are limited, with small studies reporting *cpb2* in 17% to 32% of isolates from diarrheic dogs.[60]

Other types are less commonly encountered. Type C has been implicated in peracute fatal hemorrhagic enteritis in dogs, and this strain may be more pathogenic; however, it can also be (rarely) found in healthy individuals.

The true role of *C perfringens* in enteritis in dogs and cats is unclear. Clinically, *C perfringens*–associated diarrhea is often described mainly as large bowel disease, with diarrhea, increased fecal mucus, increased defecation frequency, tenesmus, and hematochezia; however, signs consistent with small intestinal or mixed disease may also be present.[35,36] Clinical signs are by no means pathognomonic nor are they even suggestive of *C perfringens* over other pathogens, and a wide range of disease phenotypes has been attributed to this bacterium, from mild self-limiting diarrhea to rapidly fatal necrohemorrhagic enteritis.

Diagnosis

Definitive diagnosis is difficult because of the high prevalence of *C perfringens* shedding in healthy dogs and cats, the wide range of toxins that can be produced, limited knowledge about the role of different toxins in disease, and limited fecal assays for different *C perfringens* toxins.

Fecal Cytology

Microscopic detection of clostridial endospores has been used by some clinicians as a means of diagnosing *C perfringens* infection, yet there is no evidence indicating that this is an effective technique. Endospores can be produced by many different clostridia, including harmless commensals. *C perfringens* spores can be found in feces from both healthy and diarrheic dogs, and no studies have reported a correlation between the presence or number of spores and disease.[16,35,64] Similarly, identification of organisms with the typical appearance of *C perfringens* is nondiagnostic because other organisms can appear similarly, *C perfringens* is often found in healthy individuals, and no association between *C perfringens* number and disease has been reported.[35]

Fecal Culture

Because of the high prevalence of *C perfringens* in healthy dogs and cats, fecal culture is of limited utility.[64] The most useful aspect of culture might be to rule out disease, because failure to isolate *C perfringens* by a good diagnostic laboratory from a properly handled sample probably indicates an extremely low likelihood of infection. Isolation of *C perfringens* from a diarrheic individual provides little information.

Toxigenic Culture

Toxigenic culture involves testing *C perfringens* isolates for the presence of toxin genes. The main use for toxigenic culture is to support CPE ELISA, with detection of a strain containing *cpe* providing greater confidence that an ELISA-positive result is not a false positive. The relevance of B2 toxin gene identification is currently unclear. Detection of uncommon strains, such as type C, in the presence of severe disease is suggestive but far from definitive. Unless studies showing an association between disease and the presence of a specific *C perfringens* strain or toxin gene become available, toxigenic culture will not be a useful sole test.

Fecal Enterotoxin (CPE) Detection

Currently, the only commercially available tests for detection of *C perfringens* in feces are CPE immunoassays: a reverse passive latex agglutination assay (RPLAA) and an ELISA. Neither has been adequately scrutinized in dogs and cats. The RPLAA is generally considered inferior because of poor specificity, but both tests suffer from limitations in sensitivity and specificity and can yield positive results in nondiarrheic individuals.[35,64] Whether or not that indicates poor specificity or the potential that toxins can be present in the gut without any disease is unknown, but it highlights the difficulties in interpreting results. Positive results can only be considered suggestive of CPE-associated disease. Concurrent detection of strains possessing *cpe* by toxigenic culture or PCR from feces supports the presumptive diagnosis, and this is considered the optimal approach to diagnosis of CPE-associated diarrhea in veterinary patients at this time. An important aspect to consider is that these tests only detect CPE, not any of the many other *C perfringens* toxins.

Molecular Diagnostic Testing

Fecal PCR is available from various diagnostic laboratories; however, there are many potential limitations. As with culture, the high prevalence of *C perfringens* in healthy animals is a major limitation. Most commercial PCR assays target the alpha toxin gene, which is present in all *C perfringens* strains and which is of questionable virulence. Therefore, given the prevalence of *C perfringens* in dogs and cats, positive results are expected, regardless of the health status of the animal. This is why alpha toxin gene PCR provides essentially no useful information. Assays targeting less common genes and those of potentially greater relevance (eg, *cpe, cbp2,* and *etx*) might be more useful, but there is inadequate evidence at this point that PCR can be a viable sole diagnostic test. Its most useful role is as an adjunctive test, with *cpe*-positive PCR results supporting a positive CPE ELISA.

Treatment

There is little objective information guiding decisions regarding when and how to treat. Specific therapy is presumably indicated in animals with acute and moderate to severe disease (eg, hemorrhagic gastroenteritis) or chronic diarrhea. The usefulness of specific treatment in mild diarrhea is unknown and is difficult to assess given the difficulties in definitively diagnosing *C perfringens*–associated disease and the often self-limiting nature of disease.

Metronidazole and tylosin are the most commonly recommended specific treatments, although ampicillin, erythromycin, tetracycline, and cephalexin, among other antimicrobials, are also used (**Table 4**).[65] Antimicrobial resistance is a concern but has received limited investigation, and most has focused on tetracycline resistance.[66]

Zoonotic Implications

Little is known about the potential for transmission from pets to people, and pets probably play little to no role in human disease. The incidence of nonfoodborne *C perfringens*–associated disease in people in the community seems low, despite the high prevalence of *C perfringens* in healthy companion animals. *C perfringens*–associated food poisoning is caused by contamination of food with enterotoxigenic strains of *C perfringens* with subsequent growth of *C perfringens* and production of enterotoxin in improperly stored food. There is a theoretic possibility that *C perfringens* from

Table 4
Treatment options for *Clostridium perfringens*–associated diarrhea

Drug	Dose
Metronidazole	Dogs: 10–15 mg/kg PO q8-12h Cats: 62.5 mg PO q12h
Tylosin	10–20 mg/kg PO q12-24h
Amoxicillin-clavulanic acid	12.5–22 mg/kg PO q12h
Ampicillin	22 mg/kg PO q8-12h
Cephalexin	Dogs: 22 mg/kg PO q12h

dogs and cats could be inadvertently inoculated into food through poor hygiene practices; however, this is probably rare to nonexistent.

SALMONELLA
Introduction

Salmonella is a gram-negative bacterial genus that includes more than 2400 different serotypes. The majority of these are serotypes of *S enterica* subspecies *enterica*. Some *Salmonella* serotypes are highly host adapted, such as S Typhi in humans, but most have the ability to infect many species.

Salmonella is uncommonly found in the intestinal tract of healthy dogs and cats, with recent studies reporting prevalences of only 0 to 2.9% in household or shelter dogs,[36,54,67–70] 6.3% in stray dogs,[70] and 0.4% to 1.7% in healthy cats.[71–73] Much higher rates can be identified in dogs fed raw meat[74–76] and eating a single meal of *Salmonella*-contaminated meat can result in fecal shedding for up to 1 week in healthy dogs.[77] Outdoor cats may also have higher colonization rates from ingestion of colonized or infected birds, in particular songbirds.

Infection with *Salmonella* can result in colonization or infection, with disease manifestations ranging from mild self-limited diarrhea to severe hemorrhagic gastroenteritis and septicemia. Young and old dogs are most commonly affected, and fever, vomiting, diarrhea, abdominal pain, and lethargy are common.[78,79]

Diagnosis

Diagnosis of salmonellosis (disease caused by *Salmonella*) involves detection of the organism in feces (or other sites in animals with invasive disease) along with appropriate clinical signs. Detection of *Salmonella* in feces does not necessarily indicate that disease is, or will be, present, because colonization can occur. Detection of the organism in feces of an animal with clinical signs consistent with salmonellosis provides as good presumptive diagnosis but is not definitive. Isolation of *Salmonella* from blood or other typically sterile sites in the presence of disease is diagnostic.

Culture

Culture has been the standard method for diagnosis. There are a variety of culture methods and there is no consensus as to optimal procedures; however, one or two enrichment steps are almost always used to increase sensitivity.

Isolation of *Salmonella* from feces simply indicates the presence of the organism, not necessarily the role of the organism in disease. Given the low prevalence of *Salmonella* shedding in most dog and cat populations (ie, those not fed raw meat), however, isolation of *Salmonella* in an animal with signs consistent with salmonellosis provides a relatively confident diagnosis. Interpretation of results is more difficult in animals at higher risk of colonization, particular those fed raw meat, and this can create a diagnostic conundrum because those individuals are potentially at increased risk of developing salmonellosis because of a higher risk of exposure, but the high baseline rate of *Salmonella* shedding decreases the confidence in a positive result. Isolation of *Salmonella* from feces of an animal fed raw meat and with clinical signs of salmonellosis, ideally with exclusion of other causes, is a reasonable presumptive diagnosis but is far from definitive.

It is generally accepted that testing of a single fecal sample underestimates the prevalence of *Salmonella,* whether or not from low test sensitivity, low-level shedding, intermittent shedding, or other reasons. In horses, testing of at least 5 serial samples is recommended, but inadequate information is available to make recommendations for dogs and cats. Multiple samples would almost certainly increase the yield; however, the need for enhanced sensitivity for clinical diagnosis (as opposed to epidemiologic prevalence studies of animals with normal feces) could also be questioned because it is reasonable to suspect that relatively large numbers of *Salmonella* would be present during disease and detection of low levels could actually decrease the specificity. This area has not been adequately investigated.

PCR

Conventional and real-time PCR assays are widely available but suffer from a lack of validation for use with dog and cat feces. The sensitivity and specificity are unclear. These tests have the potential to be highly sensitive; however, high sensitivity cannot be assumed because of the presence of fecal PCR inhibitors and other factors; therefore, specific validation is needed. Use of an overnight enrichment in nonselective culture broth has been recommended for optimal sensitivity, with confirmation of positive PCR results by culture. This allows for a more-rapid preliminary results with confirmation of results and recovery of an isolate for susceptibility testing and typing.[80] Until tests are specifically evaluated in dogs and cats, the role of this methodology for diagnosis of salmonellosis will remain unclear.

As with culture, positive PCR results merely indicate the presence of *Salmonella* in feces, not necessarily the presence of salmonellosis.

Treatment

Management of salmonellosis depends on the nature and severity of disease. Supportive therapy is the mainstay of treatment. Antimicrobial use in salmonellosis is controversial and there is no evidence that antimicrobials are effective against enteric salmonellae or that they decrease the severity or duration of diarrhea. The main reason to consider antimicrobials is to treat or prevent bacteremia associated with bacterial translocation. The incidence of clinically relevant bacterial translocation in dogs and cats is not known and is probably low in immunocompetent adults. Antimicrobials are not typically recommended for uncomplicated gastroenteritis but may be indicated in animals with severe disease as well as young and old animals, immunosuppressed animals, or animals with significant comorbidities. Drug choice should be based on in vitro susceptibility testing.

There is no indication to treat healthy carriers, because there is no evidence that antimicrobials are effective for eradication of *Salmonella* colonization. Colonization is typically transient and treatment could increase the risk of antimicrobial resistance and antimicrobial-associated diarrhea.

Zoonotic Implications

Salmonella is a zoonotic pathogen. The incidence of nontyphoidal salmonellosis (disease caused by serotypes other than the human serotypes S Typhi or S Paratyphi) seems to be increasing in many countries. It is estimated that cases have doubled in the United States over the past 2 decades[81] and 1.4 million cases are estimated to occur annually.[82] Most infections, however, are foodborne. The incidence of disease attributable to dogs and cats is not known and pet reptiles are presumably of much greater risk.

Transmission of *Salmonella* from cats, and to a lesser extent dogs, to people has been documented in households, shelters, and veterinary clinics.[83–86] Outbreaks of salmonellosis have also been linked to people handling *Salmonella*-contaminated raw animal–based treats, such as pig ears[87,88] and dry pet foods,[89–91] with similar but unconfirmed concerns about exposure to *Salmonella* from raw pet food diets.

OTHER PATHOGENS

Many other bacterial pathogens probably play a role in bacterial enteritis in dogs and cats. Limited understanding of the nature of the intestinal flora, the complexity and variability of the intestinal flora, and lack of specific diagnostic tests limit the ability to identify a broader range of pathogens on a routine basic. Some of these known or suspected pathogens are outlined in **Table 5**.

DIAGNOSTIC PANELS

It is increasingly common for diagnostic laboratories to offer fecal panels—collections of tests that are run in parallel or series. The usefulness of such an approach compared with individual tests selected by a clinician is unclear, but fecal panels offer a few potential advantages. Testing multiple organisms increases the diagnostic yield compared with only evaluating certain pathogens, as long as all of the included pathogens are relevant to the animal species and geographic region. Testing multiple organisms at once also allows for detection of coinfection, something that may be overlooked if serial testing is performed and testing stopped after identifying a positive result. Fecal panels also tend to be more cost effective compared with performing many individual tests. Consistency in testing also facilitates gathering better epidemiologic data both within practices and within regions.

There are a few limitations of panels. Tests with moderate to poor specificity can result in frequent misdiagnosis, particularly in very low prevalence areas because positive results are more likely to be false-positive results. Although more cost effective than running a full series of individual tests, fecal panels are more expensive than single tests, which might be appropriate for more targeted testing in situations where there is particular risk of an individual pathogen. Panels based on PCR (as discussed previously for individual pathogens) have the potential to be more sensitive and have a shorter turnaround time; however, proper validation is often lacking and the clinical relevance of results requires clarification for many tests.

Another approach is the combination of panels with subsequent tests to further investigate positive results. For example, *C difficile* antigen ELISA, a highly sensitive but poorly specific test, can be run as part of the fecal panel, with toxin ELISA (a less sensitive but more specific method) performed only on positive samples. Similarly, combining CPE ELISA and CPE gene PCR, with either one as the initial screening test, can be useful because a sample that is positive with both methods is more likely to indicate disease than a sample positive with only one.

Table 5
Other bacterial pathogens potentially involved in enteritis in dogs and cats

Organism	Disease	Diagnosis	Comments
Enterotoxigenic *Escherichia coli*	Diarrhea in adult dogs and puppies[93–96]	Isolation of *E coli* and detection of enterotoxin genes	
Enteropathogenic *E coli*	Diarrhea in dogs and cats[96–98]	Isolation of *E coli* and detection of attaching and effacing gene (*eaeA*)	Can also be found in 6%–17% of healthy dogs and cats[99,100]
Enterohemorrhagic (verotoxigenic) *E coli*	Diarrhea in dogs and cats.[99,101,102] Hemolytic uremia in dogs.[103,104]	Isolation of *E coli* and detection of EHEC strains (ie, O157:H7) and/or PCR detection of Shiga toxin genes	Can be found in 0–5.9% of healthy pets.[105–107] Potentially zoonotic.
Histiocytic ulcerative colitis (granulomatous colitis of Boxer dogs)	Colitis, predominantly in young Boxers, associated with adherent and invasive *E coli* strains	Colonic biopsy and histopathology. Isolation and characterization of *E coli*. Fluorescence in situ hydridization with a specific *E coli* probe.	
Yersinia enterocolitica	Unclear relevance but has been implicated in large bowel diarrhea in dogs, in particular dogs fed raw pork.[108]	Isolation from feces. Can be found in <1%–5% of normal dogs and cats.[109–111]	Zoonotic pathogen.

Given the inherent weaknesses in many tests and the lack of canine- and feline-specific validation for many, there is currently no standard recommendation regarding whether or not panels should be used. Further research regarding the epidemiology and diagnosis of these microorganisms is required to make definitive recommendations. Clinicians who are considering using fecal panels should ensure that the pathogens are relevant to their patient population and that they understand the limitations of all of the included tests.

SUMMARY

Diagnosing bacterial enteritis in the dog and cat is, at best, an inexact science. Limitations in understanding of the incredibly complex intestinal microflora and inadequate investigation of many potential pathogens and diagnostic tests create significant clinical challenges. Although the inherent limitations should be acknowledged and considered during test interpretation, these limitations should not preclude use of certain tests or combinations of tests that can provide useful information regarding the potential etiology of infection, to allow for specific treatment and understanding of disease trends and to indicate potential zoonotic disease risks (Appendix 1).

APPENDIX 1: SUMMARY OF DIAGNOSTIC TESTS FOR MAJOR CANINE AND FELINE ENTEROPATHOGENS

Organism	Test	Advantages	Disadvantages	Comments
Campylobacter	Fecal cytology	None	Nonspecific	Not useful
	Culture	Allows confirmation of the organism and speciation.	Requires specialized media and culture conditions. False-negative results can occur from poor sample handling.	Currently the standard for diagnosis but has limitations in both sensitivity and specificity.
	PCR from feces	Potentially more sensitive. Some tests may be able to speciate. Not affected by death of bacteria during shipping.	Increased sensitivity may not be desirable. Validated assays not widely available. No isolates obtained for susceptibility testing. Not all tests can adequately speciate.	Role in diagnosis currently unclear.
C difficile	Fecal cytology	None	Nonspecific.	Not useful.
	Fecal culture	Gold standard for identification of the organism. Highly sensitive with experienced laboratory.	Difficult for many laboratories. Nonspecific: does not differentiate colonization from infection and can detect irrelevant nontoxigenic strains. Requires a few days.	Potentially useful adjunctive test. Good negative predictive value with a good laboratory. Not diagnostic alone.
	Toxigenic culture[a]	As for fecal culture plus differentiates toxigenic and nontoxigenic strains.	Slow. Not readily available. Does not differentiate colonization from infection	Good adjunctive test. Good negative predictive value with a good laboratory. Not diagnostic alone.
	Antigen ELISA	Rapid. Cost effective. Highly sensitive.	Does not differentiate colonization from infection. Can detect irrelevant nontoxigenic strains.	Excellent negative predictive value. Limited positive predictive value when used alone. Good as screening test, with positive results tested for toxins.

(continued on next page)

Appendix 1
(continued)

Organism	Test	Advantages	Disadvantages	Comments
	Toxin A ELISA	Rapid, inexpensive.	Questionable sensitivity and specificity. Does not detect disease caused by toxin A–negative, toxin B–positive strains	Need validated tests for dogs and cats. Toxin A/B tests preferable.
	Toxin A/B ELISA	Rapid, inexpensive. Can detect either toxin.	Questionable sensitivity and specificity of available human tests in dogs and cats.	Clinical standard in humans. Need tests validated for use in dogs and cats.
	Cell cytotoxicity assay	Gold standard. Relatively sensitive, highly specific.	Time consuming. Technically demanding. Expensive. Not readily available.	Ideal but impractical.
	PCR from feces	Rapid. Detects toxin B gene so only identifies toxigenic strains. Potentially very sensitive.	Does not differentiate infection from colonization. Validated assays not available.	Not useful for diagnosis as a sole test. Possibly useful as an adjunctive test to support positive toxin tests.
C perfringens	Fecal cytology	None	Poor specificity. No evidence of usefulness.	Not useful
	Fecal culture	Relatively easy.	Healthy animals usually positive. Does not differentiate types.	Perhaps useful to rule out disease.
	Toxigenic culture	Allows determination of toxin genes possessed by strains.	Healthy animals usually positive. Relevance of finding most genes unclear.	Not useful alone, except perhaps with uncommon strains (ie, type C). Best used to support positive CPE ELISA, through concurrent detection of isolate possessing *cpe*.

	Test	Advantages	Disadvantages	Comments
	Enterotoxin ELISA	Quick. Identifies actual toxin, not potential to produce toxin.	Limitations in sensitivity and specificity. Does not detect other *C perfringens* toxins	Positive ELISA presumptive diagnosis. Best with concurrent detection of isolates carrying *cpe*.
	PCR from feces	Potentially rapid and sensitive. Potentially able to identify specific, more relevant, toxin genes.	Relevance varies with target. Most assays target alpha toxin gene, which should be present in many (or most) healthy animals. Need validated tests.	Alpha toxin gene PCR not particularly useful because of high expected rates in healthy animals. Tests targeting other genes might be more useful.
Salmonella	Culture	Definitively identifies organism. Allows typing and antimicrobial susceptibility testing.	Time consuming. False-negative results can result from low-level or intermittent shedding.	Clinical standard.
	PCR from enrichment broth	More sensitive.	More expensive and time consuming than direct PCR. No isolates obtained for susceptibility testing.	Probably most sensitive method. Good for surveillance but unclear whether needed for clinical testing. Best to confirm with culture.
	PCR from feces	Variable sensitivity.	Need validated tests. No isolates obtained for susceptibility testing.	Role unclear.

a Isolation of the organism with subsequent testing to demonstrate either the ability to produce toxins in vitro or the presence of toxin genes.

REFERENCES

1. Acke E, McGill K, Golden O, et al. A comparison of different culture methods for the recovery of *Campylobacter* species from pets. Zoonoses Public Health 2009;56:490–5.
2. Acke E, McGill K, Golden O, et al. Prevalence of thermophilic *Campylobacter* species in household cats and dogs in Ireland. Vet Rec 2009;164(2):44–7.
3. Hald B, Pedersen K, Wainø M, et al. Longitudinal study of the excretion patterns of thermophilic *Campylobacter* spp. in young pet dogs in Denmark. J Clin Microbiol 2004;42(5):2003–12.
4. Parsons BN, Porter CJ, Ryvar R, et al. Prevalence of *Campylobacter* spp. in a cross-sectional study of dogs attending veterinary practices in the UK and risk indicators associated with shedding. Vet J 2009;184:66–70.
5. Chaban B, Ngeleka M, Hill JE. Detection and quantification of 14 Campylobacter species in pet dogs reveals an increase in species richness in feces of diarrheic animals. BMC Microbiol 2010;10:73.
6. Westgarth C, Porter CJ, Nicolson L, et al. Risk factors for the carriage of *Campylobacter upsaliensis* by dogs in a community in Cheshire. Vet Rec 2009;165(18):526–30.
7. Moreno GS, Griffiths PL, Connerton IF, et al. Occurrence of campylobacters in small domestic and laboratory animals. J Appl Bacteriol 1993;75(1):49–54.
8. Baker J, Barton MD, Lanser J. *Campylobacter* species in cats and dogs in South Australia. Aust Vet J 1999;77(10):662–6.
9. Engvall EO, Brändstrom B, Andersson L, et al. Isolation and identification of thermophilic *Campylobacter* species in faecal samples from Swedish dogs. Scand J Infect Dis 2003;35(10):713–8.
10. Hald B, Madsen M. Healthy puppies and kittens as carriers of *Campylobacter* spp., with special reference to *Campylobacter upsaliensis*. J Clin Microbiol 1997;35(12):3351–2.
11. Chaban B, Musil K, Himsworth CG, et al. Development of cpn60-based real-time quantitative PCR assays for the detection of 14 *Campylobacter* species and application to screening of canine fecal samples. Appl Environ Microbiol 2009;75(10):3055–61.
12. Koene MG, Houwers DJ, Dijkstra JR, et al. Strain variation within *Campylobacter* species in fecal samples from dogs and cats. Vet Microbiol 2008;133:199–205.
13. Rossi M, Hänninen ML, Revez J, et al. Occurrence and species level diagnostics of *Campylobacter* spp., enteric *Helicobacter* spp. and *Anaerobiospirillum* spp. in healthy and diarrheic dogs and cats. Vet Microbiol 2008;129(3–4):304–14.
14. Acke E, Whyte P, Jones BR, et al. Prevalence of thermophilic *Campylobacter* species in cats and dogs in two animal shelters in Ireland. Vet Rec 2006; 158(2):51–4.
15. Fox JG, Hering AM, Ackerman JI, et al. The pet hamster as a potential reservoir of human campylobacteriosis. J Infect Dis 1983;147(4):784.
16. Marks S, Kather E, Kass P, et al. Genotypic and phenotypic characterization of *Clostridium perfringens* and *Clostridium difficile* in diarrheic and healthy dogs. J Vet Intern Med 2002;16(5):533–40.
17. Sandberg M, Bergsjø B, Hofshagen M, et al. Risk factors for *Campylobacter* infection in Norwegian cats and dogs. Prev Vet Med 2002;55(4):241–53.
18. Burnens AP, Angéloz-Wick B, Nicolet J. Comparison of *Campylobacter* carriage rates in diarrheic and healthy pet animals. Zentralbl Veterinarmed B 1992;39(3): 175–80.

19. Prescott JF, Barker IK, Manninen KI, et al. *Campylobacter jejuni* colitis in gnoto-biotic dogs. Can J Comp Med 1981;45(4):377–83.
20. Prescott JF, Karmali MA. Attempts to transmit *Campylobacter* enteritis to dogs and cats. Can Med Assoc J 1978;119(9):1001–2.
21. Macartney L, Al-Mashat RR, Taylor DJ, et al. Experimental infection of dogs with *Campylobacter jejuni*. Vet Rec 1988;122(11):245–9.
22. Blaser MJ, Allos BM. *Campylobacter jejuni* and related species. In: Mandell GL, Bennett JE, Dolin R, editors. 6th edition, Principles and practice of infectious diseases, vol. 2. Philadelphia: Elsevier; 2005. p. 2548–57.
23. Salazar-Lindo E, Sack RB, Chea-Woo E, et al. Early treatment with erythromycin of *Campylobacter jejuni*-associated dysentery in children. J Pediatr 1986; 109(2):355–60.
24. Anders BJ, Lauer BA, Paisley JW, et al. Double-blind placebo controlled trial of erythromycin for treatment of *Campylobacter* enteritis. Lancet 1982;1(8264): 131–2.
25. Fox JG. *Campylobacter* infections. In: Greene CE, editor. Infectious diseases of the dog and cat. 3rd edition. Philadelphia: Elsevier; 2006. p. 339–43.
26. Adak GK, Cowden JM, Nicholas S, et al. The public health laboratory service national case-control study of primary indigenous sporadic cases of *Campylobacter* infection. Epidemiol Infect 1995;115(1):15–22.
27. Fullerton KE, Ingram LA, Jones TF, et al. Sporadic *Campylobacter* infection in infants: a population-based surveillance case-control study. Pediatr Infect Dis J 2007;26(1):19–24.
28. Gillespie IA, O'Brien SJ, Adak GK, et al. Point source outbreaks of *Campylobacter jejuni* infection–are they more common than we think and what might cause them? Epidemiol Infect 2003;130(3):367–75.
29. Tam CC, Higgins CD, Neal KR, et al. Chicken consumption and use of acid-suppressing medications as risk factors for Campylobacter enteritis, England. Emerg Infect Dis 2009;15(9):1402–8.
30. Tenkate TD, Stafford RJ. Risk factors for *Campylobacter* infection in infants and young children: a matched case-control study. Epidemiol Infect 2001;127(3): 399–404.
31. Damborg P, Olsen KE, Møller Nielsen E, et al. Occurrence of *Campylobacter jejuni* in pets living with human patients infected with *C. jejuni*. J Clin Microbiol 2004;42(3):1363–4.
32. Labarca JA, Sturgeon J, Borenstein L, et al. *Campylobacter upsaliensis*: another pathogen for consideration in the United States. Clin Infect Dis 2002;34(11): E59–60.
33. Goossens H, Vlaes L, Butzler JP, et al. *Campylobacter upsaliensis* enteritis associated with canine infections. Lancet 1991;337(8755):1486–7.
34. Gurgan T, Diker KS. Abortion associated with *Campylobacter upsaliensis*. J Clin Microbiol 1994;32(12):3093–4.
35. Weese JS, Staempfli HR, Prescott JF, et al. The roles of *Clostridium difficile* and enterotoxigenic *Clostridium perfringens* in diarrhea in dogs. J Vet Intern Med 2001;15(4):374–8.
36. Cave NJ, Marks SL, Kass PH, et al. Evaluation of a routine diagnostic fecal panel for dogs with diarrhea. J Am Vet Med Assoc 2002;221(1):52–9.
37. Weese J, Armstrong J. Outbreak of Clostridium difficile-associated disease in a small animal veterinary teaching hospital. J Vet Intern Med 2003;17(6):813–6.
38. al Saif N, Brazier JS. The distribution of *Clostridium difficile* in the environment of south wales. J Med Microbiol 1996;45(2):133–7.

39. Borriello S, Honour P, Turner T, et al. Household pets as a potential reservoir for *Clostridium difficile* infection. J Clin Pathol 1983;36(1):84–7.

40. Clooten J, Kruth S, Arroyo L, et al. Prevalence and risk factors for *Clostridium difficile* colonization in dogs and cats hospitalized in an intensive care unit. Vet Microbiol 2008;129(1–2):209–14.

41. Madewell BR, Bea JK, Kraegel SA, et al. *Clostridium difficile*: a survey of fecal carriage in cats in a veterinary medical teaching hospital. J Vet Diagn Invest 1999;11(1):50–4.

42. Riley TV, Adams JE, O'Neill GL, et al. Gastrointestinal carriage of *Clostridium difficile* in cats and dogs attending veterinary clinics. Epidemiol Infect 1991; 107(3):659–65.

43. Berry AP, Levett PN. Chronic diarrhoea in dogs associated with *Clostridium difficile* infection. Vet Rec 1986;118(4):102–3.

44. Chouicha N, Marks SL. Evaluation of five enzyme immunoassays compared with the cytotoxicity assay for diagnosis of *Clostridium difficile*-associated diarrhea in dogs. J Vet Diagn Invest 2006;18(2):182–8.

45. Poutanen S, Simor A. *Clostridium difficile*-associated diarrhea in adults. CMAJ 2004;171(1):51–8.

46. Lefebvre SL, Reid-Smith RJ, Waltner-Toews D, et al. Incidence of acquisition of methicillin-resistant *Staphylococcus aureus, Clostridium difficile*, and other health-care-associated pathogens by dogs that participate in animal-assisted interventions. J Am Vet Med Assoc 2009;234(11):1404–17.

47. Lyerly DM, Neville LM, Evans DT, et al. Multicenter evaluation of the Clostridium difficile TOX A/B TEST. J Clin Microbiol 1998;36(1):184–90.

48. Russmann H, Panthel K, Bader RC, et al. Evaluation of three rapid assays for detection of Clostridium difficile toxin A and toxin B in stool specimens. Eur J Clin Microbiol Infect Dis 2007;26(2):115–9.

49. Peterson LR, Manson RU, Paule SM, et al. Detection of toxigenic *Clostridium difficile* in stool samples by real-time polymerase chain reaction for the diagnosis of *C. difficile*-associated diarrhea. Clin Infect Dis 2007; 45(9):1152–60.

50. Anderson M, Weese J. Evaluation of a real-time polymerase chain reaction assay for rapid identification of methicillin-resistant *Staphylococcus aureus* directly from nasal swabs in horses. Vet Microbiol 2007;122(1–2):185–9.

51. Weese JS, Cote NM, DeGannes RVG. Evaluation of *in vitro* properties of di-tri-octahedral smectite on clostridial toxins and growth. Equine Vet J 2003;35:638–41.

52. Dendukuri N, Costa V, McGregor M, et al. Probiotic therapy for the prevention and treatment of *Clostridium difficile*-associated diarrhea: a systematic review. CMAJ 2005;173(2):167–70.

53. Arroyo LG, Kruth SA, Willey BM, et al. PCR ribotyping of *Clostridium difficile* isolates originating from human and animal sources. J Med Microbiol 2005;54(Pt 2):163–6.

54. Lefebvre SL, Waltner-Toews D, Peregrine AS, et al. Prevalence of zoonotic agents in dogs visiting hospitalized people in Ontario: implications for infection control. J Hosp Infect 2006;62(4):458–66.

55. Weese J, Finley R, Reid-Smith R, et al. Evaluation of *Clostridium difficile* in dogs and the household environment. Epidemiol Infect 2010;138:1100–4.

56. Songer J. Clostridial enteric diseases of domestic animals. Clin Microbiol Rev 1996;9(2):216–34.

57. Cassutto BH, Cook LC. An epidemiological survey of *Clostridium perfringens*-associated enterotoxemia at an army veterinary treatment facility. Mil Med 2002;167(3):219–22.

58. McKenzie E, Riehl J, Banse H, et al. Prevalence of diarrhea and enteropathogens in racing sled dogs. J Vet Intern Med 2010;24(1):97–103.
59. Weese JS, Staempfli HR, Prescott JF. A prospective study of the roles of *Clostridium difficile* and enterotoxigenic *Clostridium perfringens* in equine diarrhoea. Equine Vet J 2001;33(4):403–9.
60. Thiede S, Goethe R, Amtsberg G. Prevalence of beta2 toxin gene of Clostridium perfringens type A from diarrhoeic dogs. Vet Rec 2001;149(9):273–4.
61. Garmory HS, Chanter N, French NP, et al. Occurrence of *Clostridium perfringens* beta2-toxin amongst animals, determined using genotyping and subtyping PCR assays. Epidemiol Infect 2000;124(1):61–7.
62. Waters M, Raju D, Garmory H, et al. Regulated expression of the beta2-toxin gene (*cpb2*) in *Clostridium perfringens* type A isolates from horses with gastrointestinal diseases. J Clin Microbiol 2005;43(8):4002–9.
63. Herholz C, Miserez R, Nicolet J, et al. Prevalence of beta2-toxigenic *Clostridium perfringens* in horses with intestinal disorders. J Clin Microbiol 1999;37(2):358–61.
64. Marks SL, Melli A, Kass PH, et al. Evaluation of methods to diagnose *Clostridium perfringens*-associated diarrhea in dogs. J Am Vet Med Assoc 1999;214(3):357–60.
65. Weese J, Greenwood S, Staempfli H. Recurrent diarrhea associated with enterotoxigenic *Clostridium perfringens* in 2 dogs. Can Vet J 2001;42(4):292–4.
66. Marks S, Kather E. Antimicrobial susceptibilities of canine *Clostridium difficile* and *Clostridium perfringens* isolates to commonly utilized antimicrobial drugs. Vet Microbiol 2003;94(1):39–45.
67. Bagcigil AF, Ikiz S, Dokuzeylu B, et al. Fecal shedding of *Salmonella* spp. in dogs. J Vet Med Sci 2007;69(7):775–7.
68. Hackett T, Lappin MR. Prevalence of enteric pathogens in dogs of north-central Colorado. J Am Anim Hosp Assoc 2003;39(1):52–6.
69. Sokolow S, Rand C, Marks S, et al. Epidemiologic evaluation of diarrhea in dogs in an animal shelter. Am J Vet Res 2005;66(6):1018–24.
70. Tsai HJ, Huang HC, Lin CM, et al. Salmonellae and campylobacters in household and stray dogs in northern Taiwan. Vet Res Commun 2007;31(8):931–9.
71. Spain CV, Scarlett JM, Wade SE, et al. Prevalence of enteric zoonotic agents in cats less than 1 year old in central New York State. J Vet Intern Med 2001;15(1):33–8.
72. Van Immerseel F, Pasmans F, De Buck J, et al. Cats as a risk for transmission of antimicrobial drug-resistant *Salmonella*. Emerg Infect Dis 2004;10(12):2169–74.
73. Zhao S, McDermott PF, White DG, et al. Characterization of multidrug resistant *Salmonella* recovered from diseased animals. Vet Microbiol 2007;123(1–3):122–32.
74. Joffe DJ, Schlesinger DP. Preliminary assessment of the risk of *Salmonella* infection in dogs fed raw chicken diets. Can Vet J 2002;43(6):441–2.
75. Morley P, Strohmeyer R, Tankson J, et al. Evaluation of the association between feeding raw meat and *Salmonella enterica* infections at a Greyhound breeding facility. J Am Vet Med Assoc 2006;228(10):1524–32.
76. Lefebvre SL, Reid-Smith R, Boerlin P, et al. Evaluation of the risks of shedding Salmonellae and other potential pathogens by therapy dogs fed raw diets in Ontario and Alberta. Zoonoses Public Health 2008;55(8–10):470–80.
77. Finley R, Ribble C, Aramini J, et al. The risk of salmonellae shedding by dogs fed *Salmonella*-contaminated commercial raw food diets. Can Vet J 2007;48(1):69–75.

78. Venter BJ. Epidemiology of salmonellosis in dogs—a conceptual model. Acta Vet Scand Suppl 1988;84:333–6.

79. Choudhary SP, Kalimuddin M, Prasad G, et al. Observations on natural and experimental salmonellosis in dogs. J Diarrhoeal Dis Res 1985;3(3):149–53.

80. Ward MP, Brady TH, Couëtil LL, et al. Investigation and control of an outbreak of salmonellosis caused by multidrug-resistant Salmonella Typhimurium in a population of hospitalized horses. Vet Microbiol 2005;107(3–4):233–40.

81. Pegues DA, Ohl ME, Miller SI. Salmonella species, including Salmonella Typhi. In: Mandell GL, Bennett JE, Dolin R, editors, Principles and practice of infectious diseases, vol. 2. Philadelphia: Elsevier; 2005. p. 2636–54.

82. Mead PS, Slutsker L, Dietz V, et al. Food-related illness and death in the United States. Emerg Infect Dis 1999;5(5):607–25.

83. Wright JG, Tengelsen LA, Smith KE, et al. Multidrug-resistant Salmonella Typhimurium in four animal facilities. Emerg Infect Dis 2005;11(8):1235–41.

84. Wall PG, Threlfall EJ, Ward LR, et al. Multiresistant Salmonella Typhimurium DT104 in cats: a public health risk. Lancet 1996;348(9025):471.

85. Centers for Disease Control and Prevention (CDC). Outbreaks of multidrug-resistant Salmonella typhimurium associated with veterinary facilities–Idaho, Minnesota, and Washington, 1999. MMWR Morb Mortal Wkly Rep 2001; 50(33):701–4.

86. Tauni MA, Osterlund A. Outbreak of Salmonella Typhimurium in cats and humans associated with infection in wild birds. J Small Anim Pract 2000;41(8): 339–41.

87. Clark C, Cunningham J, Ahmed R, et al. Characterization of Salmonella associated with pig ear dog treats in Canada. J Clin Microbiol 2001;39(11):3962–8.

88. Pitout JD, Reisbig MD, Mulvey M, et al. Association between handling of pet treats and infection with Salmonella enterica serotype newport expressing the AmpC beta-lactamase, CMY-2. J Clin Microbiol 2003;41(10):4578–82.

89. Centers for Disease Control and Prevention (CDC). Multistate outbreak of human Salmonella infections caused by contaminated dry dog food–United States, 2006–2007. MMWR Morb Mortal Wkly Rep 2008;57(19):521–4.

90. Centers for Disease Control and Prevention (CDC). Update: recall of dry dog and cat food products associated with human Salmonella Schwarzengrund infections–United States, 2008. MMWR Morb Mortal Wkly Rep 2008;57(44):1200–2.

91. Schotte U, Borchers D, Wulff C, et al. Salmonella Montevideo outbreak in military kennel dogs caused by contaminated commercial feed, which was only recognized through monitoring. Vet Microbiol 2007;119(2–4):316–23.

92. Fernández H, Martin R. Campylobacter intestinal carriage among stray and pet dogs. Revista de saúde pública 1991;25(6):473–5.

93. Fox JG, Maxwell KO, Taylor NS, et al. "Campylobacter upsaliensis" isolated from cats as identified by DNA relatedness and biochemical features. J Clin Microbiol 1989;27(10):2376–8.

94. López CM, Giacoboni G, Agostini A, et al. Thermotolerant Campylobacters in domestic animals in a defined population in Buenos Aires, Argentina. Prev Vet Med 2002;55(3):193–200.

95. Hammermueller J, Kruth S, Prescott J, et al. Detection of toxin genes in Escherichia coli isolated from normal dogs and dogs with diarrhea. Can J Vet Res 1995;59(4):265–70.

96. Olson P, Hedhammar A, Faris A, et al. Enterotoxigenic Escherichia coli (ETEC) and Klebsiella pneumoniae isolated from dogs with diarrhoea. Vet Microbiol 1985;10(6):577–89.

97. Olson P, Hedhammar A, Wadstrom T. Enterotoxigenic *Escherichia coli* infection in two dogs with acute diarrhea. J Am Vet Med Assoc 1984;184(8):982–3.
98. Drolet R, Fairbrother JM, Harel J, et al. Attaching and effacing and enterotoxigenic *Escherichia coli* associated with enteric colibacillosis in the dog. Can J Vet Res 1994;58(2):87–92.
99. Pospischil A, Mainil JG, Baljer G, et al. Attaching and effacing bacteria in the intestines of calves and cats with diarrhea. Vet Pathol 1987;24(4):330–4.
100. Turk J, Maddox C, Fales W, et al. Examination for heat-labile, heat-stable, and Shiga-like toxins and for the eaeA gene in *Escherichia coli* isolates obtained from dogs dying with diarrhea: 122 cases (1992–1996). J Am Vet Med Assoc 1998;212(11):1735–6.
101. Sancak AA, Rutgers HC, Hart CA, et al. Prevalence of enteropathic *Escherichia coli* in dogs with acute and chronic diarrhoea. Vet Rec 2004;154(4):101–6.
102. Krause G, Zimmermann S, Beutin L. Investigation of domestic animals and pets as a reservoir for intimin- (eae) gene positive Escherichia coli types. Vet Microbiol 2005;106(1/2):87–95.
103. Smith KA, Kruth S, Hammermueller J, et al. A case-control study of verocytotoxigenic *Escherichia coli* infection in cats with diarrhea. Can J Vet Res 1998;62(2): 87–92.
104. Abaas S, Franklin A, Kuhn I, et al. Cytotoxin activity on Vero cells among *Escherichia coli* strains associated with diarrhea in cats. Am J Vet Res 1989;50(8): 1294–6.
105. Chantrey J, Chapman PS, Patterson-Kan JC. Haemolytic-uraemic syndrome in a dog. J Vet Med 2002;49(9):470–2.
106. Holloway S, Senior D, Roth L, et al. Hemolytic uremic syndrome in dogs. J Vet Intern Med 1993;7(4):220–7.
107. Roopnarine RR, Ammons D, Rampersad J, et al. Occurrence and characterization of verocytotoxigenic *Escherichia coli* (VTEC) strains from dairy farms in Trinidad. Zoonoses and Public Health 2007;54(2):78–85.
108. Fredriksson-Ahomaa M, Korte T, Korkeala H. Transmission of *Yersinia enterocolitica* 4/O:3 to pets via contaminated pork. Lett Appl Microbiol 2001;32(6):375–8.
109. Bucher M, Meyer C, Grötzbach B, et al. Epidemiological data on pathogenic *Yersinia enterocolitica* in Southern Germany during 2000–2006. Foodborne Pathog Dis 2008;5(3):273–80.
110. Fukushima H, Nakamura R, Iitsuka S, et al. Presence of zoonotic pathogens (*Yersinia* spp., *Campylobacter jejuni, Salmonella* spp., and *Leptospira* spp.) simultaneously in dogs and cats. Zentralblatt für Bakteriologie, Mikrobiologie und Hygiene 1 Abt Originale B. Hygiene 1985;181(3–5):430–40.
111. Wooley RE, Shotts EB, McConnell JW. Isolation of *Yersinia enterocolitica* from selected animal species. Am J Vet Res 1980;41(10):1667–8.

Laboratory Tests for the Diagnosis and Management of Chronic Canine and Feline Enteropathies

Nora Berghoff, Dr med vet*, Jörg M. Steiner, Dr med vet, PhD

KEYWORDS

- Enteropathy • Canine • Feline • Function tests
- Diarrhea • Gastrointestinal

DIAGNOSIS OF CHRONIC ENTEROPATHIES

Chronic enteropathies are commonly encountered in both cats and dogs. Although definitive diagnosis often requires the collection and histopathologic evaluation of gastrointestinal biopsies, less invasive laboratory tests are also helpful in the diagnosis and should be performed before considering the collection of biopsies.

Before evaluating the patient for a primary gastrointestinal disorder, it is crucial to rule out secondary gastrointestinal diseases, which could be associated with hepatic, pancreatic, renal, adrenal, and thyroid disorders, or other underlying diseases. This procedure is best accomplished by collecting a minimum database, which should include a complete blood count (CBC), a serum biochemistry profile, and a urinalysis. CBC is often unremarkable but may show abnormalities such as eosinophilia in patients with parasitic infestation or eosinophilic gastroenteritis. Neutrophilia is occasionally observed, and lymphopenia may be found in patients with protein-losing enteropathies (PLEs). Anemia may be observed if gastrointestinal bleeding is present.

A serum biochemistry profile helps assess possible hepatic or renal failure, both of which may cause clinical signs of gastrointestinal disease. Mild to moderate increases in serum or plasma liver enzyme activities (ie, alkaline phosphatase, alanine aminotransferase) because of a reactive hepatopathy may be observed in some patients with chronic intestinal disease, even in the absence of primary liver disease.[1,2]

Disclosure: The authors are affiliated with the Gastrointestinal Laboratory at Texas A&M University, which provides specialized gastrointestinal function testing for cats and dogs.
Gastrointestinal Laboratory, Department of Small Animal Clinical Sciences, Texas A&M University, 4474 TAMU, College Station, TX 77843, USA
* Corresponding author.
E-mail address: nberghoff@cvm.tamu.edu

Vet Clin Small Anim 41 (2011) 311–328
doi:10.1016/j.cvsm.2011.01.001
0195-5616/11/$ – see front matter

Concurrent intestinal inflammation, cholangiohepatitis, and pancreatitis (triaditis) may be observed particularly in cats and might also be accompanied by increased liver enzyme activities. Hypoalbuminemia is an important indicator of PLE, particularly if it is associated with hypoglobulinemia. Moreover, serum albumin concentration should always be measured because hypoalbuminemia has been shown to be a negative prognostic indicator in dogs with chronic enteropathies.[3] Hypocholesterolemia can be frequently observed in dogs with lymphangiectasia because cholesterol is lost in the lymphatic fluid, and malabsorption is also common in these patients.

In addition to the required minimum database collected for each patient, serum concentrations of canine and feline pancreatic lipase immunoreactivity (PLI, now measured as Spec cPL and Spec fPL [IDEXX Laboratories, Westbrook, ME, USA], respectively) may help diagnose or rule out pancreatitis in a patient with clinical signs of gastrointestinal disease. Furthermore, increased PLI concentrations in dogs with inflammatory bowel disease (IBD) have been shown to be associated with a poor response to steroid treatment and a negative outcome.[4] Therefore, measurement of PLI may be warranted in dogs with IBD. In cats with IBD, hypocobalaminemia and hypoalbuminemia have been reported more frequently in those patients who had a concurrently increased serum fPLI concentration.[5] It may therefore be advisable to measure serum fPLI concentration in these patients to detect potential concurrent pancreatic inflammation.[5]

Exocrine pancreatic insufficiency (EPI) often represents an important differential diagnosis in patients with chronic enteropathies because EPI usually manifests itself as chronic weight loss and loose stools, although liquid diarrhea is uncommon. The test of choice for diagnosing EPI in both cats and dogs is the serum trypsin-like immunoreactivity (TLI) assay.[6,7] Other tests for EPI, such as fecal elastase or fecal proteolytic activity assays, are not recommended because they are less reliable and may have false-positive or negative test results.[8]

In cats, particularly those of an older age, serum concentration of total T4 or free T4 should also be determined to rule out hyperthyroidism as a potential cause for gastrointestinal signs. If these data are unknown, cats should also be assessed for feline leukemia virus and feline immunodeficiency virus status.

Furthermore in dogs, atypical hypoadrenocorticism with no abnormalities of serum electrolytes may cause clinical signs of gastrointestinal disease and should therefore be ruled out. Basal serum or plasma cortisol concentrations of more than 2 µg/dL allow to rule out hypoadrenocorticism. However, in dogs with a serum or plasma basal cortisol concentration less than 2 µg/dL, the possibility of hypoadrenocorticism should be further evaluated with an adrenocorticotropic hormone stimulation test, which remains to be the gold standard test for hypoadrenocorticism.[9]

Various additional laboratory tests are available and can be classified into 2 groups based on their purpose. The first group represents tests that help determine a causative agent, such as fecal examination for parasites or fecal cultures for enteropathogens. The second group comprises tests that assess gastrointestinal function and disease, which include measurement of serum concentrations of cobalamin, folate, and C-reactive protein (CRP), and fecal α_1-proteinase inhibitor (α_1-PI) concentration.

LABORATORY TESTS THAT ASSESS THE CAUSE
Diagnostic Tests for Helminths

Fecal examination
Patients presenting with clinical signs of chronic intestinal disease should be evaluated for endoparasitic infestation before more elaborate diagnostic tests are initiated.

Infections with hookworms (ie, *Ancylostoma* spp, *Uncinaria* spp), roundworms (ie, *Toxocara* spp, *Toxascaris leonina*), and whipworms (ie, *Trichuris vulpis*, rarely observed in cats) may all cause chronic diarrhea.

The diagnostic technique of choice for detecting a wide range of parasitic ova is fecal flotation with centrifugation. The centrifugation step has been shown to lead to superior recovery of parasite eggs when compared with simple bench-top flotation methods and can greatly decrease the number of false-negative test results.[10] Different flotation solutions can be used. A recent study determined that a modified Sheather's sugar solution (specific gravity [SG] of 1.27) was the most sensitive method for detection of various helminthic ova.[11] A 33% zinc sulfate solution ($ZnSO_4$, SG of 1.18) is also frequently used but has been shown to be less sensitive for recovery of heavy parasite eggs, such as *Taenia* or *Physaloptera*, because of a lower SG of the solution.[11] Commercial test kits with $ZnSO_4$ are available for benchtop analysis (eg, OVASSAY *Plus* Kit, Synbiotics Corp, San Diego, CA, USA), and can be modified for use in conjunction with centrifugation.[12] In all cases, it is advisable to measure the SG of the solution after preparation by use of a hydrometer and adjust it as necessary because a correct SG is paramount to a successful fecal examination.[11] Fecal smears are not recommended for the diagnosis of helminths because of high false-negative rates of 72% to more than 90%.[10]

Heterobilharzia americana

Heterobilharzia americana is a trematode that causes schistosomiasis in dogs and can be found along the US Gulf Coast and the Southern Atlantic Coast.[13] The parasite requires a freshwater snail as an intermediate host. Therefore, exposure is highest in areas with marshland and other types of open water access. Infection occurs when the cercariae penetrate the host's skin. They migrate first to the lungs, and then to the liver, where they develop into adult flukes, which then mate and lay eggs into the mesenteric veins. The eggs penetrate the mesenteric vein and travel into the intestinal wall and finally into the lumen, which may lead to granulomatous inflammation.[13,14] Clinical signs are often nonspecific and may include chronic diarrhea, hematochezia, weight loss, vomiting, and anorexia. The severity of the diarrhea presumably depends on the number of eggs being shed.[14] Hypoalbuminemia, hyperglobulinemia, eosinophilia, hypercalcemia, and increased liver enzyme activities are also frequently noted.

A diagnosis of *H americana* infection in the dog can be made based on polymerase chain reaction (PCR), a direct fecal smear (**Fig. 1**), or sodium chloride sedimentation. In contrast, commonly used flotation methods usually fail to identify this parasite.[13] A miracidia hatching technique has been described, which is performed by resuspending fecal sediment in distilled water, causing miracidia to hatch if eggs are present in the sediment, thus facilitating identification.[15] The fecal PCR assay can detect as few as 1 to 2 parasite eggs per gram of feces (Gastrointestinal Laboratory at Texas A&M University; www.vetmed.tamu.edu/gilab). Because eggs are frequently shed intermittently, it may be advisable to collect 2 to 3 fecal samples from different days for analysis.

Diagnostic Tests for Protozoal Infections

Giardia spp

Infections with *Giardia duodenalis* are a common cause of chronic diarrhea in dogs and cats. *Giardia* oocysts can be detected using fecal flotation, but the experience of the person performing the examination seems to have a significant effect on the outcome because of difficulties in recognizing this pathogen (**Fig. 2**).[11] If flotation is

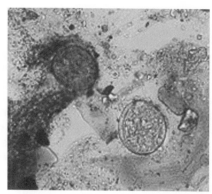

Fig. 1. In this fecal smear, 2 subspherical to oval *Heterobilharzia americana* ova are visible (unstained fecal smear, original magnification ×400). (*Courtesy of* Dr Micah Bishop, Texas A&M University.)

used, ZnSO$_4$ (SG of 1.18) with centrifugation is recommended because the SG of the solution ensures flotation of the cysts, while maintaining cyst morphology.[11] Solutions with a higher SG can lead to distortion of the cysts, thus making cyst identification more challenging.[11] Sensitivity of this technique has been reported to be as low as 49% if a single fecal sample is examined[16] but can be greatly improved to more than 90% by examining 3 fecal samples from different days because *Giardia* species is often shed intermittently.[11,17] In fact, as much as a 10-fold difference in cyst shedding can be observed between samples collected 3 days apart.[18]

Direct immunofluorescence assays (IFAs; eg, MeriFluor Cryptosporidium/Giardia, Meridian Bioscience, Inc, Cincinnati, OH, USA) performed on fecal samples are considered to be the gold standard for the diagnosis of *Giardia* organisms, with a reported sensitivity and specificity of more than 90% each.[16,19] These tests are widely available at veterinary diagnostic laboratories. Other diagnostic tests for *Giardia* organisms include qualitative enzyme immunoassays (eg, ProSpecT Giardia Microplate assay, Remel Inc, Lenexa, KS, USA; GIARDIA II, Techlab, Blacksburg,

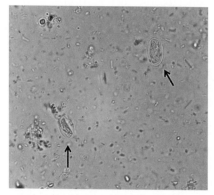

Fig. 2. In this fecal smear, 2 *Giardia duodenalis* cysts (*arrows*) can be observed (unstained fecal smear, original magnification ×1000). (*Courtesy of* Dr Yasushi Minamoto, Texas A&M University.)

VA, USA), and a SNAP test (SNAP *Giardia* Test, Idexx Laboratories, Westbrook, ME, USA). All of these assays have good specificities (>90%), whereas the reported sensitivities vary. Sensitivity for the ProSpecT *Giardia* Microplate assay has been shown to be very good at 93% to 100%,[17,20] whereas the GIARDIA II assay appears to be less sensitive at about 51%.[16] The SNAP *Giardia* test has been evaluated in several studies, with a mean sensitivity of about 73% (range 50%–100%). As with fecal flotation, examination of at least 2 different fecal samples may yield higher accuracies for *Giardia* detection when using any of these tests.[19] The SNAP test may be particularly useful for fast in-house screening for *Giardia* organisms and may increase diagnostic yield, especially if used in combination with fecal flotation.[11]

Cryptosporidium spp

Most infections with *Cryptosporidium parvum*, as well as *Cryptosporidium canis* in the dog and *Cryptosporidium felis* in the cat, are subclinical or cause only mild clinical signs.[21,22] In some animals, especially those that are immunosuppressed, the organism may cause intermittent chronic diarrhea and a malabsorption syndrome because of villus atrophy, villus fusion, and inflammation.[21,22]

A recent study determined that an enzyme immunoassay (ProSpecT Cryptosporidium microplate assay, Remel Inc, Lenexa, KS, USA) is the most sensitive test (sensitivity of 89%) for the diagnosis of *C parvum* infections if only 1 fecal sample is evaluated.[22] The 2 gold standard techniques, a modified Ziehl-Neelsen acid-fast staining procedure, and an IFA test (Merifluor Cryptosporidium/Giardia, Meridian Bioscience, Inc, Cincinnati, OH, USA) required examination of at least 2 or 3 different fecal samples to reach the same sensitivity.[22] Further studies may be warranted to investigate the effect of antigenic diversity of the different *Cryptosporidium* species on assay performance.

Tritrichomonas foetus

In recent years, *Tritrichomonas foetus* has been recognized as an important enteric pathogen in cats. Contrary to cattle, in which it is a venereal pathogen, *T foetus* colonizes the large intestine in cats, causing clinical signs of chronic large bowel diarrhea. However, in some cats, the infection may be asymptomatic. Affected cats are usually younger than 1 year, although infections have been documented in cats as old as 13 years.[23] Dense housing conditions, as encountered in catteries and shelters, are associated with a prevalence of up to 31%.[24]

Diagnosis of *T foetus* can be attempted by identifying the trophozoites on a direct fecal smear prepared from a fresh fecal sample, although the reported sensitivity of this technique is only 14% (**Fig. 3**).[24] Furthermore, *T foetus* may be mistaken for *Giardia* spp or the nonpathogenic *Pentatrichomonas hominis*.[25] *T foetus* can also be cultured from a rectal swab or a fresh fecal sample using a specific *Tritrichomonas* culture system (InPouch TF-Feline, Biomed Diagnostics Inc, White City, OR, USA). The pouch system allows for direct microscopic examination and concurrent culture of the organism, while it inhibits the growth of *Giardia* spp and *P hominis*, thereby increasing the specificity of this method. Cultures are incubated at room temperature and microscopically inspected for growth of *T foetus* on a daily basis up to 12 days. One study reported a sensitivity of 56% for the InPouch culture system.[24] Several laboratories offer a PCR-based assay that represents the most sensitive and specific method of detection currently available, with a reported sensitivity of 94%.[24,26] PCR also offers a faster turnaround time than the culture system and simplified sample handling because fecal samples for PCR do not need to be freshly voided and are stable at various storage temperatures.

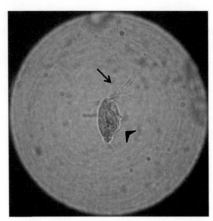

Fig. 3. *Tritrichomonas foetus* organism. Note the 3 anterior flagellae (*arrow*) as well as the lateral undulating membrane (*arrowhead*) (Lugol's iodine, original magnification ×400). (*Reproduced from* www.fabcats.org, Dr Andy Sparkes; with permission.)

Diagnostic Tests for Bacterial Infections

Intestinal bacterial infections may cause clinical signs of gastrointestinal disease in dogs and cats that are most often characterized by diarrhea, which may be acute or chronic and of small and/or large bowel origin.[27] The bacterial species described in the following section are of particular interest at present. An in-depth review on the topic of bacterial enteritis, including diagnosis of organisms, is described by J. Scott Weese elsewhere in this issue.

Campylobacter spp and Clostridium spp

Several different species of *Campylobacter* (*Campylobacter jejuni, Campylobacter coli, Campylobacter upsaliensis,* and *Campylobacter helveticus*) have previously been associated with diarrheal disease in dogs and cats.[28] However, a recent study has shown that *C upsaliensis* is commonly identified in healthy dogs, and *C helveticus* appears to be part of the normal intestinal microbiota of cats.[29] *C jejuni* was identified in dogs with gastrointestinal disease, but not in healthy animals, and *C coli* was not found in any of the dogs or cats investigated.[29] For diagnosis, both culture and PCR-based diagnostics are available. However, evaluation of fecal smears for the presence of spiral bacteria is not useful because pathogenic *Campylobacter* spp cannot be distinguished from nonpathogenic strains or other spiral organisms, such as *Helicobacter* spp.

Clostridium perfringens and Clostridium difficile have also been associated with diarrhea in dogs and cats and are both capable of producing potentially harmful toxins. However, these toxin-producing clostridial strains have also been identified in feces from many healthy nondiarrheic animals. Thus, it is difficult to define a clear causal relationship between these bacteria and clinical signs, and it is at present unknown whether *C perfringens* and *C difficile* are a major cause of enteritis or whether they represent secondary or commensal organisms.[30–32]

At present, PCR-based assays for the *C perfringens* enterotoxin or *C difficile* toxin genes are not considered to be specific for clostridial enteropathies, and only the detection of the actual toxins by enzyme-linked immunosorbent assay (ELISA) is thought to be of diagnostic value. However, the sensitivies and specificities of available toxin ELISAs are variable when used in dogs, and results should be interpreted with caution. Positive test results may be suggestive of a clostridial enteropathy, whereas a negative test result does not definitively rule it out (see the article by J. Scott Weese elsewhere in this issue for further exploration of this topic).

Escherichia coli

Recently, studies have found an association between histiocytic ulcerative colitis (granulomatous colitis) in Boxer dogs and strains of Escherichia coli that are of an adherent and invasive (AIEC) phenotype.[33] Several studies have demonstrated a response to treatment with enrofloxacin, and eradication of the E coli leads to clinical remission, suggesting a causal relationship.[33–35] Similarly, it has been shown that cats with IBD have a higher number of mucosa-associated E coli and other Enterobacteriaceae in the duodenum than healthy cats, and that the presence of E coli is associated with an abnormal mucosal architecture.[36] A diagnosis of AIEC can be made using fluorescent in-situ hybridization (FISH) on endoscopically obtained colonic biopsies. This FISH method (available through the College of Veterinary Medicine at Cornell University; http://www.vet.cornell.edu/labs/simpson/FISHFAQS.cfm) uses eubacterial probes to detect invasive organisms on and within the intestinal mucosa. Positive samples are then further analyzed to identify which specific genera of Enterobacteriaceae are present.

Tests for Other Infectious Diseases

Histoplasma

In dogs, disseminated Histoplasma capsulatum infections frequently involve the gastrointestinal tract, causing chronic diarrhea. The diarrhea may be of large and/or small intestinal origin, depending on the primary location of the granulomatous infiltrates caused by H capsulatum. If the small bowel is affected, a PLE may be present as well.[37] Clinical signs of feline disseminated histoplasmosis are usually nonspecific and may include lethargy, weight loss, fever, anorexia, and pale mucous membranes, whereas gastrointestinal signs such as vomiting and diarrhea are observed only rarely.[37]

For diagnosis, a peripheral blood smear may, in some cases, reveal the organism within monocytes, neutrophils, and rarely eosinophils.[37,38] However, a cytology specimen obtained via fine needle aspirate or scraping from affected tissues, is usually required to reach a diagnosis. In dogs with Histoplasma infection of the gastrointestinal tract, rectal scrapings or imprint cytology specimens from colonic mucosal biopsies may be helpful for a diagnosis. Lymph node and bone marrow aspirates have been shown useful in both cats and dogs. Staining with Wright-Giemsa–type stains visualizes the organisms within cells of the mononuclear phagocyte system on cytology specimens.[37,38] If cytology does not reveal any organisms, a tissue biopsy for histologic evaluation with special fungal stains may be required.[37,38]

Serologic tests for the diagnosis of histoplasmosis in cats or dogs using complement fixation or agar-gel immunodiffusion generally yield disappointing results because of possible false-negative or false-positive results. An enzyme immunoassay is available for Histoplasma antigen detection in serum or urine (MVista Histoplasma capsulatum Quantitative Antigen EIA; MiraVista Diagnostics, Indianapolis, IN, USA). However, cross-reactivity between Blastomyces and Histoplasma antigens has been described for this assay.[37] Therefore, a positive test result is not diagnostic for histoplasmosis but may aid in early diagnosis of a fungal infection.[38] Fungal culture from various body fluids and tissues may also be used for diagnosis, and a positive result confirms an infection.[37]

Pythium

Pythium insidiosum is an aquatic oomycete of the kingdom Stramenopila. Infection with Pythium may affect any part of the gastrointestinal tract, as well as surrounding organs, and clinical signs can therefore vary according to the location of the lesions. Obstructions and palpable masses can be found in some patients presenting with pythiosis.[39] Furthermore, pythiosis seems to be more prevalent in young large-breed dogs, and should thus be considered as a differential diagnosis in these patients that present with chronic clinical signs of gastrointestinal disease, especially if a palpable mass, obstruction, or evidence of an eosinophilic or pyogranulomatous enteritis and/or colitis can be found.[39,40]

There are 2 noninvasive serologic tests, an immunoblot assay and an ELISA, available for diagnosis of pythiosis. Both tests are highly sensitive and specific for use in dogs and cats.[39,41] In addition, ELISA may be used to monitor treatment because dramatic decreases in titers have been observed after successful surgical resection, whereas patients with a clinical recurrence retain high antibody titers.[39] The organism can also be cultured from tissue samples, if available, but culture and subsequent identification are often difficult because of bacterial contamination and challenging morphologic features, respectively. Infected tissues may also be analyzed using a PCR assay, which provides a very sensitive and specific test for P insidiosum.[39] In histologic tissue specimens, Pythium can be visualized using Gömöri methenamine silver.[39] Because Pythium tends to more commonly be associated with the submucosal and muscular layers of the intestinal wall, a diagnosis may be missed on endoscopic biopsies that do not reach deep tissue layers. Thus, pythiosis should be suspected if pyogranulomatous inflammation is found, yet a causative organism cannot be identified.[39] Tissue sections may also be analyzed using immunohistochemical methods. For this use, a polyclonal antibody against P insidiosum that does not cross-react with other species such as Lagenidium or Conidiobolus has been developed. This technique has been shown to be highly specific for the identification of Pythium hyphae in biopsies.[39,42]

LABORATORY TESTS THAT ASSESS THE SMALL INTESTINE FOR FUNCTION AND DISEASE
Cobalamin

Cobalamin (Vitamin B_{12}) is a water-soluble vitamin that is of both diagnostic and therapeutic importance, particularly if low serum concentrations are determined in a patient. Cobalamin is abundant in most commercial pet foods. Therefore, a dietary deficiency is uncommon, and low serum cobalamin concentrations more likely result from a disturbance within the absorptive mechanism of cobalamin.

Absorption of cobalamin is a complex process.[43] Dietary cobalamin is bound to animal protein in the diet and as such cannot be absorbed. After partial digestion of the protein in the stomach, cobalamin is released and immediately bound to R binder protein. On entering the small intestine, the R binder protein is digested by pancreatic proteases. Free cobalamin now binds to intrinsic factor (IF), the majority of which is secreted by the pancreas in cats and dogs.[44,45] This cobalamin-IF complex is subsequently absorbed by specialized receptors in the ileum.

It is obvious that this mechanism can be disturbed by a variety of factors. Chronic severe disease of the ileal mucosa may lead to destruction or reduced expression of the cobalamin-IF receptors on ileal enterocytes, causing cobalamin malabsorption. Eventually, body stores of cobalamin become depleted and a cobalamin deficiency ensues. Thus, a low serum cobalamin concentration indicates severe and long-standing disease involving the distal small intestine.

Another frequent cause of cobalamin deficiency in both cats and dogs is EPI.[46,47] Most of the IF in dogs and virtually the entire IF in cats is of pancreatic origin.[44,45]

Thus, a lack of exocrine pancreatic secretory products is accompanied by a decrease or absence of IF, leading to decreased absorption of cobalamin. The absence of pancreatic proteases in patients with EPI may further inhibit cobalamin absorption because cobalamin can no longer dissociate from R binder proteins. Because EPI is a major cause of cobalamin deficiency in both cats and dogs, it is recommended to determine a patient's serum TLI concentration at the time of cobalamin measurement to rule out EPI.

Cobalamin coupled to IF can also be absorbed by anaerobic intestinal bacteria.[48] Thus, when the numbers of these bacteria are increased, they may compete for cobalamin, which can also lead to decreased serum cobalamin concentrations. However, although a decreased serum cobalamin concentration may be associated with small intestinal dysbiosis (formerly also known as small intestinal bacterial overgrowth), it is neither a very sensitive nor specific test for this condition.

Lastly, a portion of the cobalamin that is absorbed by the ileal enterocytes undergoes enterohepatic circulation and is excreted in the bile.[49] This physiologic process may further reduce the amount of cobalamin that is actually retained by the body in an animal with compromised cobalamin absorption and can thus further aggravate cobalamin deficiency.

Serum cobalamin concentrations can be measured by several commercial immunoassays. Concentrations below the lower end of the reference range warrant supplementation with cobalamin, and it is recommended to supplement parenterally to bypass the impaired enteric absorptive mechanism (for more information on cobalamin supplementation, see www.vetmed.tamu.edu/gilab). Dosages are administered over the course of 4 months, and the serum cobalamin concentration should be rechecked 1 month after the last injection. Supplementation should only be discontinued if the underlying condition is fully resolved and the patient's cobalamin concentration has returned into the upper normal or supranormal range. In many patients, malabsorption of cobalamin is ongoing, and continued substitution with cobalamin is necessary.

Many dogs and especially cats with chronic small intestinal disease may show decreased serum cobalamin concentrations. However, a serum cobalamin concentration within the reference interval does not rule out presence of small intestinal disease because it is possible that the patient's body stores of cobalamin are still sufficient to maintain a normal serum cobalamin concentration despite ongoing malabsorption. The serum cobalamin concentration should be measured in all patients with chronic small intestinal disease because a recent study has determined cobalamin to be a risk factor for negative outcome in dogs with chronic enteropathies and may be an indicator for the patient to be refractory to treatment.[3]

Folate

Folic acid (Vitamin B_9, folate) is a water-soluble vitamin that is produced by plants and many bacterial species. Most commercial pet foods contain sufficient amounts and dietary deficiencies are uncommon. Thus, similar to cobalamin, changes in serum folate concentrations are more likely caused by either a decreased absorption of folate or possible alterations in the intestinal microbiota. While cobalamin can be regarded as a marker for distal small intestinal disease, folate represents an indicator of proximal intestinal disease. Thus, measurements of these 2 vitamins complement each other, and serum folate concentrations are generally determined in a panel with cobalamin when assessing small intestinal function.

Most of the dietary folate is present as folate polyglutamate, which the body cannot easily absorb. Folate conjugase, an enzyme produced by the jejunal brush border, hydrolyzes folate polyglutamate to folate monoglutamate by removing all but 1 of the glutamate residues. The monoglutamate form of folate can then be absorbed by specific folate carriers in the proximal small intestine.[50]

In patients with disease involving the proximal small intestine, mucosal damage may have a 2-fold effect on folate absorption. First, folate polyglutamate hydrolysis may be reduced if folate conjugase activity is impaired, leaving folate in its unabsorbable polyglutamate form. Secondly, folate absorption may be decreased if the mucosal carriers are damaged.[51] Both scenarios can lead to a decreased serum folate concentration, and folate deficiency if the condition is chronic and body stores become depleted.

Many bacterial species, including some species that are part of the physiologic bacterial ecosystem of the small intestine, are capable of synthesizing folate. Folate produced by these bacteria is released into the intestinal lumen and is available for absorption by the host. It is therefore possible that patients with small intestinal dysbiosis (formerly known as small intestinal bacterial overgrowth) might have an increased serum folate concentration.[51,52] However, serum folate measurements are not a sensitive test for small intestinal dysbiosis, and similarly, a folate concentration within the reference interval should not be used to rule out possible bacterial overgrowth of the small intestine.

In a patient with cobalamin deficiency, serum folate concentrations may be falsely normal or increased. This may happen because cobalamin is a cofactor for an enzymatic pathway in which folate is used. If the supply of cobalamin is insufficient, folate is not used in this reaction and it accumulates, which may cause serum folate concentrations to be normal in the face of folate malabsorption.[53] In these patients, a decrease in serum folate concentrations may be observed after cobalamin supplementation is initiated, because normalized cobalamin concentration may increase folate consumption. Therefore, reevaluation of the serum folate concentration after initiation of cobalamin supplementation may be beneficial to obtain a more accurate picture of folate metabolism.

Fecal α1-PI

The fecal α_1-PI assay is a test for PLE and is available for both cats and dogs. The α_1-PI is a plasma protein of similar size as albumin. If the intestinal mucosal barrier is compromised and leakage of plasma proteins into the intestinal lumen occurs, α_1-PI is lost at approximately the same rate as albumin. Unlike albumin, however, α_1-PI's properties protect it from being digested by intestinal proteases. Therefore, it is able to persist throughout the intestinal transit and is passed undamaged in the feces, in which it can then be measured (**Fig. 4**).[54]

Prompt diagnosis of PLE in a patient is of importance because hypoalbuminemia is a risk factor for negative outcome,[3] and the cause should be treated aggressively to improve survival. Presence of hypoalbuminemia, particularly if it is associated with hypoglobulinemia, in a patient with diarrhea is suggestive, but not diagnostic, of PLE. If renal protein loss or hepatic failure can be ruled out, and the patient does not have evidence of gastrointestinal bleeding or exudative skin disease, intestinal protein loss is most likely. The α_1-PI assay is especially valuable in patients without clinical signs of gastrointestinal disease in which other causes of hypoalbuminemia have been ruled out. Assessment of fecal α_1-PI concentrations may identify patients that have ongoing intestinal protein loss before clinical signs of gastrointestinal disease develop.

Fecal samples from 3 different defecations need to be collected into special sample tubes and frozen immediately after collection. For more information, it is recommended

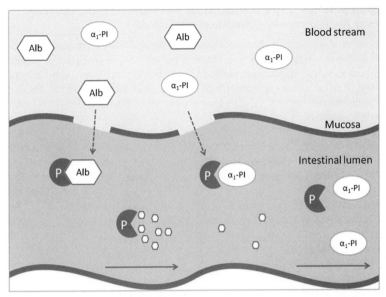

Fig. 4. Principle of the fecal α_1-PI assay. In patients with disturbed mucosal integrity, plasma proteins such as albumin and α_1-PI can be lost into the intestinal lumen. Unlike albumin and many other proteins, which are degraded by proteases, α_1-PI is resistant to proteolytic degradation. It can be measured using an immunoassay and can serve as a marker for gastrointestinal protein loss. Alb, albumin; P, protease.

to contact the Gastrointestinal Laboratory at Texas A&M University (www.vetmed. tamu.edu/gilab).

CRP

CRP is a positive acute-phase protein, therefore its serum concentration increases in response to an inflammatory stimulus. Although this response is not specific to the intestinal tract, a study has shown significantly increased serum CRP concentrations in dogs with moderate to severe IBD when compared with a group of healthy dogs.[55] Furthermore, the authors of that study were able to demonstrate that CRP concentrations decreased significantly after successful treatment. This suggests that determination of serum CRP concentrations may be beneficial in evaluating the response to treatment in canine patients with chronic enteropathies.

Serum CRP is most commonly measured as an ELISA. This assay is currently only available for dogs.

Tests for Intestinal Permeability and Absorptive Function

Intestinal permeability may be tested by oral administration of a non-metabolizable probe, such as ^{51}Cr-EDTA, iohexol, or a combination of lactulose and rhamnose (L/R ratio), and subsequent measurement of these probes in serum or urine. Similarly, tests for assessment of mucosal absorptive function have been performed using xylose or a combination of xylose and methylglucose (X/M ratio).[56–58] However, these tests have not been shown to be very sensitive or specific for gastrointestinal disorders in cats or dogs. Therefore, these tests are no longer used clinically.

PROMISING NEW TESTS FOR DIAGNOSIS OF GASTROINTESTINAL DISEASE
Perinuclear Antineutrophilic Cytoplasmic Antibodies

Perinuclear antineutrophilic cytoplasmic antibodies (pANCAs) are autoantibodies that result in a characteristic perinuclear staining pattern in granulocytes when used with immunofluorescence detection methods.[59] In human patients with IBD, pANCAs have been used as serologic markers of disease, and can be found in about 50% to 80% of patients with ulcerative colitis, whereas most patients (70%–90%) with Crohn disease are negative.[59,60]

Assays for measurement of pANCA have also been evaluated in dogs, and have shown variable sensitivities from 23% to 51%, and a specificity of 83% to 95% for canine IBD.[59–61] Thus, the detection of pANCA appears to be associated with IBD, but because of the poor sensitivity, appears not to be useful as a screening test for IBD.[59] One study found a higher rate of pANCA positive samples in dogs with diet-responsive diarrhea (62%) compared with dogs with idiopathic IBD (23%).[60] Recently, the use of the pANCA assay for early detection of PLE and protein-losing nephropathy (PLN) in Soft-Coated Wheaten Terriers has been studied.[62] In this group of dogs, the pANCA assay was able to predict PLE and/or PLN with a sensitivity of 95% and specificity of 80%. Furthermore, in most of these dogs, the first abnormal test result was obtained 1 or 2 years before onset of hypoalbuminemia, which may prove helpful in early diagnosis and more successful treatment of affected dogs.[62]

Calprotectin and S100A12

Calprotectin (S100A8/A9) and S100A12 are calcium-binding proteins that are highly abundant in neutrophils, and to a lesser extent in macrophages and monocytes.[63,64] Fecal concentrations of these proteins have been shown to be increased in human patients with IBD, when compared with healthy controls.[63–65] Furthermore, fecal concentrations of calprotectin correlate with endoscopic and histologic indices of disease activity.[66] IBD in humans is commonly associated with a neutrophilic infiltrate; therefore an increase in S100 proteins in this species is not surprising. In contrast, in dogs and cats with IBD, inflammatory infiltrates are most often lymphocytic-plasmacytic in nature, or less commonly eosinophilic. Thus, at initial consideration the increase of a marker for mainly neutrophilic inflammation in dogs and cats with IBD may be counterintuitive. However, one study has documented an increased number of cells staining positive for calprotectin in dogs with IBD compared with control dogs.[67] Another study found significantly increased mucosal S100-mRNA expression in dogs with IBD.[68] Furthermore, expression of calprotectin is inducible in various cell types, including epithelial cells.[69] Therefore, despite the lack of an obvious neutrophilic infiltrate in dogs and cats with IBD, an increase in S100 protein concentrations may still be expected.

An immunoassay for measurement of canine calprotectin in serum and fecal samples has recently been developed and analytically validated.[70] This assay is currently being extensively evaluated in dogs with various gastrointestinal diseases. Because of cross-reactivity with feline calprotectin, future use of this assay for cats with gastroenteropathies may also be possible.[70] Similarly, an assay for measurement of S100A12 has been developed and is being assessed for its usefulness in canine gastroenteropathies.[71,72]

If their clinical relevance is confirmed, canine-specific and feline-specific assays for calprotectin and S100A12 may become valuable tools for clinicians, as there is currently a lack of laboratory tests for markers of intestinal inflammation in small animals.

N-methylhistamine

Mast cells may participate in inflammatory processes of the intestine through the release of a variety of inflammatory mediators, such as histamine.[73–76] Increased numbers of intestinal mucosal mast cells have been observed in human patients with IBD, mainly at sites of active inflammation.[74,76–79] Furthermore, an increased release of histamine into the intestinal mucosa and the intestinal lumen has been documented at these sites with increased mast cell density.[76] Because histamine mediates pro-inflammatory effects on other immune cells as well as nerve and smooth muscle cells, it may contribute to the pathophysiology and clinical signs observed in patients with IBD.[76] As a stable metabolite of histamine, N-methylhistamine (NMH) has been suggested as a marker for mast cell degranulation and gastrointestinal inflammation. Increased urinary NMH concentrations have been documented in patients with active Crohn Disease and ulcerative colitis, and have been shown to correlate with endoscopic severity indices, clinical disease activity and C-reactive protein.[76,80,81]

An assay for measurement of NMH in canine urine and fecal samples has recently been developed.[82] Because the methodology is not species specific, this assay may also be used for feline samples. Fecal NMH concentrations have been shown to be increased in Norwegian Lundehunds with chronic gastrointestinal disease.[83] Preliminary data also show increased fecal NMH concentrations in some Soft-Coated Wheaten Terriers with gastrointestinal disease. In these dogs, increased mast cell degranulation has been implicated as a potentially contributing factor to the development of PLE and PLN.[84]

At present, the NMH assay is being evaluated for its potential diagnostic use in dogs with IBD and other gastroenteropathies.

SUMMARY

A variety of laboratory tests can be useful in the diagnosis and management of patients with chronic enteropathies. They are all minimally invasive and generally only require either a blood or fecal sample for analysis. Therefore, performing these tests before initiating more invasive procedures is recommended in the diagnostic approach of patients with chronic enteropathies.

Many of these tests have inherent limitations that need to be considered. For example, a negative test result may not rule out presence of an infectious agent. Likewise, a positive result does not necessarily imply causality because the infectious organism may be an opportunist. Thus, appropriate use and interpretation of the available tests is encouraged. It is apparent that we are currently lacking specific markers and tests to aid in diagnosis of chronic canine and feline enteropathies. Novel tests, such as pANCA, fecal S100 proteins, and NMH may prove to be such markers. However, these tests are still being investigated, and their overall clinical usefulness in the diagnosis of chronic enteropathies in dogs and cats needs to be clearly defined.

REFERENCES

1. Hall E, German A. Inflammatory bowel disease. In: Steiner J, editor. Small animal gastroenterology. Hanover (Germany): Schluetersche; 2008. p. 312–29.
2. Webster C. History, clinical signs, and physical findings in hepatobiliary disease. In: Ettinger S, Feldman E, editors. Textbook of veterinary internal medicine. St Louis (MO): Saunders Elsevier; 2010. p. 1612–25.

3. Allenspach K, Wieland B, Grone A, et al. Chronic enteropathies in dogs: Evaluation of risk factors for negative outcome. J Vet Intern Med 2007;21(4):700–8.
4. Kathrani A, Steiner JM, Suchodolski J, et al. Elevated canine pancreatic lipase immunoreactivity concentration in dogs with inflammatory bowel disease is associated with a negative outcome. J Small Anim Pract 2009;50(3):126–32.
5. Bailey S, Benigni L, Eastwood J, et al. Comparisons between cats with normal and increased fPLI concentrations in cats diagnosed with inflammatory bowel disease. J Small Anim Pract 2010;51(9):484–9.
6. Williams DA, Batt RM. Sensitivity and specificity of radioimmunoassay of serum trypsin-like immunoreactivity for the diagnosis of canine exocrine pancreatic insufficiency. J Am Vet Med Assoc 1988;192:195–201.
7. Steiner JM, Williams DA. Serum feline trypsin-like immunoreactivity in cats with exocrine pancreatic insufficiency. J Vet Intern Med 2000;14(6):627–9.
8. Steiner JM, Rehfeld JF, Pantchev N. Evaluation of fecal elastase and serum cholecystokinin in dogs with a false positive fecal elastase test. J Vet Intern Med 2010; 24(3):643–6.
9. Lennon EM, Boyle TE, Hutchins RG, et al. Use of basal serum or plasma cortisol concentrations to rule out a diagnosis of hypoadrenocorticism in dogs: 123 cases (2000–2005). J Am Vet Med Assoc 2007;231(3):413–6.
10. Dryden MW, Payne PA, Ridley R, et al. Comparison of common fecal flotation techniques for the recovery of parasite eggs and oocysts. Vet Ther 2005;6(1): 15–28.
11. Dryden MW, Payne PA, Smith V. Accurate diagnosis of Giardia spp and proper fecal examination procedures. Vet Ther 2006;7(1):4–14.
12. Zajac AM, Johnson J, King SE. Evaluation of the importance of centrifugation as a component of zinc sulfate fecal flotation examinations. J Am Anim Hosp Assoc 2002;38(3):221–4.
13. Johnson E. Canine schistosomiasis in North America: an underdiagnosed disease with an expanding distribution. Compend Contin Educ Vet 2010;32(3): E1–4.
14. Fradkin J, Braniecki A, Craig T, et al. Elevated parathyroid hormone-related protein and hypercalcemia in two dogs with schistosomiasis. J Am Anim Hosp Assoc 2001;37(4):349–55.
15. Goff WL, Ronald NC. Miracidia hatching technique for diagnosis of canine schistosomiasis. J Am Vet Med Assoc 1980;177(8):699–700.
16. Rishniw M, Liotta J, Bellosa M, et al. Comparison of 4 Giardia diagnostic tests in diagnosis of naturally acquired canine chronic subclinical giardiasis. J Vet Intern Med 2010;24(2):293–7.
17. Decock C, Cadiergues MC, Larcher M, et al. Comparison of two techniques for diagnosis of giardiasis in dogs. Parasite 2003;10(1):69–72.
18. Payne PA, Ridley RK, Dryden MW, et al. Efficacy of a combination febantel-praziquantel-pyrantel product, with or without vaccination with a commercial Giardia vaccine, for treatment of dogs with naturally occurring giardiasis. J Am Vet Med Assoc 2002;220(3):330–3.
19. Geurden T, Berkvens D, Casaert S, et al. A Bayesian evaluation of three diagnostic assays for the detection of Giardia duodenalis in symptomatic and asymptomatic dogs. Vet Parasitol 2008;157(1–2):14–20.
20. Rimhanen-Finne R, Enemark HL, Kolehmainen J, et al. Evaluation of immunofluorescence microscopy and enzyme-linked immunosorbent assay in detection of Cryptosporidium and Giardia infections in asymptomatic dogs. Vet Parasitol 2007;145(3–4):345–8.

21. Palmer CS, Traub RJ, Robertson ID, et al. Determining the zoonotic significance of Giardia and Cryptosporidium in Australian dogs and cats. Vet Parasitol 2008; 154(1–2):142–7.
22. Marks SL, Hanson TE, Melli AC. Comparison of direct immunofluorescence, modified acid-fast staining, and enzyme immunoassay techniques for detection of *Cryptosporidium* spp in naturally exposed kittens. J Am Vet Med Assoc 2004;225(10):1549–53.
23. Gookin JL, Breitschwerdt EB, Levy MG, et al. Diarrhea associated with trichomonosis in cats. J Am Vet Med Assoc 1999;215(10):1450–4.
24. Gookin JL, Stebbins ME, Hunt E, et al. Prevalence of and risk factors for feline *Tritrichomonas foetus* and Giardia infection. J Clin Microbiol 2004;42(6):2707–10.
25. Gookin JL, Foster DM, Poore MF, et al. Use of a commercially available culture system for diagnosis of *Tritrichomonas foetus* infection in cats. J Am Vet Med Assoc 2003;222(10):1376–9.
26. Gookin JL, Birkenheuer AJ, Breitschwerdt EB, et al. Single-tube nested PCR for detection of *Tritrichomonas foetus* in feline feces. J Clin Microbiol 2002;40(11):4126–30.
27. Marks S, Kather E. *Clostridium perfringens*- and *Clostridium difficile*-associated diarrhea. In: Greene CE, editor. Infectious diseases of the dog and cat. 3rd edition. St Louis (MO): Saunders Elsevier; 2006. p. 363–9.
28. Fox JG. Campylobacter infections. In: Greene CE, editor. Infectious diseases of the dog and cat. 3rd edition. St Louis (MO): Saunders Elsevier; 2006. p. 339–43.
29. Suchodolski JS, Gossett NM, Aicher KM, et al. Molecular assay for the detection of *Campylobacter* spp. in canine and feline fecal samples. J Vet Intern Med 2010; 24:748–9.
30. Chouicha N, Marks SL. Evaluation of five enzyme immunoassays compared with the cytotoxicity assay for diagnosis of *Clostridium difficile*-associated diarrhea in dogs. J Vet Diagn Invest 2006;18(2):182–8.
31. Weese JS, Staempfli HR, Prescott JF, et al. The roles of *Clostridium difficile* and enterotoxigenic *Clostridium perfringens* in diarrhea in dogs. J Vet Intern Med 2001;15(4):374–8.
32. Marks SL, Kather EJ, Kass PH, et al. Genotypic and phenotypic characterization of *Clostridium perfringens* and *Clostridium difficile* in diarrheic and healthy dogs. J Vet Intern Med 2002;16(5):533–40.
33. Mansfield CS, James FE, Craven M, et al. Remission of histiocytic ulcerative colitis in Boxer dogs correlates with eradication of invasive intramucosal *Escherichia coli*. J Vet Intern Med 2009;23(5):964–9.
34. Hostutler RA, Luria BJ, Johnson SE, et al. Antibiotic-responsive histiocytic ulcerative colitis in 9 dogs. J Vet Intern Med 2004;18(4):499–504.
35. Davies DR, O'Hara AJ, Irwin PJ, et al. Successful management of histiocytic ulcerative colitis with enrofloxacin in two Boxer dogs. Aust Vet J 2004;82(1–2):58–61.
36. Janeczko S, Atwater D, Bogel E, et al. The relationship of mucosal bacteria to duodenal histopathology, cytokine mRNA, and clinical disease activity in cats with inflammatory bowel disease. Vet Microbiol 2008;128:178–93.
37. Greene CE. Histoplasmosis. In: Greene CE, editor. Infectious diseases of the dog and cat. 3rd edition. St Louis (MO): Saunders Elsevier; 2006. p. 577–84.
38. Taboada J, Grooters A. Histoplasmosis, blastomycosis, sporotrichosis, candidiasis, pythiosis, and lagenidiosis. In: Ettinger S, Feldman E, editors. Textbook of veterinary internal medicine. St Louis (MO): Elsevier Saunders; 2010. p. 971–88.
39. Grooters AM, Foil CS. Miscellaneous fungal infections. In: Greene CE, editor. Infectious diseases of the dog and cat. 3rd edition. St Louis (MO): Saunders Elsevier; 2006. p. 637–50.

40. Berryessa NA, Marks SL, Pesavento PA, et al. Gastrointestinal pythiosis in 10 dogs from California. J Vet Intern Med 2008;22(4):1065–9.
41. Rakich PM, Grooters AM, Tang KN. Gastrointestinal pythiosis in two cats. J Vet Diagn Invest 2005;17(3):262–9.
42. Grooters A, Lopez M, Brown A, et al. Production of polyclonal antibodies for the immuno-histochemical identification of Pythium insidiosum. J Vet Intern Med 2001;15:315.
43. Markle HV. Cobalamin. Crit Rev Clin Lab Sci 1996;33(4):247–356.
44. Fyfe JC. Feline intrinsic factor (IF) is pancreatic in origin and mediates ileal cobalamin (CBL) absorption. J Vet Intern Med 1993;7:133.
45. Batt RM, Horadagoda NU, McLean L, et al. Identification and characterization of a pancreatic intrinsic factor in the dog. Am J Physiol 1989;256:G517–23.
46. Simpson KW, Morton DB, Batt RM. Effect of exocrine pancreatic insufficiency on cobalamin absorption in dogs. Am J Vet Res 1989;50:1233–6.
47. Thompson KA, Parnell NK, Hohenhaus AE, et al. Feline exocrine pancreatic insufficiency: 16 cases (1992–2007). J Feline Med Surg 2009;11:935–40.
48. Singh VV, Toskes PP. Small bowel bacterial overgrowth: presentation, diagnosis, and treatment. Curr Gastroenterol Rep 2003;5(5):365–72.
49. Simpson KW, Fyfe J, Cornetta A, et al. Subnormal concentrations of serum cobalamin (Vitamin B_{12}) in cats with gastrointestinal disease. J Vet Intern Med 2001; 15(1):26–32.
50. Rosenberg IH. Absorption and malabsorption of folates. Clin Haematol 1976;5(3): 589–618.
51. Ruaux CG. Laboratory tests for the diagnosis of intestinal disorders. In: Steiner JM, editor. Small animal gastroenterology. Hanover (Germany): Schluetersche; 2008. p. 50–5.
52. Batt RM, Morgan JO. Role of serum folate and Vitamin B_{12} concentrations in the differentiation of small intestinal abnormalities in the dog. Res Vet Sci 1982;32:17–22.
53. Donnelly JG. Folic acid. Crit Rev Clin Lab Sci 2001;38(3):183–223.
54. Melgarejo T, Williams DA, Asem EK. Enzyme-linked immunosorbent assay for canine a_1-protease inhibitor. Am J Vet Res 1998;59(2):127–30.
55. Jergens AE, Schreiner CA, Frank DE, et al. A scoring index for disease activity in canine inflammatory bowel disease. J Vet Intern Med 2003;17(3):291–7.
56. Rodriguez H, Suchodolski JS, Berghoff N, et al. Development and analytic validation of a gas chromatography-mass spectrometry method for the measurement of sugar probes in canine serum. Am J Vet Res 2009;70(3):320–9.
57. Klenner S, Frias R, Coenen M, et al. Estimation of intestinal permeability in healthy dogs using the contrast medium iohexol. Vet Clin Pathol 2009;38(3):353–60.
58. Hall E, German A. Diseases of the small intestine. In: Ettinger S, Feldman E, editors. Textbook of veterinary internal medicine. St Louis (MO): Elsevier Saunders; 2010. p. 1527–72.
59. Allenspach K, Luckschander N, Styner M, et al. Evaluation of assays for perinuclear antineutrophilic cytoplasmic antibodies and antibodies to Saccharomyces cerevisiae in dogs with inflammatory bowel disease. Am J Vet Res 2004;65(9): 1279–83.
60. Luckschander N, Allenspach K, Hall J, et al. Perinuclear antineutrophilic cytoplasmic antibody and response to treatment in diarrheic dogs with food responsive disease or inflammatory bowel disease. J Vet Intern Med 2006;20(2):221–7.
61. Mancho C, Sainz A, Garcia-Sancho M, et al. Detection of perinuclear antineutrophil cytoplasmic antibodies and antinuclear antibodies in the diagnosis of canine inflammatory bowel disease. J Vet Diagn Invest 2010;22(4):553–8.

62. Allenspach K, Lomas B, Wieland B, et al. Evaluation of perinuclear anti-neutrophilic cytoplasmic autoantibodies as an early marker of protein-losing enteropathy and protein-losing nephropathy in soft coated wheaten terriers. Am J Vet Res 2008;69(10):1301–4.

63. Sidler MA, Leach ST, Day AS. Fecal S100A12 and fecal calprotectin as noninvasive markers for inflammatory bowel disease in children. Inflamm Bowel Dis 2008; 14(3):359–66.

64. Konikoff MR, Denson LA. Role of fecal calprotectin as a biomarker of intestinal inflammation in inflammatory bowel disease. Inflamm Bowel Dis 2006;12(6):524–34.

65. Bunn SK, Bisset WM, Main MJ, et al. Fecal calprotectin as a measure of disease activity in childhood inflammatory bowel disease. J Pediatr Gastroenterol Nutr 2001;32(2):171–7.

66. Roseth AG, Aadland E, Jahnsen J, et al. Assessment of disease activity in ulcerative colitis by faecal calprotectin, a novel granulocyte marker protein. Digestion 1997;58(2):176–80.

67. German AJ, Hall EJ, Day MJ. Immune cell populations within the duodenal mucosa of dogs with enteropathies. J Vet Intern Med 2001;15(1):14–25.

68. Jergens A, Nettleton D, Suchodolski J, et al. Interplay of commensal bacteria, host gene expression, and clinical disease activity in the pathogenesis of canine inflammatory bowel disease. J Vet Intern Med 2010;24:1570–1.

69. Ehrchen JM, Sunderkotter C, Foell D, et al. The endogenous Toll-like receptor 4 agonist S100A8/S100A9 (calprotectin) as innate amplifier of infection, autoimmunity, and cancer. J Leukoc Biol 2009;86(3):557–66.

70. Heilmann R, Suchodolski J, Steiner J. Development and analytic validation of a radioimmunoassay for the quantification of canine calprotectin in serum and feces from dogs. Am J Vet Res 2008;69(7):845–53.

71. Heilmann RM, Suchodolski JS, Steiner JM. Purification and partial characterization of canine S100A12. Biochimie 2010;92:1914–22.

72. Heilmann R, Lanerie D, Suchodolski J, et al. A method for the quantification of serum and fecal canine S100A12. J Vet Intern Med 2010;24:751–2.

73. Peters L, Kovacic J. Histamine: metabolism, physiology, and pathophysiology with applications in veterinary medicine. J Vet Emerg Crit Care 2009;19(4): 311–28.

74. He SH. Key role of mast cells and their major secretory products in inflammatory bowel disease. World J Gastroenterol 2004;10(3):309–18.

75. Kumar V, Sharma A. Mast cells: emerging sentinel innate immune cells with diverse role in immunity. Mol Immunol 2010;48:14–25.

76. Winterkamp S, Weidenhiller M, Otte P, et al. Urinary excretion of N-methylhistamine as a marker of disease activity in inflammatory bowel disease. Am J Gastroenterol 2002;97(12):3071–7.

77. Schwab D, Raithel M, Hahn EG. Evidence for mast cell activation in collagenous colitis. Inflamm Res 1998;47(Suppl 1):S64–5.

78. Fox CC, Lichtenstein LM, Roche JK. Intestinal mast cell responses in idiopathic inflammatory bowel disease. Histamine release from human intestinal mast cells in response to gut epithelial proteins. Dig Dis Sci 1993;38(6):1105–12.

79. Le Berre N, Heresbach D, Kerbaol M, et al. Histological discrimination of idiopathic inflammatory bowel disease from other types of colitis. J Clin Pathol 1995;48(8):749–53.

80. Weidenhiller M, Raithel M, Winterkamp S, et al. Methylhistamine in Crohn's disease (CD): increased production and elevated urine excretion correlates with disease activity. Inflamm Res 2000;49(Suppl 1):S35–6.

81. Kimpel S, Nagel A, Kestler C, et al. Evaluation of urinary N-methylhistamine excretion during a long-term follow up of patients with inactive Crohn's disease. Inflamm Res 2007;56(Suppl 1):S61–2.

82. Ruaux C, Wright J, Steiner J, et al. Gas chromatography-mass spectrometry assay for determination of N-tau-methylhistamine concentration in canine urine specimens and fecal extracts. Am J Vet Res 2009;70(2):167–71.

83. Berghoff N, Suchodolski J, Steiner J. Fecal N-methylhistamine concentrations in Norwegian Lundehunds with gastrointestinal disease. J Vet Intern Med 2008; 22(3):748.

84. Vaden S, Hammerberg B, Orton S, et al. Mast cell degranulation responses in Soft-Coated Wheaten Terriers with protein-losing enteropathy and/or nephropathy. J Vet Intern Med 2000;14:348.

Ultrasonography of Small Intestinal Inflammatory and Neoplastic Diseases in Dogs and Cats

Lorrie Gaschen, PhD, DVM, Dr med vet

KEYWORDS

- Inflammatory bowel disease • Food allergy • Lymphoma
- Intestinal hemodynamics • Intestinal neoplasia
- Fungal infection

Ultrasonography has become a mainstay of diagnosing intestinal diseases in dogs and cats. Using ultrasonography to differentiate inflammatory from neoplastic infiltrative disease has been the focus of recent investigations.[1–5] Abdominal radiography remains an important part of screening patients with vomiting and diarrhea, and should be performed in conjunction with the ultrasonographic examination in most instances. Barium studies of the gastrointestinal tract remain important for the diagnosis of foreign bodies in vomiting animals and for assessing gastrointestinal emptying and transit times. However, for detecting infiltrative intestinal diseases the ultrasonographic examination is superior. Computed tomography and magnetic resonance imaging for the detection of infiltrative small intestinal diseases in dogs and cats have not yet been investigated.

Differentiating inflammatory from neoplastic infiltration of the small intestine is crucial to choosing appropriate treatment strategies in dogs and cats. Ultrasonography is often one of the first diagnostic tools used for that purpose. Although overlap in the sonographic appearances of inflammatory and neoplastic infiltration make a definitive diagnosis difficult, awareness of features of both diseases is important for the accurate interpretation of the sonographic findings. Full-thickness intestinal biopsy remains the gold standard for differentiating inflammatory from neoplastic disease of the small intestine.

The author has nothing to disclose and no funding sources to note.

Veterinary Clinical Sciences, School of Veterinary Medicine, Louisiana State University, Skip Bertman Drive, Baton Rouge, LA 70803, USA

E-mail address: lgaschen@vetmed.lsu.edu

Vet Clin Small Anim 41 (2011) 329–344
doi:10.1016/j.cvsm.2011.01.002
0195-5616/11/$ – see front matter. Published by Elsevier Inc.

EQUIPMENT

High-resolution images are necessary for the recognition of detailed features of intestinal wall abnormalities in dogs and cats (**Fig. 1**). Therefore, high-frequency curved or linear array transducers with a minimum of 7.5 MHz are required for accurate examination of the small intestinal wall and its associated layering. Color and spectral Doppler are important for the detection of intestinal ischemia or increased vascularization, such as observed with some neoplastic infiltrations.[6] Spectral Doppler has also been used to assess intestinal blood flow in chronic enteropathies. Contrast-enhanced harmonic ultrasound imaging of the small intestine is not yet established for detection of intestinal disease in veterinary medicine.

EXAMINATION TECHNIQUE FOR THE SMALL INTESTINE

Dogs and cats should be fasted and have the ventral abdomen clipped as for any routine ultrasound examination. The animals can be examined in dorsal, right, or left lateral recumbency. A combination of different positions can be advantageous for evaluating intestinal segments not visible in one of the recumbencies. Furthermore, gas and fluid contents move to different portions of the intestine when the animal is repositioned, which can aid in visualization of the intestinal wall. Small intestinal segments should be traced throughout the entire abdomen from the pylorus to the ileocecocolic junction.

The entire intestinal tract should be assessed for:

- Wall thickness
- Wall layering
- Layer echogenicity
- Motility
- Peri-intestinal echogenicity
- Presence of free fluid

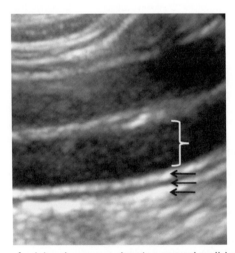

Fig. 1. Sagittal image of a jejunal segment showing normal wall layering, thickness, and echogenicity. The bracket shows the mucosa and the outer 3 arrows point to the submucosa, muscularis, and serosa, starting from the mucosa moving outwards. The mucosa is practically anechoic, and the outer 3 layers are thin and approximately the same thickness relative to each other.

- Regional lymphadenomegaly
- Focal, multifocal, or diffuse distribution of disease.

Table 1 lists ultrasound parameters for normal small intestines.[7-9] Involvement of other organ systems is also important for prioritizing a differential diagnosis list, and a complete sonographic examination of the abdomen should be performed in patients with gastrointestinal signs. In addition, the presence of peri-intestinal hyperechoic mesentery or free fluid can alert the sonographer to regional inflammation, neoplastic invasion, or perforation.

The descending duodenum, jejunum, and ileum can be differentiated from one another ultrasonographically based on their location, wall layering, and communication with adjacent intestinal segments (see **Table 1**). In dogs the duodenum is the most lateral intestinal segment in the right abdomen. The duodenum follows a straight course along the right body wall cranially to the cranial duodenal flexure, where it abruptly turns toward the left to join the pylorus. The flexure is usually visible in all dogs, but may be difficult to locate in deep-chested animals. A right intercostal approach may be necessary to examine the pyloroduodenal junction in some dogs.[10,11] In cats, the pyloroduodenal junction has a more midline location, immediately caudal to the hilus of the liver, and the duodenum courses laterally to the right kidney. Focal, hyperechoic structures that appear like outpouchings of the lumen into the mucosa can often be detected at the antimesenteric border of the duodenal wall. These normal structures are associated with Peyer patches, are only present on the duodenum, and should not be misdiagnosed as ulcerations. The duodenum

Table 1
Normal ultrasonographic features of the small intestine

Ultrasound Parameter	Location	Wall Thickness	Specific Features
Dogs			
Duodenum	Right lateral abdomen	<20 kg: ≤5.1 mm 20–29 kg: ≤5.3 mm >30 kg: ≤6 mm	Peyer patches at the antimesenteric border Major and minor duodenal papilla
Jejunum	Mid and caudal abdomen	<20 kg: ≤4.1 mm 20–29 kg: ≤4.4 mm >30 kg: ≤4.7 mm	—
Ileum	Right mid abdomen, medial to the duodenum	—	Thicker submucosa Ileocecocolic junction Rosette appearance in cross section
Cats			
Duodenum	Pylorus mid abdomen at liver hilus Duodenum right lateral abdomen	1.3–3.8 mm	Major duodenal papilla more prominent (2.9–5.5 mm) than in the dog and can be identified in most cats
Jejunum	Mid and caudal abdomen	1.6–3.6 mm	—
Ileum	Right mid abdomen, medial to the duodenum	2.5–3.2 mm	Thicker submucosa Wagon wheel appearance in cross section Ileocolic junction

and jejunum should be observed for peristalsis, which occurs at the rate of approximately one contraction wave per minute in normal animals.

INFLAMMATORY DISEASES

Inflammatory diseases of the small intestines are common in dogs and cats. Causes include lymphoplasmacytic enteritis (most common), eosinophilic enteritis, granulomatous enteritis (rare), protein-losing enteropathy and lymphangiectasia, food allergy, and chronic infection (giardia, histoplasma, pythium, mycobacterium, toxoplasma, prototheca).[12] These diseases do not always induce changes that can be detected with ultrasonography, and intestinal biopsy is required to confirm the diagnosis and assess the severity of lesions in many cases.

Chronic Inflammatory Disease

Although generally diffuse, inflammatory disease can also cause focal or segmental changes. It often leads to mild to moderate transmural thickening of the intestinal wall with preserved wall layering (**Fig. 2**).[3–5] In some instances the wall layering can be indistinct or completely lost if ulcerative enteritis, fibrosis, edema, hemorrhage, and/or severe lymphoplasmacytic infiltration are present.[13] The relative thickness of the layers may also change while the total wall thickness remains normal. Selective muscularis thickening can be caused by idiopathic muscular hypertrophy of the smooth muscle layer of the intestine, and has been commonly observed in inflammatory conditions.[14] The echogenicity of the mucosa may be altered in both lymphangiectasia and lymphoplasmacytic enteritis.[3] Hyperechoic mucosal speckles and striations can be identified in inflammatory disease but are nonspecific for the cause and severity (**Fig. 3**).

The sonographic abnormalities of inflammatory bowel disease (IBD) in cats are similar to those of dogs. Poor intestinal wall layer definition, focal thickening, and large hypoechoic mesenteric lymph nodes are consistent with IBD.[1] In cats the muscular layer is often selectively thickened in IBD, due to lymphoplasmacytic and eosinophilic infiltration (**Fig. 4**).[13] However, a thickened muscularis layer in the cat has also been associated with other disorders such as mechanical obstruction and lymphoma.[13] Marked thickening of the muscularis layer may also be observed in cats with eosinophilic enteritis,[15] a condition that has been reported to occur in association with feline

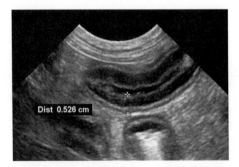

Fig. 2. Sagittal image of a jejunal segment from a dog with chronic diarrhea that had a histopathological diagnosis of lymphocytic, plasmacytic enteritis. The wall is thickened at 5.3 mm and there is a small amount of fluid in the lumen. The segment has a stiffened appearance but the wall layering is normal.

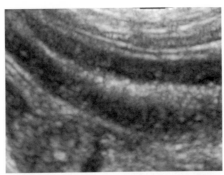

Fig. 3. Sagittal image of a jejunal segment from a dog with chronic diarrhea and a histopathological diagnosis of lymphocytic, plasmacytic enteritis. There are multifocal, pin-point, hyperechoic foci throughout the mucosa. These speckles were found to be diffuse throughout the small intestines, but no wall thickening or altered layering was found.

hypereosinophilic syndrome (**Fig. 5**). Although the changes are diffuse in most instances, a focal intestinal mass has been reported in one cat.[16] Histopathologically the mucosa of affected cats shows an increased number of eosinophils, and the muscularis is hypertrophic. Feline gastrointestinal eosinophilic sclerosing fibroplasia is another eosinophilic disorder that has recently been described in 25 cats.[17] All cats had an intestinal mass at the pylorus, jejunum, ileum, ileocecocolic junction, or colon, with the pyloric location being most common. The lesions were usually transmural, but they were limited to the mucosa in some cases; however, they never extended beyond the serosa.

Chronic inflammatory disease in cats may also produce a distinct, thin, hyperechoic line within the mucosa, which has been associated with fibrosis histopathologically.[18] The clinical relevance of this sonographic abnormality is uncertain, as it can also be found incidentally in cats without gastrointestinal disease.

Lymphangiectasia can occur in dogs with IBD or a primary idiopathic disorder.[19,20] The ultrasonographic diagnosis usually rests on the ability to demonstrate hyperechoic striations that are aligned parallel to one another and perpendicular to the

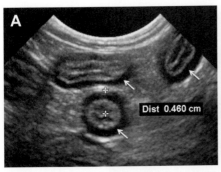
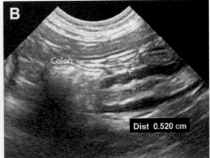

Fig. 4. (A) Transverse image of jejunal segments in a cat with a histopathological diagnosis of cholangiohepatitis and lipidosis and lymphocytic, plasmacytic, and eosinophilic enteritis. The cat also had a clinical diagnosis of pancreatitis. The muscularis (*arrowed*) is diffusely thickened throughout the jejunum, and the walls are thickened at 4.6 mm. (B) The ileum from the same cat as in A is shown in the sagittal plane. The muscularis layer of the ileum is markedly thickened.

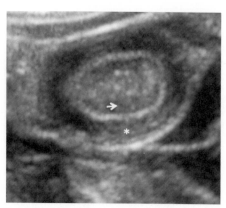

Fig. 5. Hypereosinophilic syndrome in a cat. A transverse image of the jejunum shows mild intestinal wall thickening, and a selectively thickened and relatively hyperechoic muscularis (*asterisk*). The arrow shows the mucosa, which is not as thick as the muscularis but has a diffusely increased echogenicity.

long axis of the intestine (**Fig. 6**).[20] The most common sonographic findings in dogs with histopathologically confirmed lymphangiectasia are abdominal effusion, intestinal thickening, hyperechoic mucosa, and wall corrugation.[19] However, the intestine may also appear normal. Sonographic abnormalities are typically not specific enough to differentiate lymphangiectasia from other inflammatory diseases, and they usually do not correlate with histologic severity.[19] Generalized mild dilation of the intestines and fluid content is also commonly observed, and regional lymph nodes may or may not be enlarged. Lymphangiectasia, IBD (including lymphocytic, plasmacytic, and eosinophilic forms), alimentary lymphoma, ulcer, and histoplasmosis can all cause protein-losing enteropathy.[21] Because of the overlap in the sonographic appearance of these diseases, histopathology is required for differentiation. Although in most instances abnormalities associated with lymphangiectasia are diffuse, a dog with

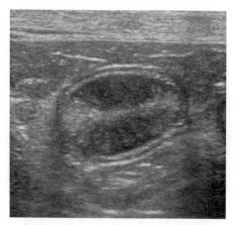

Fig. 6. Transverse image of a jejunal segment in a Yorkshire Terrier with chronic diarrhea and weight loss. There are multiple, parallel arranged hyperechoic striations throughout the mucosa. This finding was present throughout the entire jejunum and duodenum. Lymphangiectasia and lymphocytic, plasmacytic inflammation were diagnosed histopathologically.

a focal mass lesion due to lymphangiectasia has also been described. However, this presentation should be considered a rare form.[20]

Corrugation of the small intestine can be seen with inflammatory disease within or surrounding the intestinal wall. Dogs with enteritis of any type can show signs of corrugation.[22] In dogs with pancreatitis, the duodenum can commonly become corrugated due to the surrounding peritonitis. Hemo- and uroabdomen can result in similar findings in the small intestines.[22,23] Ultrasonography also allows the sonographer to detect intestinal spasms in real time. These spasms appear as intermittent contractions, resulting in a corrugated appearance of the wall that resolves after the spasm.

Few data are available concerning the monitoring of chronic enteropathies sonographically. A 2-dimensional ultrasound score has been established for canine chronic enteropathies. The ultrasound score correlates to the canine inflammatory bowel disease clinical activity index (CIBDAI) at initial presentation of the patient when the disease is clinically active.[3] However, improvement in the CIBDAI after treatment does not correlate with improvement of the ultrasound score on follow-up examinations.

Infectious Diseases

Infectious causes of intestinal wall infiltration have sonographic findings similar to neoplasia. Non-neoplastic causes of intestinal masses include fungal infections with pythium and histoplasma, abscesses, cysts, hematomas, ulcers, intussusceptions, and foreign body granulomas.[24] A focal mass with loss of wall layering is most commonly associated with neoplasia; however, fungal infections may cause similar lesions. Pythiosis and histoplasmosis can lead to either intestinal wall thickening with pseudolayering, transmural loss of layering, or a focal mass (**Fig. 7**).[25] Pseudolayering appears as alternating bands of hyper- and hypoechoic tissue within the intestinal wall that does not correspond to the normal wall layers. The distribution of fungal infection in the intestine can be focal or multifocal, but is usually not diffuse. Regional lymph nodes are often enlarged, rounded, or irregularly shaped, and hypoechoic or heterogeneous sonographically. These nodes can also grow to immense proportions, creating a large mass in the mid-abdomen. Histoplasmosis has been

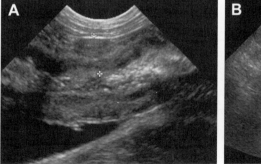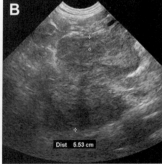

Fig. 7. (A) Sagittal image of the duodenum in a 2-year-old dog with severe weight loss. The wall is thickened (8 mm) and there is a complete, transmural loss of normal layering. The wall appears heterogeneous and stiff. Diagnosis: pythiosis. (B) A large, 5.5-cm sized, complex and heterogeneous mass was present in the mid-abdomen of the dog in A. This finding is common in pythium infections and represents infiltration of the jejunal lymph nodes.

reported in the cat, and can spread to the entire abdomen and lungs.[26] Abdominal ultrasonography of dogs and cats with intestinal histoplasmosis can reveal lymph node enlargement, a mass of uncertain origin, thickening of the muscularis layer of the small bowel, focal thickening of the ileum with loss of layering, and free peritoneal fluid. These changes are sonographically similar to those of lymphoma and other neoplasms. Histology is required for differentiation between neoplastic and non-neoplastic masses of the intestines and lymph nodes.

INTESTINAL NEOPLASIA

Focal intestinal wall thickening can be caused by neoplastic and non-neoplastic lesions. Sonographic parameters such as lesion symmetry, distribution, degree of thickening, and wall layering are most commonly used to distinguish inflammation from neoplasia.[4] In dogs, wall thickness of neoplastic infiltrative lesions is statistically greater than that of nonspecific inflammatory disease (0.5–7.9 mm vs 0.2–2.9 mm, respectively).[4] When loss of wall layering is identified sonographically, there is a 50-times greater likelihood of a diagnosis of neoplasia than of nonspecific inflammation.[4] Neoplastic masses may have concentric or eccentric wall thickening with loss of wall layering. **Table 2** lists the types of abnormal wall layering patterns that can be detected with ultrasonography, with a description of their appearances.[4] Neoplastic infiltration of the small intestine is also statistically shown to be more likely focal than diffuse, which is more common in inflammatory disease.[4]

The most common intestinal wall tumors in dogs are carcinomas, lymphoma, leiomyoma, and leiomyosarcoma.[27–30] Ileal hemangioma with a large mass detected sonographically is rare but can occur in dogs.[31] In cats, the most common causes of neoplastic intestinal disease are lymphoma, mast cell tumor, and adenocarcinomas. Visceral hemangiosarcoma involving the small intestine and colon has also been reported recently in cats; however, the sonographic characteristics have not been established.[32]

Alimentary lymphoma can be diffuse in both dogs and cats but most commonly occurs as a solitary, hypoechoic intestinal mass with transmural loss of wall layering (**Fig. 8**).[13,29] Furthermore, it is the most common neoplastic cause of diffuse infiltration

Table 2
Ultrasonographic patterns of abnormal small intestinal wall layering

Pattern	Commonly Associated With
Altered	
One or more layers are selectively thickened	IBD, lymphoma, eosinophilic enteritis
One or more layers have an abnormal echogenicity	Thickened muscularis in cats
	Fungal infections
Transmural Loss	
No layers are present between the mucosa and serosa	Lymphoma, adenocarcinoma
	Fungal infections
Concentric Loss of Layering	
Wall uniformly affected in cross section	Lymphoma
Eccentric Loss of Layering	
Wall not uniformly affected in cross section Can extend outward through the serosa	Leiomyosarcoma

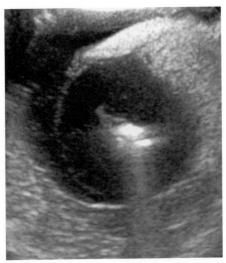

Fig. 8. Transverse image of a jejunal segment in a dog. Transmural, hypoechoic thickening with complete loss of wall layering is present. Hyperechoic material in the lumen with dirty shadowing is due to gas content. The lesion was focal. Fine-needle aspiration was diagnostic for lymphoma.

and wall thickening that can appear similar to inflammatory disease (**Fig. 9**). Lymphoma may cause partial stenosis of the intestinal lumen, but usually not complete obstruction. Regional lymph nodes are commonly enlarged, rounded, and hypoechoic. In cats, alimentary lymphoma can cause diffuse disease that infiltrates the intestinal wall without altering the wall layering. Thickening of the muscularis layer has been reported in IBD and intestinal lymphoma in that species.[33] A recent study showed a significant association between muscularis thickening and feline T-cell lymphoma (**Fig. 10**),[34] but did not show any significant difference in the prevalence of regional lymphadenopathy between cats with IBD and those with lymphoma. Cats with disease limited to the mucosa and lamina propria, based on histopathology, had no ultrasonographic abnormalities. Due to the overlap of diseases associated with muscularis thickening and lymphadenopathy in cats (see above), full-thickness intestinal biopsies are likely indicated for a definitive diagnosis.

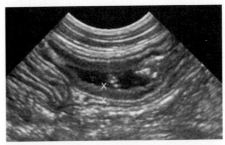

Fig. 9. Sagittal image of the jejunum in a 2-year-old Boxer with chronic diarrhea and weight loss. The wall thickness and layering are normal, but the mucosa was diffusely hyperechoic, and the intestines appeared stiff and were mildly fluid distended. Full-thickness biopsies were performed and a diagnosis of lymphoma was made histopathologically.

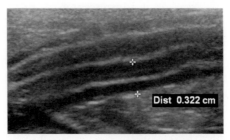

Fig. 10. Sagittal image of the jejunum in a cat. The wall thickness is normal but the muscularis is thickened. This abnormality was present throughout the jejunum and the regional lymph nodes were enlarged, rounded, and hypoechoic (not shown). Lymphoma was diagnosed.

Intestinal adenocarcinoma in dogs and cats appears sonographically as transmural thickening with complete loss of wall layering and regional lymphadenopathy (**Fig. 11**).[13,29] This appearance is very similar to that of alimentary lymphoma when it forms a mass. However, carcinomas are usually solitary whereas lymphoma can be focal, multifocal, or diffuse. Intestinal carcinoma will often cause mechanical ileus due to luminal stenosis, which is less common with lymphoma. Intestinal smooth muscle tumors such as leiomyosarcomas often become very large and have an eccentric growth out of the intestinal wall through the serosa (**Fig. 12**). These tumors can appear as extraluminal masses also.[13] Leiomyomas tend to be small, and appear as a focal intramural hypoechoic thickening with loss of wall layering (**Fig. 13**).[14] Intestinal mast cell tumors are rare and are more common in cats than dogs. Their appearance is similar to that of lymphoma, as they cause hypoechoic thickening of the wall with loss of layering.[14,35]

Widespread neoplastic infiltration throughout the mesentery and organs is referred to as carcinomatosis (**Fig. 14**). Intestinal adenocarcinoma has been associated with the development of carcinomatosis in dogs.[28] Ultrasonographic features include hypoechoic nodular foci throughout the mesentery, and often free abdominal fluid. When free fluid is present, the surface of the organs such as the liver and spleen should be carefully scanned for irregularities that may represent tumor spread.

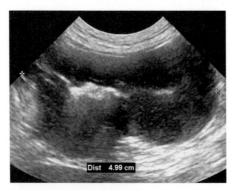

Fig. 11. Large heterogeneous jejunal mass in a dog. The mass shows transmural complete loss of wall layering and luminal stenosis. The diagnosis was carcinoma, but leiomyosarcoma and lymphoma have similar ultrasonographic features.

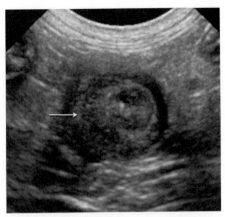

Fig. 12. Transverse image of a jejunal segment in a dog, showing an example of eccentric thickening (*arrows*) seen with leiomyosarcomas.

REGIONAL LYMPHADENOPATHY

The hepatic, gastric, pancreaticoduodenal, jejunal, and lumbar aortic lymph nodes drain the small intestine (duodenum, jejunum, and ileum) and should be assessed during the routine ultrasonographic examination. Normal lymph nodes should be slightly hypoechoic or isoechoic to the surrounding mesentery.[36] The height of jejunal lymph nodes in healthy dogs ranges from 1.6 to 8.2 mm and their width ranges from 2.6 to 14.7 mm.[36] Metastatic lymph nodes are typically enlarged, rounded, and hypoechoic in cats and dogs. Lymph nodes may be enlarged in inflammatory disease, but typically maintain a more normal shape and echogenicity (**Fig. 15**).[37] However, they may become ill defined.[38] Infectious disease will often lead to more severe lymph node enlargement with features similar to those of metastatic infiltration.[37] Regardless of the underlying cause, as the node becomes larger, necrotic, or hemorrhagic, it will appear more heterogeneous and irregular.[37] The jejunal nodes are usually readily accessible for percutaneous ultrasound-guided tissue sampling. Depending on their size and due to their close proximity to major vessels, sedation may be necessary to perform tissue sampling for cytologic analysis.

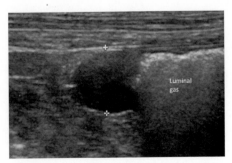

Fig. 13. Sagittal image of a jejunal segment in a dog. The dog did not present with gastrointestinal disease and a 1-cm diameter, focal, hypoechoic nodule was present at the serosal surface (between calipers). The same nodule was detected 3 months later, and cytology diagnosed a leiomyoma.

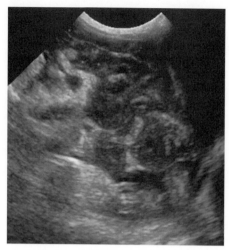

Fig. 14. Mesentery in a dog with intestinal carcinoma. Free peritoneal fluid was present and the mesentery was infiltrated with irregular, hypoechoic foci with a clumped appearance.

MOTILITY

Inflammatory, infectious, and neoplastic infiltrative diseases of the intestine can lead to functional disturbances. Functional ileus can generally be differentiated from mechanical ileus radiographically and ultrasonographically. In functional ileus, generalized, mild dilation of the intestinal lumen, which often contains fluid, is the predominant feature. Intestinal motility is decreased or absent and the intestinal walls may appear stiffened with to-and-fro movement of the fluid content.[14] This pattern can be associated with any cause of gastroenteritis, pythiosis, diffuse neoplasia, or peritoneal inflammation. It has also been reported with small intestinal infarction leading

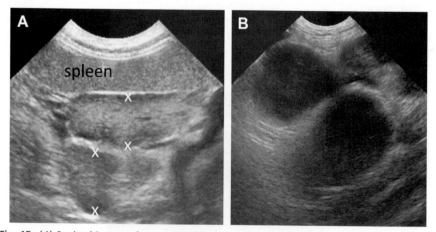

Fig. 15. (*A*) Sagittal image of two jejunal lymph nodes in a dog with lymphocytic, plasmacytic enteritis. The nodes are mildly enlarged and maintain a normal elliptical shape, but are slightly heterogeneous due to a peripheral hypoechoic rim. (*B*) Sagittal image of the jejunal lymph nodes in a dog with alimentary lymphoma. The nodes are severely enlarged, round, and markedly hypoechoic.

to segmental dilation and hypoechoic wall thickening.[39] A chronic, end-jejunal obstruction caused by a foreign body or stenosis caused by neoplasia can also lead to similar findings. Mechanical obstructions can result from tumor growth into the lumen, causing stenosis and obstruction and leading to a mixed population of intestinal diameters such as seen with foreign body obstruction. In general, the intestinal segments proximal to the obstruction show hyperperistalsis and are moderately to severely dilated, while the intestines caudal to the obstruction are of small diameter. Foreign material appears hyperechoic with shadowing, and collects proximal to the obstruction. Inflammatory and infectious infiltrative diseases typically do not cause mechanical obstructions.

GASTROINTESTINAL HEMODYNAMICS

Doppler ultrasound provides a noninvasive method of assessing gastrointestinal hemodynamics in dogs and humans.[40] Assessment of systolic and diastolic arterial blood flow in the large upstream arteries supplying the gastrointestinal tract is aimed at detecting abnormally increased or decreased resistance to flow to the intestinal capillary bed during digestion. The resistive and pulsatility indices (RI and PI, respectively) have historically been used to infer the degree of resistance to flow in downstream capillary beds. A lowered index indicates lowered resistance to flow and vice versa. The spectral waveforms of the celiac and cranial mesenteric arteries in normal dogs have been described as being of moderately high resistance in the fasted state (cranial mesenteric artery RI = 0.803 ± 0.029, celiac artery RI = 0.763 ± 0.025, cranial mesenteric artery PI = 2.290 ± 0.311, celiac artery PI = 1.962 ± 0.216).[40,41] Reference values for postprandial RI and PI have also been made available.[40,41] Vasodilation during digestion leads to decreasing Doppler indices and increasing diastolic blood flow velocity, which infer decreased resistance to flow in the downstream capillary bed of the gastrointestinal tract.

   In dogs with proven food allergies that develop gastrointestinal signs, dietary provocation with the allergen results in prolonged vasodilation at 90 minutes postprandially compared with provocation with nonallergens and the dog's regular diet.[41] Abnormal hemodynamics have also been shown in dogs with chronic enteropathies due to other causes.[42] This noninvasive ultrasonographic method shows promise for assessing hemodynamic pathophysiology in dogs with adverse reactions to food and chronic enteropathies due to other causes.

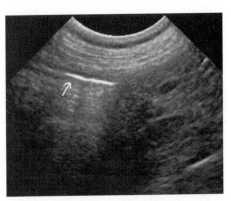

Fig. 16. Hyperechoic reverberation echoes adjacent to the peritoneum in the nondependent aspect of the abdomen (*arrow*). The free air resulted from a perforated intestinal tumor.

COMPLICATIONS

Perforation of the duodenum, jejunum, or ileum due to neoplastic infiltration is not common but can occur. Sonographic findings include bright regional mesenteric fat, peritoneal effusion, fluid-filled stomach or intestines typically caused by local peritonitis, intestinal wall thickening, free peritoneal air, loss of intestinal wall layering, and corrugated intestines (**Fig. 16**).[23] The intestines should be screened for the presence of a mass, presence of a luminal foreign body, and mechanical ileus.

SUMMARY OF IMPORTANT POINTS

- Lymphoplasmacytic enteritis and lymphoma of the small intestine share similar ultrasonographic characteristics
- Neoplastic infiltration is more often focal, shows more severe thickening, and causes loss of wall layering when compared with inflammatory disease
- Lymph nodes tend to be larger when involved in neoplastic versus inflammatory disease
- In endemic regions, fungal infections cannot be differentiated from neoplasia on the basis of ultrasonographic findings
- Due to overlap in the sonographic appearance of neoplastic and inflammatory disease, histopathology is necessary for differentiation.

REFERENCES

1. Baez JL, Hendrick MJ, Walker LM, et al. Radiographic, ultrasonographic, and endoscopic findings in cats with inflammatory bowel disease of the stomach and small intestine: 33 cases (1990–1997). J Am Vet Med Assoc 1999;215(3): 349–54.
2. Barr BS. Infiltrative intestinal disease. Vet Clin North Am Equine Pract 2006;22(1): e1–e7.
3. Gaschen L, Kircher P, Stüssi A, et al. Comparison of ultrasonographic findings with clinical activity index (CIBDAI) and diagnosis in dogs with chronic enteropathies. Vet Radiol Ultrasound 2008;49(1):56–64.
4. Penninck DG, Smyers B, Webster CR, et al. Diagnostic value of ultrasonography in differentiating enteritis from intestinal neoplasia in dogs. Vet Radiol Ultrasound 2003;44:570–5.
5. Rudorf H, van SG, O'Brien RT, et al. Ultrasonographic evaluation of the thickness of the small intestinal wall in dogs with inflammatory bowel disease. J Small Anim Pract 2005;46(7):322–6.
6. Patsikas MN, Papazoglou LG, Jakovljevic S, et al. Color Doppler ultrasonography in prediction of the reducibility of intussuscepted bowel in 15 young dogs. Vet Radiol Ultrasound 2005;46(4):313–6.
7. Delaney F, O'Brien RT, Waller K. Ultrasound evaluation of small bowel thickness compared to weight in normal dogs. Vet Radiol Ultrasound 2003;44(5): 577–80.
8. Newell SM, Graham JP, Roberts GD, et al. Sonography of the normal feline gastrointestinal tract. Vet Radiol Ultrasound 1999;40(1):40–3.
9. Goggin JM, Biller DS, Debey BM, et al. Ultrasonographic measurement of gastrointestinal wall thickness and the ultrasonographic appearance of the ileocolic region in healthy cats. J Am Anim Hosp Assoc 2000;36(3):224–8.
10. Brinkman-Ferguson EL, Biller DS. Ultrasound of the right lateral intercostal space. Vet Clin North Am Small Anim Pract 2009;39(4):761–81.

11. Brinkman EL, Biller DS, Armbrust LJ, et al. The clinical utility of the right lateral intercostal ultrasound scan technique in dogs. J Am Anim Hosp Assoc 2007; 43(4):179–86.
12. Hall EJ, German AJ. Inflammatory bowel disease. In: Steiner JM, editor. Small animal gastroenterology. 1st edition. Hannover (Germany): Schluetersche Verlagsgesellschaft mbH; 2008. p. 312–50.
13. Penninck DG. Gastrointestinal tract. In: Penninck DG, D'anjou MA, editors. Atlas of small animal ultrasonography. 1st edition. Ames (IA): Blackwell Publishing; 2008. p. 281–337.
14. Penninck DG. Gastrointestinal tract. In: Nyland TG, Mattoon JS, editors. Small animal diagnostic ultrasound. 2nd edition. Philadelphia: W.B. Saunders Co; 2002. p. 227–30.
15. Hendrick M. A spectrum of hypereosinophilic syndromes exemplified by six cats with eosinophilic enteritis. Vet Pathol 1981;18(2):188–200.
16. Wilson SC, Thomson-Kerr K, Houston DM. Hypereosinophilic syndrome in a cat. Can Vet J 1996;37(11):679–80.
17. Craig LE, Hardam EE, Hertzke DM, et al. Feline gastrointestinal eosinophilic sclerosing fibroplasia. Vet Pathol 2009;46(1):63–70.
18. Penninck DG, Webster CR, Keating JH. The sonographic appearance of intestinal mucosal fibrosis in cats. Vet Radiol Ultrasound 2010;51(4):458–61.
19. Kull PA, Hess RS, Craig LE, et al. Clinical, clinicopathologic, radiographic, and ultrasonographic characteristics of intestinal lymphangiectasia in dogs: 17 cases (1996–1998). J Am Vet Med Assoc 2001;219(2):197–202.
20. Louvet A, Denis B. Ultrasonographic diagnosis—small bowel lymphangiectasia in a dog. Vet Radiol Ultrasound 2004;45(6):565–7.
21. Peterson PB, Willard MD. Protein-losing enteropathies. Vet Clin North Am Small Anim Pract 2003;33(5):1061–82.
22. Moon ML, Biller DS, Armbrust LJ. Ultrasonographic appearance and etiology of corrugated small intestine. Vet Radiol Ultrasound 2003;44(2):199–203.
23. Boysen SR, Tidwell AS, Penninck DG. Ultrasonographic findings in dogs and cats with gastrointestinal perforation. Vet Radiol Ultrasound 2003;44(5):556–64.
24. Papazoglou LG, Tontis D, Loukopoulos P, et al. Foreign body-associated intestinal pyogranuloma resulting in intestinal obstruction in four dogs. Vet Rec 2010;166(16):494–7.
25. Graham JP, Newell SM, Roberts GD, et al. Ultrasonographic features of canine gastrointestinal pythiosis. Vet Radiol Ultrasound 2000;41(3):273–7.
26. Mavropoulou A, Grandi G, Calvi L, et al. Disseminated histoplasmosis in a cat in Europe. J Small Anim Pract 2010;51(3):176–80.
27. Monteiro CB, O'Brien RT. A retrospective study on the sonographic findings of abdominal carcinomatosis in 14 cats. Vet Radiol Ultrasound 2004;45(6):559–64.
28. Paoloni MC, Penninck DG, Moore AS. Ultrasonographic and clinicopathologic findings in 21 dogs with intestinal adenocarcinoma. Vet Radiol Ultrasound 2002;43(6):562–7.
29. Penninck DG. Characterization of gastrointestinal tumors. Vet Clin North Am Small Anim Pract 1998;28(4):777–97.
30. Yam PS, Johnson VS, Martineau HM, et al. Multicentric lymphoma with intestinal involvement in a dog. Vet Radiol Ultrasound 2002;43(2):138–43.
31. Aita N, Iso H, Uchida K. Hemangioma of the ileum in a dog. J Vet Med Sci 2010; 72(8):1071–3.
32. Culp WT, Drobatz KJ, Glassman MM, et al. Feline visceral hemangiosarcoma. J Vet Intern Med 2008;22(1):148–52.

33. Evans SE, Bonczynski JJ, Broussard JD, et al. Comparison of endoscopic and full-thickness biopsy specimens for diagnosis of inflammatory bowel disease and alimentary tract lymphoma in cats. J Am Vet Med Assoc 2006;229(9): 1447–50.

34. Zwingenberger AL, Marks SL, Baker TW, et al. Ultrasonographic evaluation of the muscularis propria in cats with diffuse small intestinal lymphoma or inflammatory bowel disease. J Vet Intern Med 2010;24(2):289–92.

35. Sato AF, Solano M. Ultrasonographic findings in abdominal mast cell disease: a retrospective study of 19 patients. Vet Radiol Ultrasound 2004;45(1):51–7.

36. Agthe P, Caine AR, Posch B, et al. Ultrasonographic appearance of jejunal lymph nodes in dogs without clinical signs of gastrointestinal disease. Vet Radiol Ultrasound 2009;50(2):195–200.

37. D'anjou MA. Abdominal cavity, lymph nodes, and great vessels. In: Penninck DG, D'anjou MA, editors. Atlas of small animal ultrasonography. 1st edition. Iowa: Blackwell Publishing; 2008. p. 445–63.

38. Nyman HT, Kristensen AT, Flagstad A, et al. A review of the sonographic assessment of tumor metastases in liver and superficial lymph nodes. Vet Radiol Ultrasound 2004;45(5):438–48.

39. Wallack ST, Hornof WJ, Herrgesell EJ. Ultrasonographic diagnosis—small bowel infarction in a cat. Vet Radiol Ultrasound 2003;44(1):81–5.

40. Kircher P, Lang J, Blum J, et al. Influence of food composition on splanchnic blood flow during digestion in unsedated normal dogs: a Doppler study. Vet J 2003;166(3):265–72.

41. Kircher PR, Spaulding KA, Vaden S, et al. Doppler ultrasonographic evaluation of gastrointestinal hemodynamics in food hypersensitivities: a canine model. J Vet Intern Med 2004;18(5):605–11.

42. Gaschen L, Kircher P. Two-dimensional grayscale ultrasound and spectral Doppler waveform evaluation of dogs with chronic enteropathies. Clin Tech Small Anim Pract 2007;22(3):122–7.

Clinical Immunology and Immunopathology of the Canine and Feline Intestine

Karin Allenspach, Dr med vet, FVH, PhD, FHEA, MRCVS

KEYWORDS

- Gut-associated lymphoid tissue • IgA • Innate immunity
- Toll-like receptors • Microbiome • Inflammatory bowel disease

GUT-ASSOCIATED LYMPHOID TISSUE

The mucosal immune system in the gut has evolved as a system that is tolerant of food antigens and commensals but is still able to respond rapidly to pathogenic microbes when they are encountered. The anatomy of the gut-associated lymphoid tissue consists of secondary lymphoid organs, which act as inductive sites of the immune response, including Peyer patches (PP) in the small intestine, isolated lymphoid follicles (ILFs) throughout the whole gastrointestinal (GI) tract, and the mesenteric lymph nodes; and the effector sites, comprised of the lamina propria (LP) mucosae. Comparatively, the GI mucosa in human beings consists of several hundred square meters of surface, which in its entirety represents the major site of daily contact with infectious agents. The two most important protective mechanisms that have evolved in mammals to prevent most of the pathogens, commensals, and food antigens from triggering an immune response are the induction of oral tolerance and the production of mucosal secretory immunoglobulin A (IgA). Both of these mechanisms critically depend on the interaction of commensals with cells of the intestinal immune system.

Production of Mucosal IgA

In the mucosa, IgA is secreted mainly in its dimeric form, where two IgA molecules are joined by a J chain and transported transepithelially to the lumenal side of the intestine.[1] Approximately 80% of the antibody production in the body occurs in this form, which emphasizes its major importance in mucosal defense mechanisms. IgA

Disclosure: The following funding agencies supported the author's research cited in this article: CEVA Santé Animale, British Biotechnology and Biosciences Research Council, Pfizer, Petsavers BSAVA, and the UK Kennel Club Charitable Trust.
Royal Veterinary College, University of London, Hawkshead Lane, North Mymms AL9 7PT, UK
E-mail address: kallenspach@rvc.ac.uk

is the main mechanism for keeping lumenal bacteria from crossing the epithelial barrier.[2] Moreover, it has recently been shown that effective IgA production is also necessary to keep the microbiome composition healthy.[3] In mice deficient in mucosal IgA production or in human beings with IgA deficiency, the microbiome undergoes a switch to a mainly anaerobic composition, which could be implicated in the occurrence of chronic inflammation.[4] To produce effective IgA, B cells undergo two genetic alterations in the imunoglobulin locus, namely somatic hypermutation and class switch recombination. Somatic hypermutation produces point mutations in the variable region of the light and heavy chains, a process that increases antibody specificity and is termed, affinity maturation. Class switch recombination alters the effector function of the antibody by replacing the $C\mu$ exon with one of several downstream CH (heavy chain) exons. This process produces different sets of IgH isotypes, such as IgG, IgE, or IgA. To undergo class switching to IgA, B cells must be induced to produce a specific enzyme called activation-induced cytidine deaminase.[5,6] How this process is triggered in the different sites of gut-associated lymphoid tissue has only recently been elucidated and is explained in the following sections.

IgA Production in Peyer Patches

The germinal centers in PP enable the interaction of antigen with B cells, dendritic cells (DCs), and follicular T-helper cells (fThs). DCs have the ability to present antigen to cells of the adaptive immune system and, therefore, play a critical role in the interface of innate and adaptive immunity at mucosal surfaces. DCs in the subepithelial dome of PP carry bacteria from the intestinal lumen and secrete interleukin (IL)-6, which induces B cells to preferentially undergo class switching to IgA. This process is aided by fThs, which, in the PP, express high levels of retinoic acid, which, together with transforming growth factor β (TGF-β), induces fThs to differentiate primarily into T-regulatory cells.[7] fThs express CD40 ligand on their surface, which interacts with CD40 expressed on the surface of B cells, which then induces class switching of B cells to IgA-producing cells. This process is, therefore, called T-cell–dependent IgA production. The B cells, which now have been primed to undergo class switching to IgA, travel to the mesenteric lymph nodes, where they are imprinted with gut-homing integrins, which guide them to leave the capillaries in the LP and produce IgA locally in the LP (**Fig. 1**).

IgA Production in Isolated Lymphoid Follicles and the Lamina Propria

In ILFs and the LP, class switching of B cells to IgA does not require the help of T cells but instead is dependent on more direct interaction with the microbiome.[8–10] The DCs in the LP have an important role in that they continuously sample antigen from the lumen by extending dendrites between the epithelial cells.[11] They recognize and respond to bacterial and viral microbe-associated molecular patterns (MAMPs) by virtue of binding of pattern-recognition receptors (PRRs) to these motifs. Toll-like receptors (TLRs) and nuclear organization domain (NOD) receptors are PRRs located on the surface or in the cytoplasm of epithelial cells and DCs.[12,13] These receptors recognize specific MAMPs, which are conserved molecules found on bacteria and other infectious agents. Different TLRs recognize different MAMPs: for example, TLR4 recognizes lipopolysaccharide (LPS) present in the cell wall of gram-negative bacteria; TLR2 recognizes lipopeptides and lipotechoic acid mainly found in the cell wall of gram-positive bacteria; and TLR5 recognizes flagellin, the main protein of bacterial flagella.[14] Binding of MAMPs by TLRs initiates a complex intracellular signaling pathway culminating in the activation of the transcription factor, nuclear factor κB.[15] DCs in the LP that have been activated by ligand binding to TLRs produce

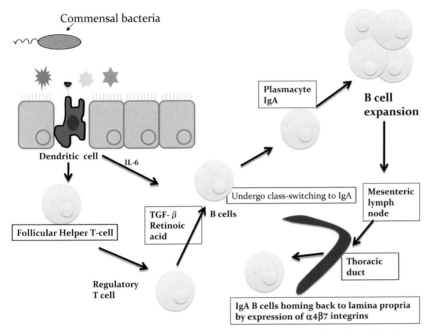

Fig. 1. IgA production in PP. DCs sample luminal antigens by extending dendrites between the epithelial cells through PRRs on their surface. They travel to the germinal centers in PP, where the interaction of DCs with fThs activates the latter to differentiate primarily into T-regulatory cells, which produce TGF-β and retinoic acid. This interaction of fThs and B cells seems crucial to IgA production in the PP, which is why this process is termed, T-cell–dependent IgA production. In this milieu, B cells undergo class switching to IgA-producing plasma cells and travel to the mesenteric lymph nodes, where they are imprinted with gut-homing integrins, such as α4β7. The B cells then travel in the thoracic duct to local capillaries in the LP mucosae where they secrete IgA. IgA is then transported transcellularly through intestinal epithelial cells to the lumen, where it is effective in coating bacteria and stopping them from penetrating the mucosal barrier as well as changing expression of surface molecules on the bacteria.

factors, such as B-cell activating factor (BAFF) belonging to the tumor necrosis factor (TNF) and a proliferation-inducing ligand (APRIL), which are cytokines that act synergistically with TNF and inducible nitric oxide synthase (iNOS) to produce class switching to IgA in plasma cells **(Fig. 2)**.[16] In mammals, ILFs only develop after birth, when the intestinal mucosa has been colonized by commensal bacteria. It is, therefore, reasonable to assume that the normal commensal flora in the gut is essential in inducing and maintaining IgA production, which presents evidence of an effective symbiosis between the host and the microbes (see **Fig. 2**).

Oral Tolerance

The second important mechanism of mucosal immunity in the GI tract is the concept of oral tolerance, which describes the fact that an antigen given orally does not elicit a systemic immune response. It is a mechanism to inhibit overreaction against innocuous luminal antigens, such as commensal microorganisms and food antigens. Oral tolerance is mediated mainly by the induction of T-regulatory cells in the mesenteric lymph nodes. Some studies have shown that several commensal bacteria can actively modulate the intracellular signaling after binding to their respective TLR. This has been

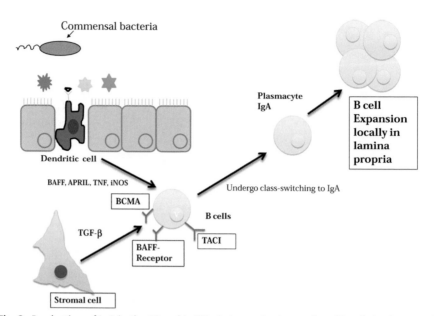

Fig. 2. Production of IgA in the LP and in ILFs. IgA can also be produced locally in the LP and in ILFs through a process independent of T cells. In this case, DCs bind pathogen-associated molecular patterns on the surface of bacteria through TLRs and produce cytokines, such as APRIL, BAFF belonging to the TNF family, TNF, and iNOS. These cytokines are essential to induce B cells to undergo class switching to IgA. With the help of TGF-β from stromal cells, IgA plasma cells secrete IgA, which is again transported transcellularly through intestinal epithelial cells to the lumen. BCMA, B-cell maturation antigen; TACI, transmembrane activator and CAML interactor.

shown the case for *Lactobacilli, Bacteroides*, nonpathogenic *Escherichia coli*, and attenuated *Salmonella* that lack flagellin.[17,18] DCs are believed to play a major role in the development of oral tolerance in the gut. They drive the differentiation of T cells to produce specific cytokines of T_H1, T_H2, or T_H17 subset, and, therefore, determine the result of the effector arm of the adaptive immune system by recruiting the appropriate inflammatory cells to eliminate the inciting antigen or infectious agent.

Recent studies have shown how DCs decide which T-helper cell response they trigger.[19,20] DCs encountering commensals or pathogens through PRRs predominantly produce either IL-23 or IL-12 and IL-27. This in turn drives T cells to differentiate from naive T cells into one of the following types of T cells: T_H1/T_H17 cells, which then produce proinflammatory cytokines, such as IL-17, IL-22, and TNF; T_H2 cells, producing IL-4, IL-5, and IL-13; or T-regulatory cells, which go on to produce IL-10, TGF-β, and lower levels of IL-17. In the presence of commensals and in normal intestinal homeostasis, a balance between effector and regulatory subpopulations of T cells is maintained through this tightly controlled cytokine network, such that the effects of T_H17 cells are counter-regulated by cytokines produced by T-regulatory cells and Th_3 cells (**Fig. 3**).

PATHOGENESIS OF CANINE INFLAMMATORY BOWEL DISEASE: THE INTERPLAY OF MUCOSAL INNATE IMMUNITY WITH THE INTESTINAL MICROBIOTA

Inflammatory bowel disease (IBD) is a complex disease that can affect any part of the GI tract in dogs and cats. Although the exact pathogenesis of IBD in small animals has not

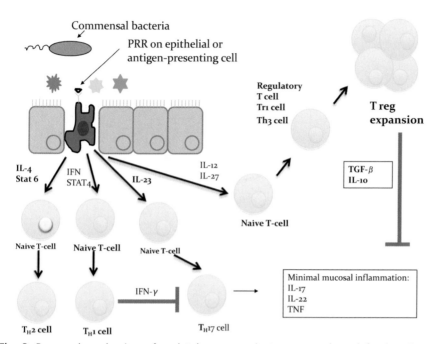

Fig. 3. Proposed mechanism of oral tolerance against commensals and food antigens. Antigen-presenting cells continuously sample antigens from the intestinal lumen through PRRs. Depending on the nature of these antigens, the signals elicited by the antigen-presenting cells drives the adaptive immune response in the appropriate direction to eradicate a pathogen. For example, in the case of a parasite, naive T cells are preferentially driven to differentiate into T_H2 cells, which recruit eosinophils, basophils, and mast cells to kill the parasites. In the case of a pathogenic virus, the naive T cells preferentially differentiate into T_H1 cells, which produce cytokines, such as IFN-γ. These cytokines recruit macrophages, which then kill intracellular viruses. In the case of pathogenic bacteria being recognized, naive T cells preferentially differentiate into T_H17 cells, which produce proinflammatory cytokines, such as IL-17 and IL-22. This recruits T cells to kill extracellular bacteria. In the case of commensal bacteria being recognized through PRRs, naive T cells preferentially differentiate into T-regulatory cells, which counteract the effect of proinflammatory cytokines produced by T_H17 cells, which is the concept of oral tolerance.

been elucidated, many scientific publications on IBD in humans and mouse models of the human disease have led to the formulation of current hypotheses (**Fig. 4**). Genetics, the mucosal immune system, and environmental factors (ie, diet and dysbalances in the intestinal microbiome) all play a role. In humans and animals affected with IBD, the inflammatory response, which is normally only seen as a reaction toward pathogenic bacteria breaching the intestinal barrier, occurs in the absence of pathogens. It is believed that the innate immune system reacts to normal commensals in the intestinal lumen as if they were pathogens. Several recent studies performed in dogs and cats lend weight to a similar molecular pathogenesis in small animals with IBD.

Evidence of Innate Immunity Hyperreactivity in the Intestine of Dogs with IBD

TLRs have been shown to be upregulated in the intestine of human beings with Crohn disease and ulcerative colitis. This may be either a consequence of the ongoing stimulation of TLRs by an altered microbiota or it may be a causal factor contributing to the pathogenesis of disease. Most studies show that the mRNA and protein

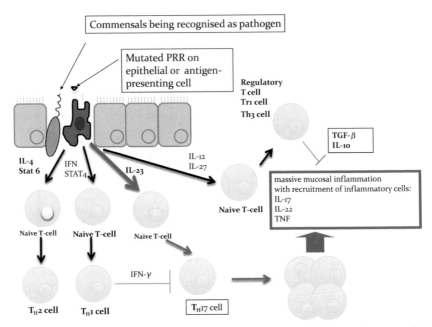

Fig. 4. Proposed pathogenesis of inflammation in canine and feline IBD. In the case of IBD, a primary defect in the recognition of commensals or pathogens by innate immunity receptors may play a role. Mutations in PRRs lead to misrepresentation of commensals as pathogens, which results in production of IL-23, driving naive T cells to differentiate into T$_H$17 cells. These T$_H$17 cells produce large amounts of proinflammatory cytokines, such as IL-17, and TNF. This leads to tissue destruction and epithelial cell injury, which lets even more antigens pass through to the LP. At that time, the inflammatory response cannot be counter-regulated anymore by T-regulatory cells, which leads to the characteristic inflammatory pattern seen in IBD.

expression of TLR2 and TLR4 are increased in the intestine of people with active IBD.[21,22] In a recent clinical study at the Royal Veterinary College of the University of London, the author and colleagues showed that dogs of any breed with clinically severe, active IBD express higher levels of TLR2 mRNA in the duodenum compared with healthy dogs as measured by real-time polymerase chain reaction (RT-PCR) in endoscopic biopsies.[23] In addition, TLR2 expression was correlated with the clinical severity of IBD using the canine chronic enteropathy clinical activity index.[24] TLR4 expression levels were similar, however, to those in healthy canine intestine. Other studies using RT-PCR have found that only a subgroup of dogs with IBD (those responding only to steroid administration) showed an increased expression of TLR2, TLR4, and TLR9 compared with healthy dogs.[25] In further studies looking at German shepherd dogs (GSDs) with IBD, the author and colleagues[26] found that TLR4 expression was 60-fold higher in the duodenum, ileum, and colon of diseased dogs compared with samples from healthy dogs; however, TLR2 and TLR9 were expressed at comparable levels to those of healthy dogs. In summary, these studies show that several innate immunity receptors are upregulated in the intestine of dogs with chronic enteropathies, which represents reasonable evidence that the innate immunity is hyperreactive in these diseases, as is the case in human beings.

The finding that TLR2 expression is highly upregulated in the intestine of dogs with IBD is particularly interesting. This receptor has recently been shown to be overexpressed in the diseased intestine in mouse models of IBD.[27] TLR2 in this context is implicated in the homeostasis and repair of intestinal tissue after injury.[28,29] It is, therefore, possible that the high expression of TLR2 the author and coworkers[26] documented in dogs with IBD could be a marker of intestinal inflammation and that its primary physiologic role is to downregulate ongoing inflammation. TLR5 expression was consistently downregulated in the intestine of GSDs with IBD when compared with healthy dogs. In mice and human beings, TLR5 is highly expressed in the healthy small intestine, with $CD11c^+$ DCs in the LP mucosae expressing most TLR5.[30] It is believed that this tolerogenic phenotype of DCs induces T-regulatory cells and stimulates the production of anti-inflammatory cytokines, such as IL-10, in response to flagellin.[31] In contrast, with intestinal inflammation characterized by the upregulation of T_H1^- and T_H17 cytokines, $CD11c^-$ DCs express low levels of TLR5 and instead high levels of TLR4. In this context, TLR4 is thought to be upregulated to compensate for the low TLR5 expression. It could be speculated that the differentially low expression of TLR5 and very high expression of TLR4 seen in the intestine in the GSDs of the author and colleagues' study indicates a similar compensatory role of TLR4, because gram-negative flagellated bacteria can also be recognized through binding of lipopolysaccharide by TLR4.

Dysbalance of the Intestinal Microbiota in Canine IBD

Molecular studies of the intestinal microbiome in dogs of different breeds with IBD have found that members of the families *Enterobacteriaceae* and *Clostridiaceae* were enriched in the diseased intestine.[32,33] These bacteria are thought to contribute to the pathogenesis of disease in dogs as well as human beings with IBD.[34–40] In the duodenum of GSDs with IBD, however, bacterial clones within the order *Lactobacillales* were found significantly more frequently than in the duodenum of healthy dogs.[26] It seems that GSDs with chronic enteropathies have a distinctly different microbiome when compared with healthy dogs and dogs from other breeds with IBD. It is characterized by over-representation of bacteria traditionally labeled as beneficial in the duodenum, specifically sequences of the order *Lactobacillales*.

Genetic Predisposition in Dogs with IBD

Over the past decade, many genes have been found to be associated with an increased risk of development of IBD in human beings, many of them implicated in the intestinal innate immune response. Mutations in PRRs, such as NOD2, TLR4, IL-23 receptor, and others, have all been associated with IBD in people.[41–44] A genetic component to IBD In dogs also has long been suspected. This is particularly evident in the boxer, a breed predisposed to histiocytic ulcerative colitis.[45,46] It has recently been discovered that a gene implicated in cellular autophagy is mutated in affected boxers.[47] This could be important in that engulfed bacteria (mainly *E coli* of the enteroadhesive type[48]) may not be efficiently destroyed intracellularly if the enzyme for fusion of the autophagosome with the lysosome is functionally defective.

Another example of a breed disposition for IBD is the GSD, which seems predisposed to antibiotic-responsive diarrhea and other forms of chronic enteropathies.[49–51] The Kathrani and colleagues[52] recently performed a mutational analysis of the canine genes for TLR2, TLR4, TLR5, and NOD2 in GSDs with IBD. One of the three polymorphisms identified in the TLR5 gene of GSDs was subsequently evaluated in a case-control study with more than 50 cases and breed controls and was found significantly associated with IBD. In addition, four nonsynonymous single nucleotide polymorphisms (SNPs) were identified in exon 4 of the canine NOD2 gene. The heterozygote genotype for all four NOD2 SNPs was found significantly more frequently in affected dogs than in controls. These results were mirrored in non-GSD breeds: the heterozygote genotype for all four SNPs was found significantly more frequently in a population of 96 dogs of different breeds with IBD compared with the non-GSD control population.

IMMUNOLOGIC MARKERS OF IBD

Noninvasive markers of disease have been available to aid the diagnosis and monitoring of human IBD for several decades. Many of them are based on knowledge gained from the discovery of the molecular events implicated in the pathogenesis of Crohn disease and ulcerative colitis. Progress in applying similar markers in dogs and cats with IBD has been comparatively slow, however. One major drawback is that to date, no validated histologic grading system correlating histologic severity with clinical activity of disease is available for use in dogs and cats. Nonetheless, some immunologic markers have been assessed for their usefulness in clinical practice and are reviewed in the following sections.

MEASUREMENTS OF INFLAMMATORY CYTOKINES AS MARKERS OF DISEASE

Cytokines, especially proinflammatory T_H1-type cytokines, such as TNF, could be a promising marker for chronic intestinal inflammation based on human studies. In people with IBD, high levels of intestinal mucosal TNF have been shown to correlate with the severity of disease.[53–55] Consequently, antibodies against TNF are a useful rescue therapy if all other treatments fail.[56,57] Several recent studies aimed to investigate the cytokine mRNA pattern in intestinal biopsies in dogs with chronic enteropathies. In an earlier study, the investigators measured cytokine expression in the mucosa semiquantitatively and found increased levels of interferon (IFN)-γ, TNF, IL-2, IL-5, IL-12, and TGF-β, suggesting a T_H1-biased cytokine profile in dogs with IBD similar to that in humans with IBD.[58] Newer studies in which RT-PCR was used to measure cytokine expression profiles in biopsies, however, found no distinct cytokine profile toward either a T_H1 or T_H2 pattern.[59,60] Furthermore, when cytokine mRNA levels were compared with total number of infiltrating cells and CD3 cells as well as clinical activity indices, no significant correlation of cytokines levels with any of these parameters was detected.[59] An even easier and less-invasive marker would be the measurement of cytokine levels in the peripheral blood of affected dogs. In a recent article, the investigators hypothesized that serum levels of TNF are elevated in dogs with IBD and that the levels would correlate with clinical severity of disease. Unfortunately, serum TNF levels were normal in all dogs with IBD in this study (16/16).[61] In chronic diseases, such as IBD, elevations in cytokine levels seem a predominantly local response that influences the microenvironment in the gut, but serum concentrations of inflammatory cytokines are rarely increased. It is reasonable to assume that T_H17 cytokines, such as IL-17, IL-23, and IL-22, could play an important role in the mucosal inflammatory response in canine and feline IBD, as they do in people. So far, however, studies demonstrating mRNA expression of these cytokines in the intestine of dogs and cats with IBD are lacking.

P-Glycoprotein

P-glycoprotein is a transmembrane protein functioning as a drug efflux pump in the intestinal epithelium. People with IBD who fail to respond to treatment with glucocorticosteroids express high levels of P-glycoprotein in LP lymphocytes.[62] In a recent article, duodenal biopsies from 48 dogs with chronic enteropathies (diet responsive, n = 24; steroid responsive, n = 24) were immunohistochemically evaluated using a mouse anti–human monoclonal antibody for expression of P-glycoprotein in LP lymphocytes (**Fig. 5**).[63] Dogs treated with prednisolone showed a significantly higher P-glycoprotein expression after treatment compared with expression before treatment. On the contrary, the group treated solely with an elimination diet showed no difference in P-glycoprotein scores before and after treatment. Moreover, a statistically significant association between a positive response to treatment and a low P-glycoprotein score was found when dogs from the glucocorticosteroid-treatment group were scored before initiation of treatment.[63] These results indicate that mucosal expression of P-glycoprotein may be a valuable tool to predict response to therapy in dogs with chronic enteropathies. Intestinal biopsies from dogs undergoing endoscopy for possible IBD could be stained immunohistochemically for expression of P-glycoprotein, because the protocol is relatively simple and antibodies are commercially available. Further studies will show if P-glycoprotein could represent a useful marker of disease. If, for example, a high expression of P-glycoprotein is found before treatment, a steroid-refractory disease may be more likely, and more aggressive therapy may be indicated, possibly with azathioprine and/or cyclosporine.

Perinuclear Antineutrophil Cytoplasmic Antibodies

Perinuclear antineutrophilic cytoplasmic autoantibodies (pANCAs) are mainly IgGs directed against antigens in the cytoplasm of neutrophil granulocytes and monocytes.[64] For decades, ANCAs have been used as diagnostic markers in several human autoimmune diseases, such as idiopathic systemic vasculitis, Wegener granulomatosis, idiopathic rapidly progressive glomerunephritis, microscopic polyangiitis, and Churg-Strauss syndrome.[65,66] Specifically, pANCAs have been useful in the diagnosis of human IBD, particularly the differentiation of Crohn disease and ulcerative colitis.[67–71] Moreover, pANCAs can be used as a prognostic marker as ulcerative colitis patients with high pANCA levels before colectomy procedures are more likely to develop pouchitis after the operation.[72,73] The application of this serum immunofluorescence test in the diagnosis of IBD in dogs was recently evaluated (**Fig. 6**).[74] Thirty-one dogs with IBD, 29 dogs with non–IBD-related diarrhea, and 42 healthy dogs were included in the study. Sensitivity for pANCAs was 0.51 (95% CI, 0.35–0.67) and specificity ranged between 0.56 (95% CI, 0.31–0.78) and 0.95 (95% CI, 0.72–1.00). Therefore, pANCAs proved a highly specific marker for IBD in dogs; however, the

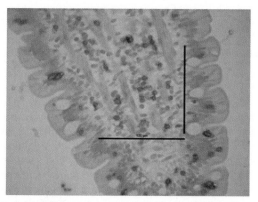

Fig. 5. Section of duodenum from a dog with chronic idiopathic enteropathy. The LP of this villus is infiltrated with P-glycoprotein–positive lymphocytes characterized by a brown-staining cytoplasm. Streptavidin-biotin immunoperoxidase technique.

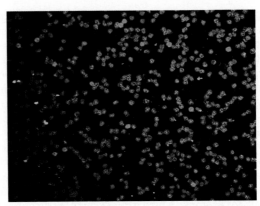

Fig. 6. Typical perinuclear staining pattern of canine granulocytes after exposure to the serum of a dog positive for pANCAs (×20).

sensitivity was too low to use it as a general screening test in the population. In another study, the specificity of pANCsA versus antinuclear antibodies (ANAs) was evaluated, because the indirect immunofluorescence test used for detection of the antibodies can also be used to evaluate ANA. In this study, a population of dogs with chronic enteropathies was evaluated for pANCAs and ANAs in the serum and pANCAs were found highly specific for IBD, because only few dogs were also positive for ANAs.[75] This is in agreement with reports from human medicine that show a specificity of up to 94% for pANCAs when distinguishing between IBD and healthy controls as well as patients with non–IBD-related diarrhea.[76] In a follow-up study in dogs with chronic enteropathies, the correlation between pANCAs and treatment response to either elimination diet alone (n = 26) or steroid-responsive disease (n = 39) was assessed.[77] A positive pANCA test before therapy was strongly associated with good response to dietary treatment, which could be helpful to guide owners toward dietary treatment options and a relatively good prognosis. There is also preliminary evidence that pANCAs could be a marker of protein-losing enteropathy and protein-losing nephropathy in familial protein-losing diseases of soft coated wheaten terriers.[78] This is not surprising, because pANCAs in dogs are likely a more general marker of immune-mediated diseases, as is the case in human medicine. Future studies will help elucidate the accuracy of this marker in a range of primary and secondary immune-mediated disease in dogs, which will be necessary to assess its usefulness in practice.

Polymerase Chain Reaction for Antigen Receptor Rearrangements

The PCR for antigen receptor rearrangements (PARR) assay amplifies the highly variable T-cell or B-cell antigen receptor genes and is used to detect the presence of a clonally expanded population of lymphocytes. The test has been used for staging and as a prognostic indicator in dogs with multicentric lymphoma[79] and has proved useful for monitoring of residual disease after remission.[80] In a recent article, PARR was investigated for its usefulness in the differentiation of intestinal lymphoma and IBD in endoscopic biopsies.[81] The sensitivity of PARR for detecting lymphoma in endoscopic biopsies from dogs with histopathologically confirmed lymphoma was 66%, which seems comparatively low for a test based on a PCR technique. In a follow-up study, the same researchers looked at PARR in endoscopic biopsies from four dogs with intestinal lymphoma, five dogs with intestinal adenocarcinomas, and 69 dogs with chronic enteritis.[82] Their gold standard was histopathologic assessment of the biopsies at the time of endoscopy; however, only one biopsy sample was used for histopathology. Sensitivity for PARR for detection of intestinal lymphoma was 100%; however, six of the enteritis cases were also positive for PARR. Cases of a positive test had significantly shorter survival than PARR negative cases, which led the investigators to conclude that the test could be a negative prognostic indicator. In a recent study at the Royal Veterinary College, the author Gajanayake[83] prospectively evaluated the accuracy of PARR in diagnosing lymphoma from endoscopically obtained biopsies compared with the gold standard of histopathology and clinical outcome (determined by follow-up information of at least 2 years). Samples from 39 dogs were included in the study. Five dogs had a diagnosis of lymphoma, of which four were positive on PARR. One dog was diagnosed with an intestinal carcinoma, three with a gastric carcinoma (with concurrent inflammation in the intestine), and 30 were diagnosed with IBD. Five dogs with IBD and two dogs with carcinoma were positive on PARR. Of the five positive dogs with IBD, four were clinically in remission at the time of follow-up, and one had been euthanized due to the development of jaundice. This indicated a sensitivity and specificity of 80% and 79%, respectively, for PARR for correct identification of canine GI lymphoma when compared with histopathology and clinical outcome as a gold standard. The data derived from this study indicate a noteworthy false-positive rate (7/36 cases or 19%) for PARR when used on endoscopic biopsies for diagnosis of canine intestinal lymphoma. Caution is, therefore, necessary, and a positive PARR test performed on an endoscopic biopsy specimen does permit to make a definitive diagnosis of lymphoma in a clinical situation.

SUMMARY

The mucosal immune system is at the forefront of defense against invading pathogens but, at the same time, must maintain tolerance toward commensals and food antigens in the intestinal lumen. Great progress has been made in identifying some of the genetic predispositions underlying the disease in certain breeds, such as the GSD. As the pathogenesis of IBD in dogs and cats is unraveled, novel therapeutic options for treatment of IBD in dogs and cats will undoubtedly become available and may include blocking of hyperreactive receptors of the innate immune system in certain breeds.

REFERENCES

1. Macpherson AJ, Lamarre A, McCoy K, et al. IgA production without mu or delta chain expression in developing B cells. Nat Immunol 2001;2:625–31.
2. Brandtzaeg P. Mucosal immunity: induction, dissemination, and effector functions. Scand J Immunol 2009;70:505–15.
3. Fagarasan S. Intestinal IgA synthesis: a primitive form of adaptive immunity that regulates microbial communities in the gut. Curr Top Microbiol Immunol 2006; 308:137–53.
4. Suzuki K, Meek B, Doi Y, et al. Aberrant expansion of segmented filamentous bacteria in IgA-deficient gut. Proc Natl Acad Sci U S A 2004;101:1981–6.
5. Fagarasan S, Muramatsu M, Suzuki K, et al. Critical roles of activation-induced cytidine deaminase in the homeostasis of gut flora. Science 2002;298:1424–7.
6. Muramatsu M, Kinoshita K, Fagarasan S, et al. Class switch recombination and hypermutation require activation-induced cytidine deaminase (AID), a potential RNA editing enzyme. Cell 2000;102:553–63.

7. Suzuki K, Ha SA, Tsuji M, et al. Intestinal IgA synthesis: a primitive form of adaptive immunity that regulates microbial communities in the gut. Semin Immunol 2007;19:127–35.

8. Suzuki K, Fagarasan S. How host-bacterial interactions lead to IgA synthesis in the gut. Trends Immunol 2008;29:523–31.

9. Suzuki K, Fagarasan S. Diverse regulatory pathways for IgA synthesis in the gut. Mucosal Immunol 2009;2:468–71.

10. Fagarasan S, Kinoshita K, Muramatsu M, et al. In situ class switching and differentiation to IgA-producing cells in the gut lamina propria. Nature 2001;413: 639–43.

11. Rescigno M, Urbano M, Valzasina B, et al. Dendritic cells express tight junction proteins and penetrate gut epithelial monolayers to sample bacteria. Nat Immunol 2001;2:361–7.

12. Gribar SC, Anand RJ, Sodhi CP, et al. The role of epithelial Toll-like receptor signaling in the pathogenesis of intestinal inflammation. J Leukoc Biol 2008;83: 493–8.

13. Gribar SC, Richardson WM, Sodhi CP, et al. No longer an innocent bystander: epithelial toll-like receptor signaling in the development of mucosal inflammation. Mol Med 2008;14:645–59.

14. Abreu MT, Fukata M, Arditi M. TLR signaling in the gut in health and disease. J Immunol 2005;174:4453–60.

15. Magalhaes JG, Tattoli I, Girardin SE. The intestinal epithelial barrier: how to distinguish between the microbial flora and pathogens. Semin Immunol 2007;19: 106–15.

16. Fagarasan S. Evolution, development, mechanism and function of IgA in the gut. Curr Opin Immunol 2008;20:170–7.

17. Tien MT, Girardin SE, Regnault B, et al. Anti-inflammatory effect of Lactobacillus casei on Shigella-infected human intestinal epithelial cells. J Immunol 2006;176: 1228–37.

18. Neish AS, Gewirtz AT, Zeng H, et al. Prokaryotic regulation of epithelial responses by inhibition of IkappaB-alpha ubiquitination. Science 2000;289:1560–3.

19. Maloy KJ. The Interleukin-23/Interleukin-17 axis in intestinal inflammation. J Intern Med 2008;263:584–90.

20. Maloy KJ, Powrie F. Regulatory T cells in the control of immune pathology. Nat Immunol 2001;2:816–22.

21. Szebeni B, Veres G, Dezsofi A, et al. Increased expression of Toll-like receptor (TLR) 2 and TLR4 in the colonic mucosa of children with inflammatory bowel disease. Clin Exp Immunol 2008;151:34–41.

22. Cario E, Podolsky DK. Differential alteration in intestinal epithelial cell expression of toll-like receptor 3 (TLR3) and TLR4 in inflammatory bowel disease. Infect Immun 2000;68:7010–7.

23. McMahon LA, House AK, Catchpole B, et al. Expression of Toll-like receptor 2 in duodenal biopsies from dogs with inflammatory bowel disease is associated with severity of disease. Vet Immunol Immunopathol 2010;135:158–63.

24. Allenspach K, Wieland B, Grone A, et al. Chronic enteropathies in dogs: evaluation of risk factors for negative outcome. J Vet Intern Med 2007;21: 700–8.

25. Burgener IA, Konig A, Allenspach K, et al. Upregulation of toll-like receptors in chronic enteropathies in dogs. J Vet Intern Med 2008;22:553–60.

26. Allenspach K, House A, Smith K, et al. Evaluation of mucosal bacteria and histopathology, clinical disease activity and expression of Toll-like receptors in

German shepherd dogs with chronic enteropathies. Vet Microbiol 2010;146(3–4): 326–35.

27. Gibson DL, Ma C, Rosenberger CM, et al. Toll-like receptor 2 plays a critical role in maintaining mucosal integrity during Citrobacter rodentium-induced colitis. Cell Microbiol 2008;10:388–403.

28. Ey B, Eyking A, Gerken G, et al. TLR2 mediates gap junctional intercellular communication through connexin-43 in intestinal epithelial barrier injury. J Biol Chem 2009;284:22332–43.

29. Cario E, Gerken G, Podolsky DK. Toll-like receptor 2 controls mucosal inflammation by regulating epithelial barrier function. Gastroenterology 2007;132: 1359–74.

30. Uematsu S, Fujimoto K, Jang MH, et al. Regulation of humoral and cellular gut immunity by lamina propria dendritic cells expressing Toll-like receptor 5. Nat Immunol 2008;9:769–76.

31. Uematsu S, Akira S. Immune responses of TLR5(+) lamina propria dendritic cells in enterobacterial infection. J Gastroenterol 2009;44:803–11.

32. Suchodolski JS, Xenoulis PG, Paddock CG, et al. Molecular analysis of the bacterial microbiota in duodenal biopsies from dogs with idiopathic inflammatory bowel disease. Vet Microbiol 2010;142(3–4):394–400.

33. Xenoulis PG, Palculict B, Allenspach K, et al. Molecular-phylogenetic characterization of microbial communities imbalances in the small intestine of dogs with inflammatory bowel disease. FEMS Microbiol Ecol 2008;66:579–89.

34. Suchodolski JS, Camacho J, Steiner JM. Analysis of bacterial diversity in the canine duodenum, jejunum, ileum, and colon by comparative 16S rRNA gene analysis. FEMS Microbiol Ecol 2008;66(3):567–78.

35. Baumgart M, Dogan B, Rishniw M, et al. Culture independent analysis of ileal mucosa reveals a selective increase in invasive Escherichia coli of novel phylogeny relative to depletion of Clostridiales in Crohn's disease involving the ileum. ISME J 2007;1:403–18.

36. Bringer MA, Glasser AL, Tung CH, et al. The Crohn's disease-associated adherent-invasive Escherichia coli strain LF82 replicates in mature phagolysosomes within J774 macrophages. Cell Microbiol 2006;8:471–84.

37. Darfeuille-Michaud A, Boudeau J, Bulois P, et al. High prevalence of adherent-invasive Escherichia coli associated with ileal mucosa in Crohn's disease. Gastroenterology 2004;127:412–21.

38. Glasser AL, Boudeau J, Barnich N, et al. Adherent invasive Escherichia coli strains from patients with Crohn's disease survive and replicate within macrophages without inducing host cell death. Infect Immun 2001;69:5529–37.

39. Lapaquette P, Glasser AL, Huett A, et al. Crohn's disease-associated adherent-invasive E. coli are selectively favoured by impaired autophagy to replicate intracellularly. Cell Microbiol 2010;12:99–113.

40. Masseret E, Boudeau J, Colombel JF, et al. Genetically related Escherichia coli strains associated with Crohn's disease. Gut 2001;48:320–5.

41. Hugot JP, Chamaillard M, Zouali H, et al. Association of NOD2 leucine-rich repeat variants with susceptibility to Crohn's disease. Nature 2001;411:599–603.

42. Franchimont D, Vermeire S, El Housni H, et al. Deficient host-bacteria interactions in inflammatory bowel disease? The toll-like receptor (TLR)-4 Asp299gly polymorphism is associated with Crohn's disease and ulcerative colitis. Gut 2004;53: 987–92.

43. Dubinsky MC, Wang D, Picornell Y, et al. IL-23 receptor (IL-23R) gene protects against pediatric Crohn's disease. Inflamm Bowel Dis 2007;13:511–5.

44. Shih DQ, Targan SR, McGovern D. Recent advances in IBD pathogenesis: genetics and immunobiology. Curr Gastroenterol Rep 2008;10:568–75.

45. Van Kruiningen HJ. Granulomatous colitis of boxer dogs: comparative aspects. Gastroenterology 1967;53:114–22.

46. Hostutler RA, Luria BJ, Johnson SE, et al. Antibiotic-responsive histiocytic ulcerative colitis in 9 dogs. J Vet Intern Med 2004;18:499–504.

47. Craven M, Mezey J, Gao C, et al. Genome-wide association scan reveals NCF2 polymorphism in boxers with adeherent invasive E.coli-associated granulomatous colitis: a potential model of chronic granulomatous disease [abstract]. Chicago: DDW; 2010.

48. Simpson KW, Dogan B, Rishniw M, et al. Adherent and invasive Escherichia coli is associated with granulomatous colitis in boxer dogs. Infect Immun 2006;74: 4778–92.

49. Batt RM, Needham JR, Carter MW. Bacterial overgrowth associated with a naturally occurring enteropathy in the German shepherd dog. Res Vet Sci 1983;35:42–6.

50. Littler RM, Batt RM, Lloyd DH. Total and relative deficiency of gut mucosal IgA in German shepherd dogs demonstrated by faecal analysis. Vet Rec 2006;158: 334–41.

51. German AJ, Hall EJ, Day MJ. Relative deficiency in IgA production by duodenal explants from German shepherd dogs with small intestinal disease. Vet Immunol Immunopathol 2000;76:25–43.

52. Kathrani A, House A, Catchpole B, et al. Polymorphisms in the tlr4 and tlr5 gene are significantly associated with inflammatory bowel disease in german shepherd dogs. PLoS One 2010;5(12):e15740.

53. Schreiber S, Nikolaus S, Hampe J, et al. Tumour necrosis factor alpha and interleukin 1beta in relapse of Crohn's disease. Lancet 1999;353:459–61.

54. Komatsu M, Kobayashi D, Saito K, et al. Tumor necrosis factor-alpha in serum of patients with inflammatory bowel disease as measured by a highly sensitive immuno-PCR. Clin Chem 2001;47:1297–301.

55. Esters N, Vermeire S, Joossens S, et al. Serological markers for prediction of response to anti-tumor necrosis factor treatment in Crohn's disease. Am J Gastroenterol 2002;97:1458–62.

56. Schreiber S, Campieri M, Colombel JF, et al. Use of anti-tumour necrosis factor agents in inflammatory bowel disease. European guidelines for 2001–2003. Int J Colorectal Dis 2001;16:1–11.

57. Sandborn WJ. Transcending conventional therapies: the role of biologic and other novel therapies. Inflamm Bowel Dis 2001;7(Suppl 1):S9–16.

58. German AJ, Helps CR, Hall EJ, et al. Cytokine mRNA expression in mucosal biopsies from German shepherd dogs with small intestinal enteropathies. Dig Dis Sci 2000;45:7–17.

59. Sauter SN, Allenspach K, Gaschen F, et al. Cytokine expression in an ex vivo culture system of duodenal samples from dogs with chronic enteropathies: modulation by probiotic bacteria. Domest Anim Endocrinol 2005;29:605–22.

60. Peters IR, Helps CR, Calvert EL, et al. Cytokine mRNA quantification in duodenal mucosa from dogs with chronic enteropathies by real-time reverse transcriptase polymerase chain reaction. J Vet Intern Med 2005;19:644–53.

61. McCann TM, Ridyard AE, Else RW, et al. Evaluation of disease activity markers in dogs with idiopathic inflammatory bowel disease. J Small Anim Pract 2007;48:620–5.

62. Farrell RJ, Menconi MJ, Keates AC, et al. P-glycoprotein-170 inhibition significantly reduces cortisol and ciclosporin efflux from human intestinal epithelial cells and T lymphocytes. Aliment Pharmacol Ther 2002;16:1021–31.

63. Allenspach K, Bergman PJ, Sauter S, et al. P-glycoprotein expression in lamina propria lymphocytes of duodenal biopsy samples in dogs with chronic idiopathic enteropathies. J Comp Pathol 2006;134:1–7.

64. Radice A, Sinico RA. Antineutrophil cytoplasmic antibodies (ANCA). Autoimmunity 2005;38:93–103.

65. Tidman M, Olander R, Svalander C, et al. Patients hospitalized because of small vessel vasculitides with renal involvement in the period 1975–95: organ involvement, anti-neutrophil cytoplasmic antibodies patterns, seasonal attack rates and fluctuation of annual frequencies. J Intern Med 1998;244:133–41.

66. Boomsma MM, Stegeman CA, van der Leij MJ, et al. Prediction of relapses in Wegener's granulomatosis by measurement of antineutrophil cytoplasmic antibody levels: a prospective study. Arthritis Rheum 2000;43:2025–33.

67. Rump JA, Scholmerich J, Gross V, et al. A new type of perinuclear anti-neutrophil cytoplasmic antibody (p-ANCA) in active ulcerative colitis but not in Crohn's disease. Immunobiology 1990;181:406–13.

68. Nakamura RM, Barry M. Serologic markers in inflammatory bowel disease (IBD). MLO Med Lab Obs 2001;33:8–15 [quiz: 16–9].

69. Bahari A, Aarabi M, Hedayati M, et al. Diagnostic value of antineutrophil cytoplasmic antibodies and anti-Saccharomyces cerevisiae antibody in Iranian patients with inflammatory bowel disease. Acta Gastroenterol Belg 2009;72: 301–5.

70. Jaskowski TD, Litwin CA, Hill HR. Analysis of serum antibodies in patients suspected of having inflammatory bowel disease. Clin Vaccine Immunol 2006;13: 655–60.

71. Homsak E, Micetic-Turk D, Bozic B. Autoantibodies pANCA, GAB and PAB in inflammatory bowel disease: prevalence, characteristics and diagnostic value. Wien Klin Wochenschr 2010;122(Suppl 2):19–25.

72. Vasiliauskas EA, Kam LY, Karp LC, et al. Marker antibody expression stratifies Crohn's disease into immunologically homogeneous subgroups with distinct clinical characteristics. Gut 2000;47:487–96.

73. Vasiliauskas EA, Plevy SE, Landers CJ, et al. Perinuclear antineutrophil cytoplasmic antibodies in patients with Crohn's disease define a clinical subgroup. Gastroenterology 1996;110:1810–9.

74. Allenspach K, Luckschander N, Styner M, et al. Evaluation of assays for perinuclear antineutrophilic cytoplasmic antibodies and antibodies to Saccharomyces cerevisiae in dogs with inflammatory bowel disease. Am J Vet Res 2004;65: 1279–83.

75. Mancho C, Sainz A, Garcia-Sancho M, et al. Detection of perinuclear antineutrophil cytoplasmic antibodies and antinuclear antibodies in the diagnosis of canine inflammatory bowel disease. J Vet Diagn Invest 2010;22:553–8.

76. Hagen EC, Daha MR, Hermans J, et al. Diagnostic value of standardized assays for anti-neutrophil cytoplasmic antibodies in idiopathic systemic vasculitis. EC/BCR project for ANCA assay standardization. Kidney Int 1998;53:743–53.

77. Luckschander N, Allenspach K, Hall J, et al. Perinuclear antineutrophilic cytoplasmic antibody and response to treatment in diarrheic dogs with food responsive disease or inflammatory bowel disease. J Vet Intern Med 2006; 20:221–7.

78. Allenspach K, Lomas B, Wieland B, et al. Evaluation of perinuclear antineutrophilic cytoplasmic autoantibodies as an early marker of protein-losing enteropathy and protein-losing nephropathy in Soft Coated Wheaten Terriers. Am J Vet Res 2008;69:1301–4.

79. Lana SE, Jackson TL, Burnett RC, et al. Utility of polymerase chain reaction for analysis of antigen receptor rearrangement in staging and predicting prognosis in dogs with lymphoma. J Vet Intern Med 2006;20:329–34.

80. Yamazaki J, Takahashi M, Setoguchi A, et al. Monitoring of minimal residual disease (MRD) after multidrug chemotherapy and its correlation to outcome in dogs with lymphoma: a proof-of-concept pilot study. J Vet Intern Med 2010; 24(4):897–903.

81. Fukushima K, Ohno K, Koshino-Goto Y, et al. Sensitivity for the detection of a clonally rearranged antigen receptor gene in endoscopically obtained biopsy specimens from canine alimentary lymphoma. J Vet Med Sci 2009;71:1673–6.

82. Kaneko N, Yamamoto Y, Wada Y, et al. Application of polymerase chain reaction to analysis of antigen receptor rearrangements to support endoscopic diagnosis of canine alimentary lymphoma. J Vet Med Sci 2009;71:555–9.

83. Gajanayake I. PARR as a diagnostic tool for endoscopic detection of intestinal lymphoma [abstract]. Presented at ECVIM Congress. Ghent (Belgium), 2008.

Adverse Food Reactions in Dogs and Cats

Frédéric P. Gaschen, Dr Med Vet, Dr Habil*, Sandra R. Merchant, DVM

KEYWORDS

- Adverse food reaction • Food allergy • Food intolerance
- Dog • Cat • Chronic enteropathies

Adverse food reactions (AFRs) are defined as reactions to an otherwise harmless dietary component, which are experienced by certain individuals on ingestion.[1] These reactions encompass disorders with an immunologic basis (food allergy [FA], also called dietary/food hypersensitivity), nonimmunologic reactions (food intolerance), and toxic reactions (intoxications) (**Fig. 1**).[1,2] Although intoxications, such as garbage can gut gastroenteritis, are encountered frequently in dogs, they are not discussed in in this review. Food intolerance may be caused by a metabolic problem such as digestive enzyme deficiency (eg, lactase deficiency in adult cats) or by a pharmacologic reaction (eg, vasoactive amines such as histidine in spoiled fish that is transformed into histamine by the intestinal flora) or can be idiosyncratic (eg, reaction to food additives, gluten-sensitive enteropathy in Irish Setter dogs).[2] FA is defined as an aberrant adverse immune response elicited by exposure to a particular food substance, most often a protein.[1–3] In general, these responses are characterized as IgE antibody dependent, cell mediated, or mixed.[1–3] In dogs and cats, all AFRs can be associated with similar inciting foods, gastrointestinal (GI) clinical signs, diagnostic test results, and responses to treatment. Thus, it may be difficult to distinguish between food intolerance and FA in the patient with primarily GI signs. Cutaneous disease is seen only in the truly FA patient.[4,5] In people, it is believed that food intolerance represents most AFR.[1]

In recent years, the importance of diet in the management of dogs and cats with chronic idiopathic intestinal disorders has received much attention.[6–8] A new term of diet-responsive or food-responsive chronic enteropathy (CE) has been coined, and it encompasses AFR as well as mild intestinal inflammatory conditions that benefit

Disclosure: The authors have nothing to disclose.
Department of Veterinary Clinical Sciences, School of Veterinary Medicine, Louisiana State University, Baton Rouge, LA 70803, USA
* Corresponding author.
E-mail address: fgaschen@lsu.edu

Vet Clin Small Anim 41 (2011) 361–379
doi:10.1016/j.cvsm.2011.02.005
0195-5616/11/$ – see front matter © 2011 Elsevier Inc. All rights reserved.
vetsmall.theclinics.com

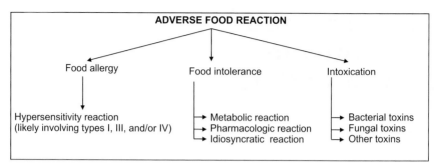

Fig. 1. Classification of AFRs in dogs and cats.

from the properties of the new diet. Dietary elimination trials are now recommended in most dogs and cats with chronic idiopathic GI signs of mild to moderate severity.[6–8]

In veterinary dermatology, further discussion has centered on the role that cutaneous AFR (CAFR) plays in canine atopic dermatitis (AD).[5] The concept that food allergens might trigger flares of AD in some dogs has been discussed in the literature. The International Task Force on Canine Atopic Dermatitis supports the concept that CAFR might manifest as AD in some canine patients.[5] However, dogs with CAFR may also experience clinical signs that are not typically associated with AD, such as GI signs. It has recently been suggested that AD be divided into food-induced atopic dermatitis (FIAD) and non–food-induced atopic dermatitis (NFIAD) or canine atopic dermatitis *sensu stricto* for cases that are not responsive to an elimination diet.[9]

Besides the GI tract, other organ systems may be affected by AFR. These systems include the central nervous system (seizures, personality changes), respiratory system (asthmalike syndrome) and lower urinary tract (cystitis). However, these organ systems are rarely involved, and subsequent clinical signs are rare.[10] One of the authors (S.R.M.) has seen young dogs in poor general condition with failure to thrive and GI signs mimicking hypoadrenocorticism, which have, in fact, FA. This misdiagnosis is usually compounded by blunting of the cortisol response to adrenocorticotropic hormone stimulation test by previous low-dose glucocorticoid administration for control of pruritus. In addition, AFR is also recognized as a cause of vasculitis with associated cutaneous manifestations.[11]

This article reviews pathophysiologic, epidemiologic, and clinical aspects of AFR in dogs and cats with added emphasis of diet-responsive chronic enteropathies.

PATHOGENESIS
GI Mucosal Barrier

The GI mucosa represents the largest surface area in contact with the external environment.[12] Although the main function of the GI mucosa is to process the ingested food into nutrients that can be absorbed and used by the body, GI mucosa is also responsible for preventing the entry of harmful pathogens into the body. The GI barrier consists of several anatomic, physiologic, and immunologic components. The single layer of mucosal epithelial cells joined by tight junctions offers an important physical barrier. It is covered by a thick mucous layer that is able to trap particles and microorganisms.[3,12] Changes in luminal pH across the different parts of the digestive tract, luminal and brush border digestive enzymes, and bile salts all contribute to destroying potential pathogens, breaking down ingested food, and rendering dietary antigens less immunogenic.[3,12] Cells and factors from the innate and adaptive immune system are additional obstacles to foreign antigens and contribute significantly to the mucosal barrier.[3,12]

Gut-associated Lymphoid Tissue

The gut-associated lymphoid tissue (GALT) is the largest and most complex part of the immune system.[13] This system can be divided into organized tissues and effector sites. Peyer patches, mesenteric lymph nodes, and intestinal lymphoid follicles are the organized tissues in charge of the induction phase of the immune response. The effector sites consist of epithelial and lamina propria lymphocytes.[13]

Oral Tolerance

Despite the large extent of exposure to dietary antigens, only a small percentage of people, dogs and cats develop FA. Oral tolerance to dietary proteins and commensal microorganisms is an active immunologic process that results in inhibition of the immune response to an antigen after prior exposure through the oral route.[12,13] Oral tolerance requires the presence of an intact GI barrier.[12,13] Antigen-presenting cells (APC), such as enterocytes and dendritic cells, and regulatory T (T_{reg}) cells are essential for the development of oral tolerance.[12,13] Several types of T_{reg} cells have been described in the GI tract of rodents and people. The T_H3 regulatory cells produce transforming growth factor β that has been shown to enhance the production of IgA in response to luminal antigens. Once released on the mucosal surface, IgAs form a complex with the antigens they bind to and prevent further interaction with the immune system.[12] Moreover, enterocytes may process luminal antigen and present it in association with major histocompatibility (MHC) class II complex, but they lack the second signal to activate the T cells.[13] Thus, antigen presentation by enterocytes results in anergy and may contribute to oral tolerance.[13] These results do not apply to cats, however, because feline crypt and villus epithelial cells do not express MHC class II complex on their surface.[14] In rodent models, priming of T cells by APC in the intestinal mucosa seems more likely to elicit a tolerogenic response, whereas priming of T cells in the mesenteric lymph node, either by migrating APC or by antigen present in the lymph, is more likely to elicit an immune response.[13]

Two mechanisms of oral tolerance are recognized that depend on the dose of GI mucosal antigen exposure. High-dose tolerance results from lymphocyte anergy, and low-dose tolerance is mediated by T_{reg} cells. Abnormalities in the development of low-dose tolerance are thought to be an important cause of FA in people.[12] Other factors that may influence oral tolerance include the normal intestinal microbiota and the genetics of the host.[12]

In FA patients, this complex balance is disrupted. Oral tolerance may be breached directly by an inflammatory process that increases mucosal barrier permeability, causing absorption of allergenic antigens and sensitization.[1] Alternatively, oral tolerance may be bypassed by presentation of antigens via the respiratory tract or the skin. In mice, epicutaneous application of food proteins may elicit a strong allergic response and inflammation.[1,3] In people, reduced exposure to microorganisms (hygiene hypothesis), increased consumption of n6 fatty acids and decreased consumption of n3 fatty acids, reduced dietary antioxidants, and excess or deficiency of vitamin D may favor a T_H2-biaised immune reaction in response to antigen exposure and lead to sensitization.[1,15]

Allergens

Most allergens are water-soluble glycoproteins that are 10 to 70 kDa in size and relatively stable to heat, acid, and proteases.[3] However, many of the allergens that are inhaled or ingested are glycosylated with oligosaccharides. These carbohydrate moieties can be present on multiple different types of protein and are prone to extensive cross-reactivity. Recent data suggest that IgE antibodies to carbohydrate epitopes can be an important factor in anaphylaxis in people.[16] There is currently no data about the existence of IgE against carbohydrate epitopes in canine and feline patients.

In dogs, the most common documented food allergens originate from beef meat, dairy products, wheat, eggs, and chicken meat.[17] Bovine IgG heavy chain found in cow's milk and meat was determined to be the target of IgE in a group of dogs with CAFR.[18] The muscle enzyme phosphoglucomutase was another target of circulating IgE in these dogs. Cross-reactivity was suspected between molecular targets of bovine and ovine origin.[18] Bovine serum albumin was the target of antibeef IgE in another dog.[19] This may have implications for vaccination of these patients because commercially available vaccines for dogs contain a large amount of bovine serum albumin. Vaccinating a dog with this molecule could sensitize the patient to this bovine allergen. In cats, the most common food allergens are beef meat, dairy products, fish, and lamb.[17]

Although type I (IgE mediated) hypersensitivity reactions are the most common mechanism associated with FA in people,[3] the situation is less clear in dogs[4] and cats. The exact mechanism leading to FA in dogs is unknown, and type I (immediate), III, and IV (delayed) hypersensitivities have been postulated to occur.[17] The clinical phenotype in small animals is, however, different from the immediate, sometimes life-threatening, reaction observed in people. In dogs, the clinical phenotypes of CAFR and AD may be remarkably similar. Although canine AD is typically associated with IgE against environmental antigens, dogs with AD frequently also exhibit high levels of food antigen–specific IgE.[20] Moreover, in a subset of dogs with skin lesions suggestive of AD, clinical remission can be induced after a food elimination trial (FIAD).[5] Thus, the division between AD and CAFR is less clear than what was previously thought.[5]

Two recent studies investigated the types of immune cells and cytokines that prevail in the skin and duodenal mucosa of dogs with well-documented CAFR and no GI signs when they were fed a challenge diet that elicited clinical signs, as well as during a successful elimination trial. The study results show a lack of changes in the expression of T_H1-, T_H2-, and T_{reg}-related genes in the duodenal mucosa, suggesting that it is not the primary site of T-cell activation that ultimately leads to cutaneous inflammation.[21] The same studies also looked at T-cell phenotypes and cytokine gene expression in the lesional and nonlesional skin of the same dog population and found that $CD8^+$ T cells were increased in lesional skin of dogs with CAFR when compared with controls. Expression of cytokines revealed a T_H2-skewed environment with increased interleukin (IL)-4, IL-13, SOC-3, and Foxp3 genes expression in lesional skin. Remarkably, these changes were not reversed during resolution of clinical signs after dietary therapy. Moreover, IL-4 and Foxp3 expression was also increased in nonlesional skin, indicating a generalized process.[22]

It is unsure why some dogs and cats with AFR develop cutaneous signs, whereas others show GI signs or a combination of both. One possible explanation is that activated T cells home to different target organs. Upregulated T cells with the skin-homing receptor cutaneous leukocyte-associated antigen are increased in people with food-responsive AD, and T cells with the $\alpha_4\beta_7$ integrin molecule are associated with the GI phenotype.[23] In dogs, T-cell homing also depends on the expression of $\alpha_4\beta_7$ ligand on mucosal lymphocytes that binds to MAdCAM-1 in the GALT endothelial cells. Other ligands are associated with intraepithelial lymphocyte localization.[14]

A gluten-sensitive enteropathy has been studied in families of Irish Setter dogs and is an example of a canine AFR with GI manifestations. This enteropathy is inherited as an autosomal recessive trait, and affected animals show chronic intermittent diarrhea and poor weight gain or weight loss between 7 and 10 months of age when fed a diet containing gluten.[24]

Many, if not most, small animals eat processed food (canned or dry). Heat treatment changes the tertiary (3-dimensional) structure of protein. This change in structure may destroy some epitopes but may also uncover previously hidden epitopes.[25]

Diet-responsive CE

Dogs and cats that respond to an elimination trial but do not relapse after provocation with their original diet or components thereof do not have true AFR, such as food intolerance or FA. It is likely that these animals have mild to moderate enteritis, colitis, or enterocolitis as a result of other causes and benefit from other advantageous properties of the special diet (**Fig. 2**). Higher bioavailability of the nutrients decreases the amount of undigested/unabsorbed substances that are otherwise metabolized by the intestinal flora and may cause changes in its composition. Likewise, prebiotics such as fructooligosaccharides also modulate the intestinal microbiome. Also, a higher n3-n6 fatty acid ratio may increase synthesis of less inflammatory eicosanoids and decrease intestinal inflammation.

EPIDEMIOLOGY

Prevalence of FA in people is thought to be between 1% and 10.8%, and children are more frequently affected than adults.[1,3] Many but not all pediatric FAs resolve before age 16 years.[1,3] There are no comparable data for dogs and cats with AFR. Based on published studies, the prevalence of AFR among dogs presented to a dermatology center with cutaneous signs is estimated between 7.6% and 12%.[26,27] Among allergic dogs, 9% to 36% are diagnosed with CAFR.[26–29] The proportion of dogs with CAFR that show GI signs varies between published case series. In a cohort of 63 dogs from Switzerland with FIAD, 20 (31%) had chronic diarrhea and/or vomiting.[29] However, earlier studies report a lower prevalence rate of 10% to 20%, with many dogs having mild GI signs, such as tendency to develop loose stool and flatulence,

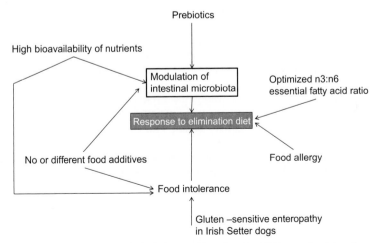

Fig. 2. Canine and feline diet-sensitive enteropathy. Possible mechanisms for positive response of the inflamed GI mucosa to an elimination trial with a commercial veterinary prescription novel protein diet or a hydrolyzed diet.

whereas few had overt diarrhea and vomiting.[26] A recent large multicenter prospective study of dogs with AD reports a GI signs prevalence of 26.3% among dogs with FIAD, whereas it was only 10.5% in dogs with NFIAD.[9]

Although there are no epidemiologic studies of canine CE, the proportion of dogs that responded completely to a 10-day elimination trial in a recent series of 70 dogs with CE from Switzerland was very high (56%). Surprisingly, 79% of these diet-responsive dogs could be switched back to their original diet after receiving a salmon, trout, and rice novel protein diet for 14 weeks. The remaining 8 dogs (21%) relapsed when the novel protein diet was discontinued and improved again when the elimination diet was resumed. These dogs were diagnosed with AFR, and 2 of them reacted to challenge with beef, lamb, chicken, or milk, suggesting FA. One dog with FA could not be successfully managed and was euthanized. This dog had initially presented with chronic GI signs and pruritus.[7] Pruritus is a parameter included in one of the scoring systems for dogs with chronic enteropathies.[7] A Dutch study published in 2010 included 26 dogs with idiopathic CE and small intestinal diarrhea. A response to an elimination trial with a hydrolyzed diet was seen in 16 of 18 dogs (complete in 12, partial in 4). Seven of 8 dogs receiving a highly digestible control diet also responded. A dietary challenge with the original food was performed in 22 of 23 responders, and 15 relapsed (65%). There was no difference in the relapse rate between dogs that received the hydrolyzed diet and those that received the control diet. Ninety percent of dogs continuously receiving the hydrolyzed diet remained in remission for up to 3 years, whereas only 12% of those on the control diet remained in remission.[8]

The prevalence of diet-responsive disease in feline CE is comparable. In a study from New Zealand, 27 (49%) of 55 cats with idiopathic CE and diarrhea and/or vomiting responded to a switch to a novel protein diet.[6] The clinical presentation of diet responders and nonresponders did not differ significantly. Challenge with the original diet triggered a recurrence of clinical signs in 16 cats (29%) that were diagnosed as food sensitive. Of these cats, 12 underwent a more detailed dietary challenge that included protein sources tailored to the cats' history. Beef, corn gluten, and wheat were the food ingredients most commonly associated with FA. Four cats had concurrent cutaneous signs, which were attributed to FA in 3 animals.[6] AFR was also diagnosed in 8 cats from a feline research colony, which exhibited vomiting and dermatitis and were responsive to an elimination trial. Dietary challenge with the original diet elicited recurrence of clinical signs within 4 weeks in 4 of 8 cats.[30]

Even though numerous canine breeds are predisposed to develop AD,[31] no definitive breed predisposition for FA has been reported in dogs, with the exception of soft-coated wheaten terriers[32] and a colony of Maltese-beagle crossbreds.[33] However, CAFR seems to occur frequently in American cocker spaniel, English springer spaniel, Labrador retriever, collie, miniature schnauzer, Chinese shar-pei, poodle, West Highland white terrier, boxer, dachshund, dalmatian, Lhasa apso, German shepherd, and golden retriever.[34,35] Specific lineages of Irish setter dogs may be at risk for gluten-sensitive enteropathy, a disease with autosomal recessive transmission.[24] In cats, Siamese and Siamese crosses may be at increased risk.[34,36]

CLINICAL SIGNS
CAFR

Dogs
Although there is no age or sex predilection for AFR, many cases occur in dogs younger than 1 year.[37] CAFR-associated allergic dermatitis is much more common than environmental allergy (AD) in dogs 6 months of age or younger. The most

common clinical sign is nonseasonal pruritus. However, in some cases, a recurrent staphylococcal folliculitis with no pruritus or resolution of the pruritus when the infection is resolved may be the main clinical manifestation. Cutaneous signs may be nonspecific and may mimic any other allergic dermatosis, such as canine AD with facial, ear, extremity, and ventral distributions as the foci of pruritus (**Figs. 3–5**). Pruritus of the ears and licking of the perianal area, "ears and rears," is a pattern attributed to AFR (**Figs. 6** and **7**). Perianal pruritus may also be seen alone. In a published case series, the ear region was involved in 80% of the cases of AFR; paws in 61%; inguinal region in 53%; and axillary, anterior foreleg, and periorbital regions in 31% to 37% of cases.[38] However, otitis externa with erythema of the pinnae and vertical canal with minimal horizontal canal involvement was the only cutaneous manifestation of AFR in 24% of dogs.[38] Otitis externa may even occur unilaterally only.

Secondary yeast/bacterial infection of the skin is a common sequel leading to a more generalized dermatitis and pruritus. A clinical presentation comparable with that of canine scabies with generalized papular pruritic dermatosis has also been associated with AFR and may be more common in Labrador retrievers (personal observation, S.R.M.). Although tail head pruritus is the classic clinical sign associated with flea allergic dermatitis in the dog, on rare occasions, tail head dermatitis may be AFR related. Secondary changes resulting from chronic pruritus to include keratinization abnormalities, lichenification, hyperpigmentation, and extensive alopecia are not uncommon. AFR dogs may show a papular dermatitis or only secondary lesions resulting from pruritus and complicating microbial infections.

Uncommon clinical signs may be the result of food-induced vasculitis,[11] food-induced urticaria,[39] and even food-induced erythema multiforme.[40] Signs consistent with vasculitis include poorly healing ulcers located in the center of the footpads, erosion, ulceration and crusting of the pinnal margin, elliptical lesions on the concave aspect of the pinna, and urticarial vasculitis.[11] Urticarial vasculitis presents as urticarialike lesions that do not blanche with diascopy and do not pit with pressure, distinguishing them from a true urticaria.[39] Erythema multiforme is a clinically distinct lesion usually consisting of erythematous polycyclic or target-shaped macules that are nonpruritic or slightly elevated papules that spread peripherally and clear centrally.[40] In rare cases, primary pustules that are associated with bacteria may be noted.

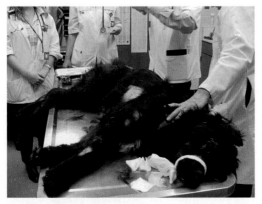

Fig. 3. Young Newfoundland with severe weight loss, lethargy, and a very poor body condition, which was later diagnosed as having FA.

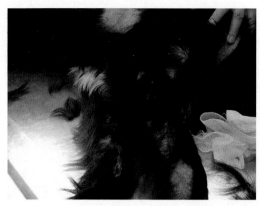

Fig. 4. Same dog as in **Fig. 3**. Papules, erythema, and alopecia were present on the distal extremity.

Cats

In cats, the mean age of onset of CAFR is 4 to 5 years.[34,36] The most consistent clinical sign is pruritus, which was reported to be present in 100% of cats with FA.[34,36] Pruritus may be localized or generalized. Miliary dermatitis is a common cutaneous reaction pattern that can be associated with AFR in its local or generalized form. Self-inflicted alopecia, the fur-mowing cat, can be observed in some cases. Pruritus most commonly affects the head and face region. Head and neck pruritus can be severe and lead to extreme self-trauma (**Figs. 8** and **9**). Some cats develop an exfoliative dermatitis. In addition, AFR may be the cause of eosinophilic plaques; indolent ulcers; and, rarely, angioedema, urticaria, and conjunctivitis.[36]

Diet-responsive CE

Dogs

Dogs with diet-responsive CE are usually relatively young. In a Swiss study describing 70 dogs with CE, the median age of dogs with diet-responsive CE was 3.4 years (range 0.6–7.6 years), whereas it was 4.8 years (range 2.1–13.0 years) in dogs that required steroid treatment.[7] Of the 38 dogs with diet-responsive CE, 27 (71%) had exclusively large bowel diarrhea (with signs such as frequent defecation, tenesmus, mucoid feces and/or hematochezia), whereas 9 dogs (24%) had mixed small and large bowel

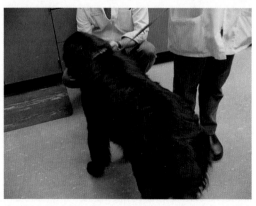

Fig. 5. Same dog as in **Figs. 3** and **4** after a successful elimination trial.

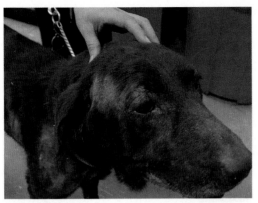

Fig. 6. Significant ear and facial pruritus with self-inflicted alopecia on a Labrador retriever.

diarrhea and 2 (5%) had only small bowel diarrhea (**Fig. 10**). Using a clinical scoring index (canine inflammatory bowel disease activity index [CIBDAI]), the severity of signs was insignificant to mild in 30%, moderate in 62%, and severe in 8% only. By comparison, most dogs requiring steroid treatment and those with protein-losing enteropathy had small bowel diarrhea, and 52% had severe clinical manifestation of disease.[7] A Dutch study that enrolled exclusively dogs with small intestinal diarrhea showed that almost 90% of dogs responded to either a highly digestible or a hydrolyzed diet over 2 to 3 months.[8]

Cats

The median age of 16 cats from New Zealand diagnosed with food sensitivity was 5 years (0.5–14.0 years). Their clinical signs included vomiting (56%), diarrhea (25%), or both (19%). Vomiting was usually infrequent (less than once a day in most cats). Nature and timing of vomitus were variable. More than half of the cats with diarrhea had large bowel signs. Weight loss was present in 69% and flatulence, in 38%. Four cats had concurrent cutaneous signs.[6]

DIFFERENTIAL DIAGNOSIS

The differential diagnoses for AFR with cutaneous and GI signs are listed in **Boxes 1–3**.

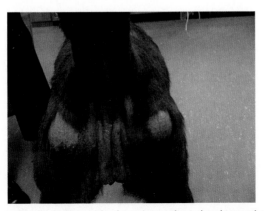

Fig. 7. Significant perianal pruritus with alopecia on the Labrador retriever in **Fig. 6.**

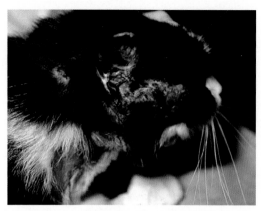

Fig. 8. Self-inflicted erosions and ulceration of the head and neck of a cat.

DIAGNOSTIC APPROACH

Diagnosis is intimately intertwined with therapy because in most cases, diagnosis is based on response to therapy. The gold standard for diagnosing AFR is abatement of clinical signs while the animal is being fed an appropriate restricted/novel diet and recurrence of clinical signs when the patient is challenged with previous food items. Other tests such as intradermal skin testing, skin patch testing, and measuring circulating food allergen–specific serum IgE are of no diagnostic value because of their low sensitivity and specificity.[41–43]

Cutaneous Form

For CAFR, a few steps should be taken before embarking on a food trial; it is preferable to treat for possible sarcoptic mange if clinical signs are suggestive. If tail head pruritus is seen, adequate flea control should be initiated and the dog should be observed for 6 to 8 weeks. Secondary bacterial and yeast infections should be appropriately treated previously. In many instances, one or more of these treatments resolve the dermatitis. If pruritus or other clinical signs persist after the earlier-listed treatments have been instituted, a food trial should be considered. Similarly, if bacterial and/or yeast dermatitis recurs after discontinuation of antimicrobial therapy, a food trial may be warranted.

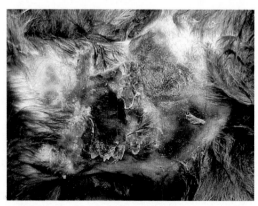

Fig. 9. Self-inflicted dorsal cervical ulcerations on a cat.

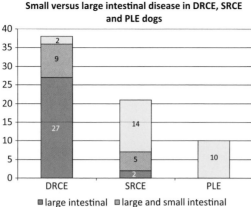

Fig. 10. Study of 70 dogs with chronic enteropathies. Numbers of dogs in each group presenting with signs of predominantly small intestinal, large intestinal, or mixed clinical signs. DRCE, diet-responsive CE; PLE, protein-losing enteropathy; SRCE, steroid-responsive CE. (*From* Allenspach K, Wieland B, Grone A, et al. Chronic enteropathies in dogs: evaluation of risk factors for negative outcome. J Vet Intern Med 2007;21(4):704; with permission.)

GI Form

In dogs and cats with CE, a systematic elimination of all possible diagnoses is required. However, a food elimination trial is usually recommended very early in this process because of the large proportion of responders. The first step consists of ruling out the presence of intestinal parasites and includes repeated (n = 3) fecal examinations, including fecal smears and fecal floatation. Fecal enzyme-linked immunosorbent assay (ELISA) delivers the most accurate results for Giardia infestation.[44] A 3- to 5-day course of fenbendazole is generally empirically prescribed (50 mg/kg once daily by mouth).

It is impossible to unequivocally differentiate dogs with diet-responsive CE from other dogs with CE by physical examination and routine laboratory investigations. However, recent studies have shown that a high percentage (62%) of dogs with diet-responsive CE had circulating antibodies against neutrophils (pANCA, perinuclear antineutrophil cytoplasmic antibodies) when compared with dogs with CE requiring steroid treatment (23%), and pANCA may therefore be a marker for diet-responsive CE.[45] The prevalence of pANCA in soft-coated wheaten terriers with

---

Box 1
Differential diagnoses of CAFR in the dog

- Nonseasonal AD
- Parasitic otitis externa or other causes of otitis externa if ear involvement only
- Drug reaction, which is a differential for any dermatosis
- Sarcoptic mange if significantly papular
- Bacterial and yeast dermatitis/hypersensitivity
- Contact dermatitis if clinical signs primarily ventral in distribution
- Flea allergy; tailhead disease is a rare manifestation of FA

Box 2
Differential diagnoses of CAFR in the cat

- Nonseasonal AD
- Flea allergy dermatitis
- Psychogenic alopecia
- Dermatophytosis
- Otodectic mange
- Other causes of otitis externa
- Other external parasites
- Drug eruption
- Feline acne

---

protein-losing nephropathy and enteropathy and AFR is high, and the test may allow early detection of the disease in this breed, although large-scale investigations are still underway.[46]

Although abdominal ultrasonography is useful to examine the GI tract of dogs and cats with CE, the technique does not distinguish diet-responsive animals from those that require other treatments. However, evaluation of blood flow through the cranial mesenteric artery and celiac artery using Doppler ultrasonography was found to be a valuable technique to document abnormal dynamics of GI perfusion after a meal. Postprandial vasodilation leads to decreasing Doppler indices and increasing diastolic blood flow velocity, which indicates decreased resistance to flow in the

---

Box 3
Differential diagnoses of chronic idiopathic enteropathies in the dog and cat

- Intestinal parasites (nematodes and protozoa)[a]
- Diet-responsive enteropathy[a]
  - AFR: food intolerance, FA
  - Mild form of IBD
- Antibiotic-responsive enteropathy [d]
- Inflammatory bowel disease (IBD)[a]
- Granulomatous colitis [d][a]
- Protein-losing enteropathy [d]
  - Intestinal lymphangiectasia [d]
  - Enteropathy of soft-coated wheaten terriers [d]
- Gluten-sensitive enteropathy of Irish Setters [d]
- Histoplasmosis [d>c]
- Alimentary lymphoma [c>d]
- Chronic idiopathic large bowel diarrhea [d][a]
- Other neoplasia

Abbreviations: d, dog; c, cat.
[a] Often associated with large bowel diarrhea

---

downstream capillary bed of the GI tract. In a colony of soft-coated wheaten terriers with FA, dietary provocation with the allergen resulted in prolonged vasodilation at 90 minutes postprandially compared with nonallergenic food (**Fig. 11**).[47] These hemodynamic changes occurred before the dogs developed clinical signs, such as diarrhea, in response to the dietary challenge.[47] This noninvasive ultrasonographic method shows promise for early detection of dogs with AFR and GI signs at the time of dietary provocation. Early detection of allergenic protein sources before the onset of GI signs may increase the acceptability of the dietary challenge among pet owners. However, in a preliminary study, the technique was not found to be as reliable for dogs with CAFR.[48] These results support the finding that no significant GI mucosal inflammation is observed in dogs with CAFR.[21]

GI endoscopy with collection of mucosal biopsy samples may be indicated in dogs and cats with CE. Dogs with diet-responsive CE could not be differentiated from those with disease requiring steroid therapy based on the severity of endoscopic or histologic lesions.[7,49] Moreover, histologic scoring was not different before and after clinically successful treatment.[7,49] Gastric or colonic antigen provocation test may be of interest in identifying the substances to which a dog is allergic, even though both tests have their limitations.[50] Moreover, these tests are not widely available at present.

A recent study describes the use of the lymphocyte blastogenic response (or lymphocyte stimulation test [LST]) to various food antigens to determine the inciting food allergen in a series of dogs with AFR and cutaneous and/or GI signs.[41] The agreement between LST and dietary elimination and provocation trials was good while the dogs were fed the allergenic diet. However, the LST was blunted in dogs receiving an elimination diet and experiencing clinical remission.[41]

TREATMENT
Dietary Elimination Trial

For maximum efficiency in performing a food trial, it is important to obtain a complete dietary history from the client concerning their pet before choosing any food for the AFR elimination diet trial. Clinical signs of GI disease usually improve within 2 weeks, whereas cutaneous clinical signs may take up to 8 to 12 weeks to respond to a dietary change.

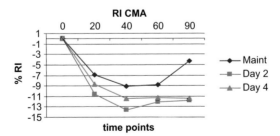

Fig. 11. Postprandial changes in the percentage of resistive index versus time in the cranial mesenteric artery in soft-coated wheaten terriers crossbreds. The dogs had been fed a meal containing an allergen that they were reactive to (see text for explanation). RI, resistive index; CMA, cranial mesenteric artery; Maint, maintenance diet that does not elicit clinical signs; Day 2 and Day 4, time between exposure to dietary allergen and examination. (*From* Kircher PR, Spaulding KA, Vaden S, et al. Doppler ultrasonographic evaluation of gastrointestinal hemodynamics in food hypersensitivities: a canine model. J Vet Intern Med 2004; 18(5):608; with permission.)

An immune response can be mounted against any substance (especially protein) to which that pet has been exposed, which has not been modified to the point of rendering it nonallergenic.

Novel protein diets

Commercially available novel protein source diets typically include proteins from venison, rabbit, duck, kangaroo, moose, elk goose, goat, ostrich, or emu and are combined with a carbohydrate source such as potatoes, sweet potatoes, rutabagas, oats, barley for the dog, and green peas for the cat. Generally, the closer the taxonomic relationship between meat sources, the higher the risk of cross-reactivity. Allergens from beef theoretically may cross-react with those from other ruminants. Thus, lamb and venison may not be the best unique ingredient protein sources because most animals have been previously exposed to beef. However, this finding has yet to be seen as a problem in veterinary medicine. There is evidence of common allergens in avian meats,[51] and the use of duck diets in patients previously exposed to chicken may not be advisable. Cross-reactivity among meats of various proveniences has not been studied yet in dogs and cats.

Controversy persists between the choices of a home-cooked diet, a commercial veterinary prescription diet, and a novel protein over-the-counter (OTC) diet for the elimination trial. The veterinary prescription diet and the OTC novel protein diet may offer the advantage of enhanced owner compliance because of minimal time in food preparation. Home-cooked diets can be unbalanced and may be inadequate in young, large breed, rapidly growing dogs if they are not carefully formulated. In addition, purchased ground meat from one animal source may be contaminated with ground meat from another meat source if the grinding machine was not completely and thoroughly cleaned between uses. However, some clients wish to home cook for their pet, and recipes for balanced formulations are available. Veterinary prescription diets or OTC novel protein diets may not be adequate for the growing puppy. Rarely, dogs have been described that tolerate home-prepared ingredients from a specific protein source but not their commercially prepared versions. This finding raises concerns that heat processing may change the food allergen configuration, substances may leech into the food during industrial processing, or food additives may be an allergen source.[38,52] In a recent study, none of the 4 OTC venison diets was considered suitable for an elimination trial because they all contained common pet food proteins, some of which were not mentioned on the label. Of the 4 OTC venison diets, 3 tested positive for soy, poultry, and/or beef using an ELISA, even though these ingredients were not listed among the ingredients.[53]

The existence of nonprotein allergens has been documented; however, these allergens are generally thought to be combined with protein allergens (glycoproteins, lipoproteins). Thus, attention should be paid to the carbohydrate and lipid sources chosen for incorporation into elimination diet because these sources may represent an important source of allergens, unless the food company has taken steps to remove any protein allergens from these components of the diet.

Hydrolyzed diets

Hydrolysates contain small peptides that are less likely to be allergenic than full size proteins. In a study by Jackson and colleagues,[54] 21% of the dogs that were hypersensitive to soy and corn reacted adversely to the hydrolyzed soy diet with return of cutaneous signs, but 79% had no problems when the diet was fed for 2 weeks. Thus, a commercially available hydrolysate soy and corn diet was tolerated by most, but not all, of the dogs sensitized to the intact compounds. In a more recent study by Ricci and colleagues[55] evaluating 12 dogs with cutaneous manifestations of allergic dermatitis after exposure to chicken meat, clinical signs improved in 11 dogs when fed a hydrolyzed chicken diet, whereas 1 animal did not significantly improve. In another study of experimental soy allergic dogs, IgE binding to hydrolyzed soy peptides was found to be significantly reduced (but not absent) compared with binding to the native soy protein.[56] In a recent systematic review of 11 studies examining the evidence in favor of reduced immunologic and clinical allergenicity of hydrolysates in dogs with CAFR, it was concluded that hydrolysate-containing diets were probably best used in dogs with no suspected hypersensitivity to the original source of hydrolyzed peptides.[57]

Oral medications

Many medications, especially OTC medications, may contain unwanted/hidden proteins. Ten of 12 dogs from a canine colony with spontaneous AFR to soy and corn displayed cutaneous signs when given a chewable tablet containing pork liver, soy, and milbemycin.[58] All flavored medication should therefore be avoided, including medication packaged in gelatin capsules. Also, coprophagic dogs may ingest undigested material that could affect a food trial. Some veterinarians even advocate the use of distilled water during the elimination trial.

Client education and compliance

Lack of client compliance is generally the biggest reason for failure of dietary trials. Often this lack of compliance is because of insufficient client education concerning expectations and especially length of the trial. It was shown that without improved client education, 52% of elimination trials would fail at the time of follow-up compared with a failure rate of 27% after better client education was instituted.[26] A food trial requires full investment and cooperation of the pet's owner, and cannot be adequately performed on a free-roaming pet. The client must have complete control of what their pet ingests. This is a particular challenge in trying to diagnose food-allergic cats. An indoor/outdoor cat or completely outdoor cat may need to be kept inside only for the duration of the food trial. Motivation can be improved by supplying the clients with a daily dietary log to fill out. Daily recording of itching level, GI signs, and honest recording of dietary violations on the log can provide extra motivation and good information as well.

The lengthy food trial required for dermatologic disease (8–12 weeks) benefits from regular motivational meetings in which pitfalls, accidents, and progress are discussed. Monthly rechecks to assess changes in cutaneous symptoms provide information on flea control, secondary infection, and other issues that can complicate interpretation of the diet trial results. If the pet is severely pruritic, a short course of oral short-acting corticosteroids or other nonsteroidal antiinflammatory medication may be warranted at the beginning of the food trial. To allow accurate evaluation of the response to the food trial, this medical manipulation must be discontinued 1 to 2 weeks before the veterinarian's assessment.

Dietary Provocation Test

A rechallenge or provocation is necessary to confirm AFR after the elimination diet has been fed for 8 to 12 weeks. Improvement over this length of time could also result from elimination of seasonal environmental allergens (change of season). In addition, successful treatment of scabies and bacterial and yeast infections and/or improved flea control may be the reason for improvement.

During the rechallenge, the initial food is reintroduced or individual ingredients from the initial food are fed one by one while continuing to feed the elimination diet to cover nutritional needs. To ensure a thorough provocation, it is important to challenge with all previous food stuffs, including flavored mediation, rawhide chews, other flavored chewable bones, treats, flavored toothpastes, and so on. The time needed to provoke a GI reaction is generally thought to be a few days after the allergen is reintroduced.[6,7] The time needed to provoke a cutaneous reaction to a food allergen is not clear. Most literature reports that clinical signs exacerbate between a few hours and 21 days.[59] In one study, the mean number of allergens to which dogs reacted to on rechallenge was 2.4, with 80% reacting to 1 or 2 proteins and 64% reacting to 2 or more of the proteins tested.[59]

However, many clients do not elect to rechallenge with the former diet, much less individual ingredients. In this scenario, the pet can either be kept on the test diet indefinitely, or other novel protein OTC diets that may be less costly can be tried. If new foods are to be tried, including treats, it is important to introduce only one food or treat at a time, so if a reaction occurs, the food stuff responsible can be more easily confirmed.

If the results of the elimination trial are negative and further allergy testing proves unrewarding or does not completely explain the clinical signs, a second food trial using a different protein/carbohydrate source or a home-cooked recipe may need to be considered. In dogs and cats with GI signs, other causes of chronic idiopathic enteropathies should be considered (see **Box 3**).

PROGNOSIS

In dogs and cats with AFR, the prognosis is excellent once the disorder is correctly identified with an appropriate food trial. However, it is difficult for many clients to maintain a strict diet without intermittent dietary violations, either knowingly (feeding a forbidden or suspect food) or unknowingly (OTC supplement with hidden food allergen, prescribed medication with food allergen, or pet scavenging food). Elimination of the forbidden food, treat, or supplement or better control of access to other foods improves the clinical signs, but treatment of a secondary bacterial or yeast infection of the skin or ears may be necessary to restore the skin to normal. In addition, a significant proportion of animals with diet-responsive CE can be switched back to their original diet after a successful treatment with an elimination diet.

SUMMARY

AFRs are common diseases that may have various clinical manifestations, including cutaneous lesions and GI signs. A systematic diagnostic and therapeutic approach centered on a dietary elimination trial followed by a dietary challenge is necessary. The prognosis is generally excellent.

REFERENCES

1. Cianferoni A, Spergel JM. Food allergy: review, classification and diagnosis. Allergol Int 2009;58(4):457–66.
2. Ortolani C, Pastorello EA. Food allergies and food intolerances. Best Pract Res Clin Gastroenterol 2006;20(3):467–83.
3. Sicherer SH, Sampson HA. Food allergy. J Allergy Clin Immunol 2010; 125(2 Suppl 2):S116–25.
4. Hillier A, Griffin CE. The ACVD task force on canine atopic dermatitis (X): is there a relationship between canine atopic dermatitis and cutaneous adverse food reactions? Vet Immunol Immunopathol 2001;81:227–31.

5. Olivry T, Deboer DJ, Prelaud P, et al. Food for thought: pondering the relationship between canine atopic dermatitis and cutaneous adverse food reactions. Vet Dermatol 2007;18(6):390–1.
6. Guilford WG, Jones BR, Markwell PJ, et al. Food sensitivity in cats with chronic idiopathic gastrointestinal problems. J Vet Intern Med 2001;15(1):7–13.
7. Allenspach K, Wieland B, Grone A, et al. Chronic enteropathies in dogs: evaluation of risk factors for negative outcome. J Vet Intern Med 2007;21(4): 700–8.
8. Mandigers PJ, Biourge V, van den Ingh TS, et al. A randomized, open-label, positively-controlled field trial of a hydrolyzed protein diet in dogs with chronic small bowel enteropathy. J Vet Intern Med 2010;24(6):1350–7.
9. Favrot C, Steffan J, Seewald W, et al. A prospective study on the clinical features of chronic canine atopic dermatitis and its diagnosis. Vet Dermatol 2010;21(1): 23–31.
10. Merchant SR, Taboada J. Food allergy and immunologic diseases of the gastrointestinal tract. Semin Vet Med Surg (Small Anim) 1991;6(4):316–21.
11. Nichols PR, Morris DO, Beale KM. A retrospective study of canine and feline cutaneous vasculitis. Vet Dermatol 2001;12(5):255–64.
12. Chehade M, Mayer L. Oral tolerance and its relation to food hypersensitivities. J Allergy Clin Immunol 2005;115(1):3–12 [quiz: 13].
13. Mowat AM. Anatomical basis of tolerance and immunity to intestinal antigens. Nat Rev Immunol 2003;3(4):331–41.
14. Stokes C, Waly N. Mucosal defence along the gastrointestinal tract of cats and dogs. Vet Res 2006;37(3):281–93.
15. Lack G. Epidemiologic risks for food allergy. J Allergy Clin Immunol 2008;121(6): 1331–6.
16. Commins SP, Platts-Mills TA. Allergenicity of carbohydrates and their role in anaphylactic events. Curr Allergy Asthma Rep 2010;10(1):29–33.
17. Verlinden A, Hesta M, Millet S, et al. Food allergy in dogs and cats: a review. Crit Rev Food Sci Nutr 2006;46(3):259–73.
18. Martin A, Sierra MP, Gonzalez JL, et al. Identification of allergens responsible for canine cutaneous adverse food reactions to lamb, beef and cow's milk. Vet Dermatol 2004;15(6):349–56.
19. Ohmori K, Masuda K, Kawarai S, et al. Identification of bovine serum albumin as an IgE-reactive beef component in a dog with food hypersensitivity against beef. J Vet Med Sci 2007;69(8):865–7.
20. Foster AP, Knowles TG, Moore AH, et al. Serum IgE and IgG responses to food antigens in normal and atopic dogs, and dogs with gastrointestinal disease. Vet Immunol Immunopathol 2003;92(3–4):113–24.
21. Veenhof EZ, Rutten VP, van Noort R, et al. Evaluation of T-cell activation in the duodenum of dogs with cutaneous food hypersensitivity. Am J Vet Res 2010; 71(4):441–6.
22. Veenhof EZ, Knol EF, Schlotter YM, et al. Characterisation of T cell phenotypes, cytokines and transcription factors in the skin of dogs with cutaneous adverse food reactions. Vet J 2011. [Epub ahead of print].
23. Sicherer SH, Sampson HA. Food allergy: recent advances in pathophysiology and treatment. Annu Rev Med 2009;60:261–77.
24. Garden OA, Manners HK, Sorensen SH, et al. Intestinal permeability of Irish setter puppies challenged with a controlled oral dose of gluten. Res Vet Sci 1998;65(1):23–8.
25. Cave NJ, Marks SL. Evaluation of the immunogenicity of dietary proteins in cats and the influence of the canning process. Am J Vet Res 2004;65(10):1427–33.

26. Chesney CJ. Food sensitivity in the dog: a quantitative study. J Small Anim Pract 2002;43:203–7.
27. Proverbio D, Perego R, Spada E, et al. Prevalence of adverse food reactions in 130 dogs in Italy with dermatological signs: a retrospective study. J Small Anim Pract 2010;51(7):370–4.
28. Wilhelm S, Favrot C. [Food hypersensitivity dermatitis in the dog: diagnostic possibilities]. Schweiz Arch Tierheilkd 2005;147(4):165–71 [in German].
29. Picco F, Zini E, Nett C, et al. A prospective study on canine atopic dermatitis and food-induced allergic dermatitis in Switzerland. Vet Dermatol 2008;19(3): 150–5.
30. Hirt R, Iben C. Possible food allergy in a colony of cats. J Nutr 1998;128(12 Suppl):2792S–4S.
31. Jaeger K, Linek M, Power HT, et al. Breed and site predispositions of dogs with atopic dermatitis: a comparison of five locations in three continents. Vet Dermatol 2010;21(1):118–22.
32. Vaden SL, Hammerberg B, Davenport DJ, et al. Food hypersensitivity reactions in Soft Coated Wheaten Terriers with protein-losing enteropathy or protein-losing nephropathy or both: gastroscopic food sensitivity testing, dietary provocation, and fecal immunoglobulin E. J Vet Intern Med 2000;14(1):60–7.
33. Jackson HA, Hammerberg B. Evaluation of a spontaneous canine model of immunoglobulin E-mediated food hypersensitivity: dynamic changes in serum and fecal allergen-specific immunoglobulin E values relative to dietary change. Comp Med 2002;52(4):316–21.
34. Carlotti DN, Remy I, Prost C. Food allergy in dogs and cats. A review of 43 cases. Vet Dermatol 1990;1:55–62.
35. Scott DW, Mille WH Jr, Griffin Skin CE. immune system and allergic skin diseases. In: Scott DW, Miller WH Jr. Griffin CE, editors. Muller and Kirk's small animal dermatology. 6th edition. Philadelphia: W.B. Saunders Co; 2001. p. 543–666.
36. Rosser EJ Jr. Food allergy in the cat: a prospective study of 13 cats. In: Ihrke PJ, editor. Advances in veterinary dermatology II. New York: Pergamon Press; 1993. p. 33.
37. Scott DW, Miller WH, Griffin CE. Skin immune system and allergic skin diseases. In: Scott DW, Miller WH, Griffin CE, editors. Muller & Kirks small animal dermatology. Philadeplphia: W.B. Saunders; 2001. p. 543–666.
38. Rosser EJ Jr. Diagnosis of food allergy in dogs. J Am Vet Med Assoc 1993; 203(2):259–62.
39. Morris DO, Beale KM. Cutaneous vasculitis and vasculopathy. Vet Clin North Am Small Anim Pract 1999;29(6):1325–35.
40. Itoh T, Nibe K, Kojimoto A, et al. Erythema multiforme possibly triggered by food substances in a dog. J Vet Med Sci 2006;68(8):869–71.
41. Ishida R, Masuda K, Kurata K, et al. Lymphocyte blastogenic responses to inciting food allergens in dogs with food hypersensitivity. J Vet Intern Med 2004;18(1):25–30.
42. Nett C. Diagnosis and management of canine cutaneous food reactions—a practical approach. Paper presented at: Sixth World Congress of Veterinary Dermatology. Hong Kong, China, November 19–22, 2008.
43. Kunkle G, Horner S. Validity of skin testing for diagnosis of food allergy in dogs. J AmVet Med Assoc 1992;200(5):677–80.
44. Rishniw M, Liotta J, Bellosa M, et al. Comparison of 4 Giardia diagnostic tests in diagnosis of naturally acquired canine chronic subclinical giardiasis. J Vet Intern Med 2010;24(2):293–7.

45. Luckschander N, Allenspach K, Hall J, et al. Perinuclear antineutrophilic cytoplasmic antibody and response to treatment in diarrheic dogs with food responsive disease or inflammatory bowel disease. J Vet Intern Med 2006;20(2):221–7.

46. Allenspach K, Lomas B, Wieland B, et al. Evaluation of perinuclear antineutrophilic cytoplasmic autoantibodies as an early marker of protein-losing enteropathy and protein-losing nephropathy in Soft Coated Wheaten Terriers. Am J Vet Res 2008;69(10):1301–4.

47. Kircher PR, Spaulding KA, Vaden S, et al. Doppler ultrasonographic evaluation of gastrointestinal hemodynamics in food hypersensitivities: a canine model. J Vet Intern Med 2004;18(5):605–11.

48. Hobbs J, Gaschen L, Merchant S, et al. Doppler ultrasound analysis of gastrointestinal blood flow for differentiating allergic from non-food allergic pruritic dogs. J Vet Intern Med 2009;23(3):732.

49. Schreiner NM, Gaschen F, Grone A, et al. Clinical signs, histology, and CD3-positive cells before and after treatment of dogs with chronic enteropathies. J Vet Intern Med 2008;22(5):1079–83.

50. Allenspach K, Vaden SL, Harris TS, et al. Evaluation of colonoscopic allergen provocation as a diagnostic tool in dogs with proven food hypersensitivity reactions. J Small Anim Pract 2006;47(1):21–6.

51. Kelso JM, Cockrell GE, Helm RM, et al. Common allergens in avian meats. J Allergy Clin Immunol 1999;104(1):202–4.

52. Rutgers HC, Batt RM, Hall EJ, et al. Intestinal permeability testing in dogs with diet-responsive intestinal disease. J Small Anim Pract 1995;36(7):295–301.

53. Raditic DM, Remillard RL, Tater KC. ELISA testing for common food antigens in four dry dog foods used in dietary elimination trials. J Anim Physiol Anim Nutr 2011;95(1):90–7.

54. Jackson HA, Jackson MW, Coblentz L, et al. Evaluation of the clinical and allergen specific serum immunoglobulin E responses to oral challenge with cornstarch, corn, soy and a soy hydrolysate diet in dogs with spontaneous food allergy. Vet Dermatol 2003;14(4):181–7.

55. Ricci R, Hammerberg B, Paps J, et al. A comparison of the clinical manifestations of feeding whole and hydrolysed chicken to dogs with hypersensitivity to the native protein. Vet Dermatol 2010. [Epub ahead of print].

56. Serra M, Brazis P, Fondati A, et al. Assessment of IgE binding to native and hydrolyzed soy protein in serum obtained from dogs with experimentally induced soy protein hypersensitivity. Am J Vet Res 2006;67(11):1895–900.

57. Olivry T, Bizikova P. A systematic review of the evidence of reduced allergenicity and clinical benefit of food hydrolysates in dogs with cutaneous adverse food reactions. Vet Dermatol 2010;21(1):32–41.

58. Jackson HA, Hammerberg B. The clinical and immunological reaction to a flavored monthly oral heartworm prophylactic in 12 dogs with spontaneous food allergy. North American Veterinary Dermatology Forum. New Orleans (LA): American College of Veterinary Dermatology; 2002. p. 60.

59. Jeffers JG, Meyer EK, Sosis EJ. Responses of dogs with food allergies to single-ingredient dietary provocation. J AmVet Med Assoc 1996;209(3):608–11.

Pitfalls and Progress in the Diagnosis and Management of Canine Inflammatory Bowel Disease

Kenneth W. Simpson, BVM&S, PhD[a],*,
Albert E. Jergens, DVM, MS, PhD[b]

KEYWORDS

• Inflammatory bowel disease • Enteropathy • Bacteria • Diet

Inflammatory bowel disease (IBD) is the collective term for a group of chronic enteropathies characterized by persistent or recurrent gastrointestinal (GI) signs and inflammation of the GI tract. It is widely accepted that IBD involves a complex interplay among host genetics, the intestinal microenvironment (principally bacteria and dietary constituents), the immune system, and the environmental triggers of intestinal inflammation.[1] However, the specific steps that lead to IBD and the basis for phenotypic variation and unpredictable responses to treatment are not known.

This article examines IBD in dogs, focusing on the interaction between genetic susceptibility and the enteric microenvironment (bacteria, diet), the utility of recently developed histologic criteria, the prognostic indicators, and the standardized approaches to treatment.

GENETIC SUSCEPTIBILITY

The predisposition of certain breeds to IBD strongly supports a role for host genetics (**Table 1**). However, causal genetic defects have not been identified to date.

The genetic basis of human IBD, principally Crohn disease (typified by granulomatous inflammation of the ileum and/or colon), ulcerative colitis (diffuse colonic

---

Disclosure: K.W.S. is a member of the Nestlé-Purina advisory council and has conducted research sponsored in part by Nestlé-Purina. A.E.J. has no conflicts of interest to disclose.
a Veterinary Clinical Sciences, College of Veterinary Medicine, Cornell University, VMC2001, Ithaca, NY 14853, USA
b Veterinary Clinical Sciences, 2446 Lloyd Veterinary Medical Center, College of Veterinary Medicine, Iowa State University, Ames, IA, USA
* Corresponding author.
E-mail address: kws5@cornell.edu

Table 1
Breed predisposition and canine IBD

Breed	Phenotype	Possible Genetic Basis
Irish setter[13]	Gluten-sensitive enteropathy	Autosomal recessive
German shepherd dog[3,10,11]	Antibiotic-responsive enteropathy	? IgA deficiency SNPs: TLR5, NOD2
Basenji[21]	Immunoproliferative small intestinal disease	—
Lundehund[23]	Protein-losing enteropathy, lymphangiectasia, atrophic gastritis, gastric carcinoma	—
Yorkshire terrier[22,37]	—	—
Rottweilers (Europe)[56,57]	Protein-losing enteropathy, lymphangiectasia, crypt lesions	—
Soft-coated wheaten terrier[14,15]	Protein-losing enteropathy, nephropathy	Common male ancestor
Shar-pei[20]	Cobalamin deficiency	Autosomal recessive, chromosome 13
Boxer dog[5,9,25]/French bulldog[58]	Granulomatous colitis (HUC)	SNPs: NCF2

Abbreviations: HUC, histiocytic ulcerative colitis; SNP, single nucleotide polymorphism.

inflammation), and celiac disease (inflammation and villous atrophy of the small intestine), is much better established. In Crohn disease, genetic susceptibility is increasingly linked to defects in innate immunity exemplified by mutations in the innate immune receptor NOD2/CARD15, which in the presence of enteric microflora may lead to upregulated mucosal cytokine production and delayed bacterial clearance or killing, thereby promoting and perpetuating intestinal inflammation.[1,2] The predisposition of certain dog breeds (see **Table 1**), along with clinical response to antibiotics, for example, in boxers and German shepherds, points to a similar interaction of host susceptibility and microflora in dogs.[3–6] In boxers with granulomatous colitis (GC), lasting remission correlates with the eradication of mucosally invasive *Escherichia coli* that have a novel adherent and invasive pathotype associated with Crohn disease,[5,7,8] and genome-wide analysis has identified disease-associated single nucleotide polymorphisms (SNPs) in a gene (*NCF2*) that is involved with killing intracellular bacteria.[9] Studies in German shepherds have identified polymorphisms in innate immunity factor TLR5, which segregates with disease, and have shown that German shepherds have increased *TLR2* and decreased *TLR5* expressions relative to healthy greyhounds.[10] In addition, 4 nonsynonymous SNPs were identified in exon 4 of the canine NOD2 gene. The heterozygote genotype for all 4 NOD2 SNPs was significantly more frequently found in the IBD population ($P = .04$; odds ratio [OR], 2.34; confidence interval [CI], 1.03–5.28) than in controls. These results were also mirrored in non–German shepherd breeds: the heterozygote genotype for all 4 SNPs was significantly more frequently found in a population of 96 dogs of different breeds with IBD than the non–German shepherd control population ($P = .0009$; OR, 3.06; CI, 1.55–6.05).[11] These results suggest that genetic abnormalities in innate immune sensing or killing enteric bacteria underlie the antibiotic responsiveness of German shepherds and boxer dogs.

In human beings, celiac disease is an inflammatory disorder of the small intestine with an autoimmune component and strong heritability. Genetic studies indicate a strong association with HLA and have identified more than 30 non-HLA risk genes, mostly immune-related.[12] Most of the celiac disease–associated regions are shared with other immune-related diseases, as well as with metabolic, hematologic, or neurologic traits, or cancer. In dogs, the interaction of genetics and diet is supported by the finding that gluten-sensitive enteropathy in Irish setters is an autosomal recessive trait, but the casual mutation has not been identifed.[13] Adverse reactions to food are also described in soft-coated wheaton terriers (SCWT) affected with protein-losing enteropathy and protein-losing nephropathy.[14] Pedigree analysis from 188 dogs demonstrated a common male ancestor, although the mode of inheritance is unknown.[15] Autoantibodies to perinuclear antineutrophil cytoplasmic antibodies (pANCA), associated with ulcerative colitis in humans,[16] have been demonstrated in 20 of 21 SCWT, and their occurrence preceded hypoalbuminemia by an average of 2.4 years.[17] Elevated pANCA levels are also described in 61% of 90 dogs of various breeds with food-responsive enteropathy versus 31% to 34% dogs with non–food-responsive IBD.[18,19] These findings suggest that immune dysregulation as evidenced by autoantibody formation is a relatively common and early feature of food-responsive enteropathies in dogs.

Shar-peis with cobalamin deficiency may present with small bowel diarrhea and also frequently weight loss and GI protein loss.[20] Two microsatellite markers (DTR13.6 and REN13N11) on canine chromosome 13 show evidence of linkage disequilibrium and support an autosomal recessive trait for cobalamin deficiency in this breed.[20] The Lundehund, Basenji, and Yorkshire terrier breeds have characteristic breed-associated GI diseases, but the genetic basis for these conditions is unknown.[21–23]

THE INTESTINAL MICROENVIRONMENT
Bacteria

Although intestinal bacteria are implicated frequently as a pivotal factor in the development of IBD in humans and animals, the specific bacterial characteristics that drive the inflammatory response have remained elusive. Advances in molecular microbiology are beginning to enable the in-depth analysis of complex bacterial communities without bacterial culture. Culture-independent analyses of bacterial 16S ribosomal DNA (rDNA) libraries in humans reveal that more than 70% of fecal flora appears uncultivable, and in healthy individuals there is significant variation in the flora in different GI segments and luminal contents compared with the mucosa.[24]

The application of 16S rDNA sequence–based analysis in combination with fluorescence in situ hybridization (FISH) has enabled the discovery of invasive E coli in the colonic mucosa of boxers with GC that is similar in pathotype to adherent and invasive E coli associated with intestinal inflammation in humans.[5,7] Eradication of the invasive E coli in boxer dogs with GC correlates with remission from disease, inferring a causal relationship.[8,25] Increasingly, studies across species show that intestinal inflammation is associated with a shift in the microbiome from gram-positive Firmicutes (eg, Clostridiales) to gram-negative bacteria, predominantly Proteobacteria, including Enterobacteriaceae.[7,26–28] Mucosa-associated Enterobacteriaceae have been found to correlate with duodenal inflammation and clinical signs in cats with signs of GI disease.[26] Studies in German shepherds with antibiotic-responsive enteropathy indicate an increased prevalence of Lactobacillales relative to greyhound controls and a complex and variable dysbiosis in dogs with tylosin-responsive enteroapthy.[10,29] It remains to be determined whether these alterations in noninvasive mucosal and luminal bacteria in dogs and cats typically diagnosed with lymphoplasmacytic IBD are a cause or a consequence of the inflammation, but their discovery has provided new opportunities for therapeutic intervention.

DIETARY CONSTITUENTS

Growing evidence supports the importance of diet in the development of canine and feline IBD. Irish setters develop an enteropathy that is related to the ingestion of gluten.[13] In SCWT, adverse reactions to corn, tofu, cottage cheese, milk, farina cream of wheat, and lamb have been described.[14] In these dogs, serum albumin concentrations decreased and fecal alpha1-protease inhibitor concentration increased when compared with baseline values 4 days after the provocative trial. Antigen-specific fecal IgE levels varied throughout the provocative trial, with peak levels after ingestion of test meals. The pANCA levels were elevated in 20 of 21 SCWT and 61% of 90 dogs of various breeds with food-responsive diarrhea (evaluated before treatment).[17,18] The underlying disease processes driving this autoantibody formation remains to be determined.

In controlled studies of 65 dogs with IBD and diarrhea of at least 6 weeks' duration, 39 responded to being fed an antigen-restricted diet of salmon and rice for 10 days.[18] The conditions relapsed in only 8 dogs when they were challenged with their original food, and none were sensitive to beef, lamb, chicken, or milk. In a recent study, 26 dogs with signs of chronic GI disease (6 had normal GI pathology) were fed either a soy and chicken hydrolysate (n = 18, Hypoallergenic diet, Royal Canin) or an intestinal diet (n = 8, Intestinal diet, Royal Canin).[30] The initial response to the diet was 88% in both groups; however, over a 3-year period, only 1 of 6 dogs on the intestinal diet was maintained in remission versus 13 of 14 on the hydrolysate. Approximately 66% of the dogs in either group relapsed in response to the original diet. In an ongoing prospective trial,[31] the authors have observed positive responses to a hydrolyzed soy diet in 59% of 27 dogs with IBD. In this study, a marked perturbation of the duodenal microbiome (dysbiosis) was detected in a majority of dogs with IBD, including those with a response to diet. From a comparative standpoint, of 55 cats with chronic GI disease 49% responded to dietary modification; signs recurred in 16 of 26 cats challenged with the original food. The dominant group of antigens eliciting a response in these cats was cereals, wheat, corn, or barley.[32]

Taken as a whole, these studies reveal responses to diet in approximately 50% of dogs with chronic GI signs and IBD.[18,30,31,33] The diagnostic terms food responsive, or dietary intolerant are more appropriate than food allergy where an immunologic basis for disease has not been identified. The observations that many patients do not relapse on rechallenge with the original diet, and that many react to cereal-based ingredients rather than animal proteins, has important implications for pathogenesis and treatment. The high response rates to diets that differ markedly in their composition (eg, hydrolyzed soy vs salmon), but are formulated from relatively few ingredients, raises the possibility that it is perhaps the absence of certain ingredients, rather than the modification or substitution of dietary protein, that has a beneficial effect. For instance, carrageenan, a common ingredient in canned pet foods, directly induces GI inflammation and inhibits apoptosis.[34]

DIAGNOSIS

A diagnosis of IBD usually involves careful integration of signalment, home environment, history, physical findings, clinicopathologic testing, diagnostic imaging, and histopathology of intestinal biopsies.

Dogs with IBD typically present for investigation of diarrhea, weight loss, or vomiting. The initial approach to chronic diarrhea or vomiting is based on determining its nature and severity and specific or localized clinical findings. The presence of additional clinical signs helps to refine the region of interest and probable cause, such as tenesmus and dyschezia, large bowel disease; melena, upper GI bleeding or ulceration; abdominal distention, difficulty breathing; or peripheral edema, enteric protein loss.

In cases in which diarrhea is present, this information is integrated to determine whether it is attributable to large bowel disease, as characterized by dyschezia, tenesmus, increased frequency of defecation, and small volume of feces with mucus and blood, or whether it is a consequence of small intestinal disease or exocrine pancreatic insufficiency, as characterized by a large volume of diarrhea, weight loss, and possible vomiting. In patients with abdominal pain, dehydration, frequent vomiting, or localized findings (eg, abdominal mass), these problems are pursued ahead of an in-depth workup for chronic diarrhea.

In patients with diarrhea and no obvious cause, it is best to adopt a systematic approach determined by the localization of diarrhea to the small or large bowel. Patients with signs of large and small bowel involvement are usually evaluated for diffuse GI disease.

Chronic small bowel diarrhea is a common presenting sign in dogs with IBD, and the diagnostic approach is summarized in **Table 2**. After exclusion of infectious and parasitic agents, non-GI disorders, exocrine pancreatic insufficiency, and intestinal structural abnormalities requiring surgery, the most common groups of intestinal diseases associated with chronic small bowel diarrhea are idiopathic IBD, diet-responsive enteropathy, antibiotic-responsive enteropathy, and lymphangiectasia.

Table 2
Initial diagnostic approach to chronic diarrhea

Integrate signalment, history, and physical examination	Breed predisposition, environment, diet, other clinical signs, localizing findings
Detect endoparasites and enteric pathogens	Fecal analysis (eg, Giardia)
Perform clinicopathologic testing	
Detect non-GI disease	CBC, biochemistry profile, UA, $\pm$ TLI, ACTH stimulation test, freeT$_4$/TSH levels, bile acid levels
Detect/characterize GI disease	Hypoproteinemia, hypocalcemia, hypocholesterolemia, leukopenia, leukocytosis, low cobalamin or folate levels[4]
Perform diagnostic imaging	
Detect non-GI disease	Radiography, ultrasonography of liver, spleen, pancreas, lymph nodes, masses, and effusions
Detect and characterize GI disease	Radiography, ultrasonography[59] to detect obstruction, intussusception, focal masses, thickening, loss of layering, hypoechoic appearance, hyperechoic striations

Abbreviations: ACTH, adrenocorticotropic hormone; CBC, complete blood cell count; T4, levorotatory thyroxine, TSH; thyroid-stimulating hormone, TLI, trypsin like immunoreactivity; UA, urinalysis.

The approach to this group of patients is usually determined by the severity of the clinical signs (ie, frequent severe diarrhea, excessive weight loss, decreased activity or appetite), along with the presence of hypoalbuminemia or hypocobalaminemia and intestinal thickening or mesenteric lymphadenopathy. In patients with these abnormalities, intestinal biopsy is required to define the cause (eg, lymphangiectasia, lymphoma) and to optimize therapy.

The clinical severity of intestinal disease can be quantified by determining the clinical disease activity index (eg, attitude, activity, appetite, vomiting, stool consistency, stool frequency, weight loss).[35] Measurement of serum C-reactive protein (CRP) levels has been shown to correlate with clinical disease activity (canine IBD activity index [CIBDAI]), and this implies that severe clinical disease is accompanied by a systemic inflammatory response.[35] Initial measurement of clinical disease activity or CRP levels may also be useful as a baseline for determining the response to treatment.

Controlled studies have shown that hypoalbuminemia is associated with a poor outcome in dogs with chronic enteropathy.[36,37] Serum concentrations of cobalamin and folate can be measured to determine whether supplementation is required, and low serum cobalamin concentration (<200 ng/L) is associated with a negative prognosis.[36]

Evaluation of hemostatic function is recommended to ascertain if hypo or hypercoagulability has developed as a consequence of enteric protein loss.

In stable patients with chronic diarrhea (ie, good attitude, appetite, mild weight loss, normal serum proteins, no intestinal thickening, or lymphadenopathy), and in those with undefined weight loss, measurement of serum cobalamin and folate concentrations can help determine the need for intestinal biopsy, localize the site of intestinal disease (eg, cobalamin is absorbed in the ileum), determine the need for cobalamin supplementation, and establish a prognosis. Stable patients with chronic diarrhea and normal cobalamin concentrations can be given the option of empirical treatment trials with diet, followed by antibiotics if there is no response to diet (see section on Minimal Change Enteropathy). Failure to respond to empirical therapy or worsening of disease is an indication for endoscopy and intestinal biopsy. In stable patients with chronic diarrhea and subnormal serum cobalamin levels, the authors pursue endoscopic evaluation and intestinal biopsy rather than empirical treatment trials.

INTESTINAL BIOPSY

Intestinal biopsies can be acquired endoscopically or surgically. In patients without an indication for surgery (eg, intestinal masses, anatomic or structural disease, perforation), the authors prefer to perform diagnostic endoscopy to visually inspect the esophageal, gastric, and intestinal mucosa and to procure endoscopic biopsy samples. It is noteworthy that in some, but not all, studies the endoscopic appearance of the small intestine correlates better with outcome than the histopathologic appearance.[30,36] If there is a suspicion of ileal involvement (eg, low cobalamin levels, ultrasonographic evidence of disease), transcolonic ileoscopy is performed in addition to the standard upper GI tract endoscopic examination.

Guidelines for biopsy acquisition have recently been published.[38] Operator experience and biopsy sample quality and number are of key importance in facilitating histopathologic evaluation. Surgical biopsy is usually preferred if involvement of the submucosa or muscularis is suspected or when endoscopic biopsy findings do not adequately explain the clinical picture.

HISTOPATHOLOGIC EVALUATION

The most common histopathologic diagnoses in dogs with chronic diarrhea are IBD, lymphangiectasia, and lymphoma. The most common histopathologic lesion found in the intestines of dogs involves increased cellularity of the lamina propria and is usually referred to as IBD. The extent of inflammation varies and ranges from focal to diffuse involvement of the small and large intestines. The type and degree of cellular accumulation is also variable and is subjectively categorized as normal, mild, moderate, or severe. The emphasis on cellularity has meant that abnormalities in mucosal architecture have been somewhat overlooked, but their correlation with proinflammatory cytokines and clinical severity of disease highlights the importance of evaluating these features.[26,39] It should be emphasized from the outset that whereas histopathologic changes can be helpful, they frequently represent a common end point of many different diseases.

Cellular Infiltrates

Intestinal infiltration with macrophages or neutrophils raises the possibility of an infectious process, and culture, special staining, and FISH are indicated.[5,26]

The presence of moderate to large numbers of eosinophils in intestinal biopsy samples, often accompanied by circulating eosinophilis, suggests possible parasitic infestation or dietary intolerance.[40]

Increased numbers of lymphocytes and plasma cells, so-called lymphoplasmacytic enteritis, is the most frequently reported form of IBD. Moderate to severe lymphoplasmacytic enteritis is often described in association with a protein-losing enteropathy.[41] Predisposed breeds include the Basenji, Lundehund, and Shar-Pei.[20,21,23] However, the appropriateness and clinical relevance of the term lymphoplasmacytic enteritis is a contentious issue, particularly in the small intestine. Dogs have similar numbers of duodenal CD3-positive T cells before and after clinical remission induced by diet or steroids,[42] and cats with and without signs of intestinal disease have similar numbers of lymphocytes and plasma cells.[43]

Mucosal Architecture

Several studies indicate that changes in mucosal architecture, such as villous morphology, lymphatic dilatation, goblet cell mucus content, and crypt lesions, are related to the presence and severity of GI disease.[8,13,26,41,44] Recent studies using quantitative observer-independent variables (eg, inflammatory cytokines) to identify histopathologic correlates of disease have shown that in cats with signs of GI disease, villus atrophy and fusion correlate with the severity of clinical signs and degree of proinflammatory cytokine upregulation in the duodenal mucosa.[26] Architectural changes in the gastric mucosa also correlate with cytokine upregulation in dogs with lymphocytic gastritis.[39]

In the colon, loss of mucus and goblet cells has been correlated with the presence of GC and severity of lymphoplasmacytic colitis.[8,44,45]

Dilation of lymphatics and the presence of crypt abscesses and cysts are most frequently encountered in dogs with protein-losing enteropathies and are often accompanied by lymphoplasmacytic inflammation of varying severity.[22,41,46,47]

Standardized Grading

The interpretation of GI histopathologic findings varies considerably among pathologists.[48] To address this problem, a working group established by the World Small Animal Veterinary Association (WSAVA) formulated a scheme to standardize the evaluation of intestinal histopathologic findings.[49] A potentially useful feature proposed in this scheme is the summing of scores in 8 predetermined categories to give an indication of disease severity, by which a score of 1 to 8 is mild, 9 to 16 is moderate, and 17 to 24 is marked. To investigate the utility of this approach, the authors have applied the WSAVA criteria to colonic biopsies from boxer dogs with GC[8] and have directly compared the WSAVA scheme to a previous one (the Roth scheme) developed for evaluating canine colitis (**Table 3**).[44] Both schemes assign an overall grade of normal, mild, moderate, or severe/marked and a final diagnosis that describes the dominant abnormalities. However, the schemes differ markedly in other respects. The Roth scheme, which was developed specifically for colitis, accounts for changes in goblet cells, which are considered of particular importance in colitis,[5,45] whereas the WSAVA scheme does not. It is evident that the final diagnosis using both schemes was concordant in 5 of 7 dogs (see **Table 3**). One of the discordant cases differed only in the degree of granulomatous inflammation assigned (Roth moderate vs WSAVA marked). However, in the other case, the Roth score assigns a final diagnosis of moderate GC, whereas the WSAVA scheme assigned a grade of no GC. This difference is because the standardized reporting form used in the WSAVA scheme only considers inflammation in the lamina propria, and not the submucosa or muscularis.[49] The WSAVA scores are readily summed and yield scores ranging from 4 to 16 in GC, with pretreatment scores decreasing in all dogs after enrofloxacin treatment (scores range from 2–8). However, because GC is a very severe form of canine colitis, it is concerning that the total scores in dogs with severe/marked GC range from 11 to 16 of 24, which corresponds to an overall severity grading of moderate. Thus it appears that the simple summing method proposed in the WSAVA scheme underestimates the severity of GC. This limitation is likely a consequence of assigning equal value to each of the 8 categories being evaluated, with the result that abnormalities

Table 3
Application of standardized grading to GC in boxer dogs

Dog	Roth[44]		WSAVA[49]		Goblet Cell Depletion	
	Pre	Post	Pre	Post	Pre	Post
1	3	2 g (2 wk), 1 lp (7 mo)	11	8[c], 2[d]	3	2[c], 0[d]
2[a]	2	NA	4	NA	0	NA
3	3	1 g	16	5	3	0
4	2	1 g	10	6	3	1
5[b]	2	1 g	12	4	2	1
6	3	NA	12	NA	3	NA
7	3	3 g	14	9	2	3

0, normal; 1, mild; 2, moderate; 3, marked/severe.
  WSAVA total: 1 to 8, mild; 9 to 16, moderate; 17 to 24, marked.
  Abbreviations: g, granulomatous infiltrate; lp, lymphocytic plasmacytic infiltrate; NA, not available.
   [a] Submucosal macrophages.
   [b] Muscularis macrophages.
   [c] 2 weeks time point.
   [d] 7 months time point.
  Data from Mansfield CS, James FE, Craven M, et al. Remission of histiocytic ulcerative colitis in Boxer dogs correlates with eradication of invasive intramucosal *Escherichia coli*. J Vet Intern Med 2009;23(5):964–9.

such as ulceration (marked epithelial change), and granulomatous or neutrophilic inflammation, are weighted similarly to lymphoplasmacytic infiltrates, which vary widely in health and disease.[1] A further limitation of the WSAVA scheme with respect to GC is that it does not consider goblet cells, which are decreased in GC and other forms of colitis and show dramatic increases after treatment (see **Table 3**).[5,44,45]

The recent finding that the WSAVA scheme, like previous standardized photographic schemes,[39] has poor agreement among pathologists[50] questions further the ability of standardized grading in its current form to translate to improved diagnosis and management of patients with IBD. Clearly, the emphasis on histopathologic evaluation has to shift from the subjective reporting of cellularity to identifying and reporting features that correlate with the presence of disease and its outcome.

THERAPEUTIC APPROACHES FOR IBD

The therapeutic approach to IBD is influenced by suspicion of a breed-related problem; the severity of disease as characterized by clinical signs, serum albumin and cobalamin concentrations, and endoscopic appearance; the type of cellular infiltrate; the presence of bacteria or fungi; and the presence of architectural changes, such as atrophy, ulceration, lymphangiectasia and/or crypt cysts. Therapeutic intervention is directed at correcting nutritional deficiencies (eg, cobalamin deficiency) and counteracting inflammation and dysbiosis (**Fig. 1**).

MINIMAL CHANGE ENTEROPATHY

Minimal change enteropathy is characterized by low clinical disease activity, normal serum albumin and cobalamin levels, and normal intestinal histopathologic findings.

Empirical Treatment

Typically, the empirical treatment for *Giardia* and endoparasitic infection is the oral administration of fenbendazole, 50 mg/kg, for 5 days.

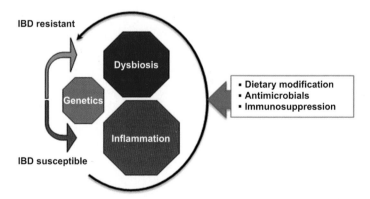

Fig. 1. Genetic susceptibility, intestinal inflammation, and the enteric microbiome are intimately related to IBD. Genetic susceptibility to IBD affects inflammation and dysbiosis. In an IBD-resistant individual, host genotype acts as a brake to limit the development and perpetuation of inflammation and dysbiosis. In an IBD-susceptible individual, disease-associated genetic polymorphisms may decrease the threshold for initiating and sustaining inflammation and dysbiosis. Therapeutic intervention is aimed at counteracting inflammation and dysbiosis.

Dietary Trial

Options for dietary trials are outlined in **Box 1**. A positive response suggests diet-responsive enteropathy, a term that includes both dietary allergy and intolerance. In dogs with GI signs related to diet, a clinical response is usually observed within 1 to 2 weeks of changing the diet.[18,30,31] If the response is good, the diet should be continued. Rechallenge with the original diet is required to confirm that clinical signs are related to the diet. However, few owners consent to rechallenge. Challenge with single dietary ingredients is necessary to define the specific components eliciting an adverse response. If dietary trials with 2 different diets are unsuccessful, the next step is usually an antibiotic trial.

Antibiotic Trial

An antibiotic trial typically involves oral administration of tylosin, 10 to 15 mg/kg, every 8 hours; oxytetracycline, 20 mg/kg, every 8 hours; or metronidazole, 10 mg/kg, every 12 hours.[3,4,6] A positive response suggests antibiotic-responsive enteropathy, which was called small intestinal bacterial overgrowth despite the absence of increase in total bacteria (for further explanation of this topic, see article by Hall elsewhere in this issue).[3,4,51] The dog is typically maintained on antibiotics for 28 days. If signs recur after stopping, long-term antibiotic therapy with tylosin, 5 mg/kg, administered orally once a day can be used to maintain dogs that are tylosin responsive (Elias Wester-marck, personal communication, 2010). If the response is poor, the patient should be carefully reappraised before considering other treatment options.

GRANULOMATOUS OR NEUTROPHILIC ENTEROPATHY

Enteropathies characterized by neutrophilic or granulomatous inflammation are described infrequently in dogs. Some may be associated either with bacterial infections, such as from E coli (GC in boxers), Streptococcus, Campylobacter, Yersinia, and Mycobacteria, or with fungal (eg, Histoplasma) or algal (eg, Prototheca) infections.

Box 1
Options for dietary trials

Global modification

- Switch to a different diet or a different manufacturer

Optimize assimilation

- Highly digestible (usually rice based)
- Fat restricted (<15% dry matter)
- Easy-to-digest fats (eg, medium-chain triglyceride oil)
- Restricted fiber

Antigenic modification

- Antigen-restricted /novel protein source
- Protein hydrolysate

Immunomodulation

- Altered fat composition (eg, ω-3 or ω-6 fatty acid, fish oil)
- Prebiotics (eg, inulin)

Culture of mucosal biopsies, intestinal lymph nodes, and other abdominal organs and imaging of chest and abdomen should be undertaken in cases of granulomatous or neutrophilic enteritis to detect infectious organisms and systemic involvement. Gomori methenamine silver, periodic acid–Schiff, Gram, and modified Steiner stains are the traditional cytochemical stains used to search for infectious agents in fixed tissues. FISH with a probe directed against eubacterial 16S ribosomal RNA is a more contemporary and sensitive method of detecting bacteria within formalin-fixed tissues.[26,42] It is imperative not to immunosuppress patients with granulomatous or neutrophilic infiltrates until infectious agents have been excluded.

Eradication of mucosally invasive *E coli* in boxers with GC is associated with clinical cure, but treatment failure associated with antibiotic resistance is increasing.[5,8,25] The prognosis for idiopathic granulomatous or neutrophilic enteropathies is regarded to be poor if an underlying cause is not identified.

LYMPHOCYTE AND PLASMA CELL PREDOMINANT ENTEROPATHY

Studies in dogs with chronic diarrhea diagnosed as lymphoplasmacytic enteritis provide reasonable evidence that various subsets of dogs will respond to treatment with diet, antibiotics, or immunosuppressive therapy (**Fig. 2**).[4,6,18,30,36] At present, because there is no reliable means for predicting which dogs will respond to which treatment, treatment consists of a series of therapeutic trials.

Response to Standardized Therapy

As mentioned earlier, in controlled studies of 65 dogs with IBD and diarrhea of at least 6 weeks' duration, 39 of 65 dogs responded to dietary modification (restricted antigen diet) and the remaining dogs were treated with corticosteroids (2 mg/kg every 24 hours for 10 days, followed by a tapering dose over 10 weeks).[18] The CIBDAI and histopathologic scores were similar (>70% moderate to severe in each group) in dogs that did and did not respond to diet. Dogs that responded to diet tended to

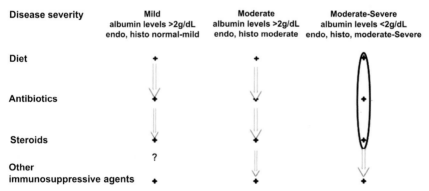

Fig. 2. Treatment by therapeutic trials in dogs with lymphocytic plasmacytic enteritis. A sequential step-up approach, starting with dietary modification is usually applied to patients with mild to moderate disease. The need and clinical confidence to step up between different treatment modalities (diet, antibiotics, steroids, other immunosuppressive therapy) is indicated by the size of the arrows. In dogs with severe disease, a step-down approach is used, with concurrent therapy with diet, antibiotics, and steroids/azathioprine given from the outset (indicated by the circle), and immunosuppressive therapy and antibiotics are withdrawn in patients with a favorable response. endo, endoscopy; histo, histopathology.

be younger and had higher serum albumin concentrations than dogs that did not respond to diet. Dogs that did not respond to diet were treated with steroids. The intestinal histopathologic findings did not differ in either diet-responsive or steroid-responsive dogs before and after treatment. Of the 21 diet-unresponsive dogs, 10 responded to prednisolone with no relapse after taper for up to 3 years. Of the 11 diet- and steroid-unresponsive dogs, 9 were euthanased after administration of steroids, with only 2of 8 steroid-refractory dogs responding to cyclosporine administered orally (5 mg/kg every 24 hours for 10 weeks).[18]

The approach outlined in **Box 2** incorporates an antibiotic trial (tylosin) into a diet (hydrolysate) and immunosuppression–based approach. In an ongoing study,[31] 26 of 27 (96%) dogs with IBD have responded to standardized treatment: 16 diet responsive, 3 steroid responsive, 3 partially responsive to food + antibiotics, 3 responsive to food + steroid + antibiotics, and 1 responsive to antibiotics alone. The response to diet in 21 dogs with normal serum protein levels was 67%, compared with 33% in 6 dogs with low serum protein levels. It is noteworthy that we observed clinical remission in response to dietary manipulation alone in 2 of 6 dogs with IBD accompanied by hypoproteinemia.

In summary, the positive response to dietary modification in 60% to 88% of dogs with lymphocyte and plasma cell dominant enteritis IBD[18,30,31,33] suggests that a dietary trial with a restricted antigen or hydrolyzed diet is a good therapeutic starting point. An unexpected positive finding of these recent studies is how few dogs require continuous treatment with corticosteroids or other immunosuppressive agents.

EOSINOPHIL-PREDOMINANT ENTERITIS

Eosinophilic enteritis is characterized by excessive accumulation of eosinophils in the lamina propria. This condition is speculated to result from an immunologic reaction to parasites or diet.[40] The disease may also involve other areas of the GI tract.

Clinical Findings

The principal clinical signs are chronic small bowel diarrhea accompanied by vomiting or weight loss. Large bowel signs or vomiting predominate in some cases. Physical findings range from normal to focally or diffusely thickened intestines and marked weight loss.

Diagnosis

Eosinophilic enteritis is diagnosed by adopting an approach similar to that described for lymphoplasmacytic enteritis. Clinicopathologic abnormalities may include peripheral eosinophilia. Mast cell neoplasms, hypoadrenocorticism, and endoparasites can produce a similar spectrum of clinical signs and should be ruled out.

Histopathology is characterized by accumulation of large numbers of eosinophils in the intestinal mucosa.

Treatment

Prophylactic administration of an anthelmintic, such as oral fenbendazole, 50 mg/kg, every 24 hours for 5 days, is warranted to treat potential visceral larva migrans, which has been associated with eosinophilic gastroenteritis. Some patients may respond to antigen-restricted or protein hydrolysate diets, and those failing dietary therapy are usually administered oral prednisolone, 2 mg/kg, every 24 hours that is tapered over an 8-week period. The prognosis for eosinophilic enteritis is typically considered good, with few patients requiring continuous immunosuppression.

Box 2
Standardized treatment of dogs with lymphoplasmacytic IBD

Mild to moderate clinical disease activity, mild to moderate histopathology (lymphocytes and plasma cells are predominant cell type), serum albumin levels greater than 2 g/L

Empirical treatment

- Treatment for *Giardia* and helminths if not already initiated. Cobalamin and folate supplementation if these are subnormal

Sequential treatment

- Dietary trial with a hydrolyzed or antigen-restricted diet for 2 weeks; if the response is good, then maintain on diet. Consider rechallenge to confirm dietary intolerance and single-ingredient challenge to define offending substrates

- Antibiotic trial, for example, tylosin for 2 weeks; if the response is good, maintain on antibiotics for 28 days and then discontinue. Consider transition to probiotics, despite the lack of evidence to support their ability to maintain remission

- Immunosuppression with glucocorticoids; for example, oral prednisolone 2 mg/kg every 24 hours for 21 days, 1 mg/kg every 24 hours for 21 days, 0.5 mg/kg every 24 hours for 21 days, 0.5 mg/kg every 48 hours for 14 days is a typical protocol. It is the authors experience that side effects of glucocorticoids are usually more marked in large than small breed dogs (this may be because of relative overdosing on the basis of body weight rather than surface area). For this reason, the authors typically initiate immunosuppression in all dogs weighing more than 31.5 kg with azathioprine ± concurrent glucocorticoid treatment at a faster taper for example, for dogs weighing more than 31.5 kg: oral azathioprine 2 mg/kg every 24 hours for 5 days, then 2 mg/kg every other day and oral prednisolone 2 mg/kg every 24 hours for 10 days, 1 mg/kg every 24 hours for 10 days, 0.5 mg/kg every 24 hours for 10 days, and 0.5 mg/kg every 48 hours for 10 days)

- If there is a poor response, reappraise before considering escalating immunosuppression (eg, add azathioprine or substitute with oral cyclosporine, 5 mg/kg, every 24 hours for 10 weeks[52] if already on azathioprine)

- If the response is good, first taper immunosuppression and then stop antibiotics

Moderate to severe clinical disease activity, moderate to severe intestinal histopathology (atrophy, fusion, lymphocytes and plasma cells are the predominant cell type), serum albumin levels less than 2 g/L

- Empirical treatment for *Giardia* and helminths if not already initiated

- Cobalamin and folate supplementation if their levels are subnormal

- Dietary modification pending biopsy result; concurrent dietary modification (hydrolyzed or antigen-restricted diet), antibiotics (eg, tylosin), and immunosuppression (glucocorticoids and/or azathioprine)

- If the response is poor, reappraise all findings before considering escalating immunosuppression (eg, cyclosporine)

- Consider failure to absorb oral prednisolone and switch to injectable corticosteroids

- Dexamethasone may be preferable to prednisolone in patients with ascites to avoid increased fluid retention

- Concurrent therapy with ultralow-dose aspirin (0.5 mg/kg) and judicious use of diuretics (furosemide [Lasix] and spironolactone are often used in patients considered at risk for thromboembolic disease and in those severely distended with tense ascites, respectively)

- The use of elemental diets and partial parenteral nutrition may be indicated in some dogs that have severe protein-losing enteropathy

- If the response is good, first taper immunosuppressive agents and then stop antibiotics

LYMPHANGIECTASIA AND CRYPT CYSTS/ABSCESSES

Intestinal lymphangiectasia is characterized by abnormal distention of lymphatic vessels within the mucosa. Lymphangiectasia is a consequence of a localized or generalized lymphatic abnormality or an increased portal pressure (eg, right-sided heart failure, caval obstruction, hepatic disease). Lymphatic abnormalities are often associated with lipogranulomatous inflammation that is visible as small white granules on the intestinal mesentery. Tumor infiltration of lymphatics or lymph nodes can also cause lymphangiectasia. In some cases, lymphangiography reveals a generalized lymphatic abnormality. Dilation of lymphatics is associated with the exudation of protein-rich lymph into the intestine and severe malabsorption of long-chain fats. Crypt cysts and abscesses may also be observed in intestinal biopsies.

The Yorkshire terrier (4.2- to 10-fold relative risk), SCWT (concurrent proteinuria), and Norwegian Lundehund seem to be overrepresented, supporting a familial cause in some dogs.[14,15,22,23,37]

Clinical Findings

Clinical findings are essentially a consequence of the intestinal loss of protein and range from weight loss to chronic diarrhea, vomiting, ascites, edema, and chylothorax. In a study of 12 Yorkshire terriers,[37] hypoalbuminemia (<3.1 g/dL) was present in all 12 dogs (median 1.6 g/dL), and hypoglobulinemia (<1.9 g/dL) in 7 dogs (median 1.7 g/dL). Additional biochemical abnormalities included hypocalcemia (n = 12), hypocholesterolemia (n = 11), hypomagnesemia (n = 9), hypokalemia (n = 5), and hypochloremia (n = 5). Hypocalcemia and hypomagnesemia have been attributed to hypovitaminosis D.[53,54] Hematologic abnormalities in 12 Yorkshire terriers included mild anemia (n = 5), thrombocytosis (n = 8), mature neutrophilia (n = 6), and neutrophilia with a left shift (n = 3).[37]

Diagnosis

Lymphangiectasia usually presents as a protein-losing enteropathy, with endoscopic appearance of white blebs on the mucosa (dilated lymphatics). Endoscopic biopsies are often adequate. Surgical biopsy should be undertaken carefully, with appropriate attention to potential for bleeding, exacerbation of hypoproteinemia by fluid therapy, and potential for dehiscence.

Treatment

The cause of lymphangiectasia is usually not determined. Treatment is supportive and symptomatic. Dietary recommendations are similar to those for other causes of small bowel diarrhea (highly digestible, restricted antigen, or hydrolysate). Fat restriction has been emphasized as a mainstay of treatment, but no controlled studies have evaluated this approach. Medium-chain triglyceride (MCT) oil, usually in the form of coconut oil, at 0.5 to 2 mL/kg body weight per day can be added to the diet, or a diet already containing MCT can be fed to provide a source of calories, that is in theory easy to assimilate. The use of MCT improves outcome in children with primary lymphangiectasia,[55] but there are no studies in dogs.

Prednisolone, 1 mg/kg, every 24 hours is often administered orally and may work by decreasing lipogranulomatous inflammation or concurrent mucosal inflammation. Prednisolone is tapered to the lowest effective dose once remission has been achieved. In patients with severe malabsorption, parenteral glucocorticoids may be required, and a switch to dexamethasone may be made in patients with ascites or edema. Escalation of immunosuppression (eg, by oral administration of cyclosporine,

5 mg/kg, every 24 hours[52]) may be tried if the patient is unresponsive. However, patients with lymphangiectasia appear more prone to sepsis than other forms of IBD. So it is imperative not to overimmunosuppress these patients, and concurrent therapy with metronidazole or tylosin is frequently initiated to decrease the risk of bacterial translocation through the markedly impaired gut. Aspirin, 0.5 mg/kg, every 24 hours is often given orally to dogs with low antithrombin III levels if they are considered at risk for thromboembolism. Diuretics are used if ascites is problematic.

Response to therapy is variable with some dogs staying in remission for several years and others pursuing a path toward fulminant hypoproteinemia or thromboembolic disease. The prognosis is always guarded. In a recent study of 12 Yorkshire terriers,[37] empirical therapy with corticosteroids (11 of 12), azathioprine (2 of 12), antibiotics (amoxicillin-clavulanate, n = 6; metronidazole, n = 6; tylosin n = 5; and enrofloxacin n = 2), plasma, and diuretics was associated with a poor outcome. Of the 12 cases, 7 died or were euthanased within 3 months of diagnosis (thromboembolism was suspected in 3). Long-term survival was achieved in 3 dogs, (36, 24, and 8 months), and 2 are alive at 3 and 4 months after diagnosis.

SUMMARY

This article has examined IBD in dogs, focusing on the interaction between genetic susceptibility and the enteric microenvironment (bacteria, diet), the utility of recently developed histologic criteria, the prognostic indicators, and the standardized approaches to treatment. It is evident that despite much effort, the histopathologic interpretation of intestinal biopsies is still a substantial pitfall in the diagnosis and management of IBD. Progress has been made in documenting the clinical determinants of outcome, such as hypoalbuminemia and hypocobalaminemia, by performing standardized therapeutic trials in dogs with lymphoplasmacytic enteritis (at least 50% respond to diet alone, without recourse to immunosuppression), by identifying and treating invasive bacteria in patients with granulomatous inflammation, and by starting to unravel the basis of host susceptibility to IBD.

REFERENCES

1. Packey CD, Sartor RB. Interplay of commensal and pathogenic bacteria, genetic mutations, and immunoregulatory defects in the pathogenesis of inflammatory bowel diseases. J Intern Med 2008;263(6):597–606.
2. Perez LH, Butler M, Creasey T, et al. Direct bacterial killing in vitro by recombinant Nod2 is compromised by Crohn's disease-associated mutations. PLoS One 2010; 5(6):e10915.
3. Batt RM, McLean L, Riley JE. Response of the jejunal mucosa of dogs with aerobic and anaerobic bacterial overgrowth to antibiotic therapy. Gut 1988; 29(4):473–82.
4. German AJ, Day MJ, Ruaux CG, et al. Comparison of direct and indirect tests for small intestinal bacterial overgrowth and antibiotic-responsive diarrhea in dogs. J Vet Intern Med 2003;17(1):33–43.
5. Simpson KW, Dogan B, Rishniw M, et al. Adherent and invasive Escherichia coli is associated with granulomatous colitis in boxer dogs. Infect Immun 2006;74(8): 4778–92.
6. Westermarck E, Skrzypczak T, Harmoinen J, et al. Tylosin-responsive chronic diarrhea in dogs. J Vet Intern Med 2005;19(2):177–86.
7. Baumgart M, Dogan B, Rishniw M, et al. Culture independent analysis of ileal mucosa reveals a selective increase in invasive Escherichia coli of novel

phylogeny relative to depletion of Clostridiales in Crohn's disease involving the ileum. ISME J 2007;1(5):403–18.

8. Mansfield CS, James FE, Craven M, et al. Remission of histiocytic ulcerative colitis in Boxer dogs correlates with eradication of invasive intramucosal Escherichia coli. J Vet Intern Med 2009;23(5):964–9.

9. Craven M. Genome wide analysis of granulomatous colitis in Boxer dogs. Anaheim (CA): ACVIM; 2010.

10. Allenspach K, House A, Smith K, et al. Evaluation of mucosal bacteria and histopathology, clinical disease activity and expression of Toll-like receptors in German shepherd dogs with chronic enteropathies. Vet Microbiol 2010;146(3–4):326–35.

11. Kathrani A. Overdominant Single Nucleotide Polymorphisms in the Nucleotide Oligomerisation Domain Two (NOD2) Gene are Significantly Associated With Canine Inflammatory Bowel Disease. Proceedings of the ACVIM symposium. Anaheim (CA): ACVIM; 2010. p. 176.

12. Trynka G, Wijmenga C, van Heel DA. A genetic perspective on coeliac disease. Trends Mol Med 2010;16(11):537–50.

13. Garden OA, Pidduck H, Lakhani KH, et al. Inheritance of gluten-sensitive enteropathy in Irish Setters. Am J Vet Res 2000;61(4):462–8.

14. Vaden SL, Hammerberg B, Davenport DJ, et al. Food hypersensitivity reactions in Soft Coated Wheaten Terriers with protein-losing enteropathy or protein-losing nephropathy or both: gastroscopic food sensitivity testing, dietary provocation, and fecal immunoglobulin E. J Vet Intern Med 2000;14(1):60–7.

15. Littman MP, Dambach DM, Vaden SL, et al. Familial protein-losing enteropathy and protein-losing nephropathy in Soft Coated Wheaten Terriers: 222 cases (1983–1997). J Vet Intern Med 2000;14(1):68–80.

16. Anand V, Russell AS, Tsuyuki R, et al. Perinuclear antineutrophil cytoplasmic autoantibodies and anti-Saccharomyces cerevisiae antibodies as serological markers are not specific in the identification of Crohn's disease and ulcerative colitis. Can J Gastroenterol 2008;22(1):33–6.

17. Allenspach K, Lomas B, Wieland B, et al. Evaluation of perinuclear antineutrophilic cytoplasmic autoantibodies as an early marker of protein-losing enteropathy and protein-losing nephropathy in Soft Coated Wheaten Terriers. Am J Vet Res 2008;69(10):1301–4.

18. Luckschander N, Allenspach K, Hall J, et al. Perinuclear antineutrophilic cytoplasmic antibody and response to treatment in diarrheic dogs with food responsive disease or inflammatory bowel disease. J Vet Intern Med 2006;20(2):221–7.

19. Mancho C, Sainz A, García-Sancho M, et al. Detection of perinuclear antineutrophil cytoplasmic antibodies and antinuclear antibodies in the diagnosis of canine inflammatory bowel disease. J Vet Diagn Invest 2010;22(4):553–8.

20. Grützner N, Bishop MA, Suchodolski JS, et al. Association study of cobalamin deficiency in the Chinese Shar Pei. J Hered 2010;101(2):211–7.

21. Breitschwerdt EB, Ochoa R, Barta M, et al. Clinical and laboratory characterization of Basenjis with immunoproliferative small intestinal disease. Am J Vet Res 1984;45(2):267–73.

22. Kimmel SE, Waddell LS, Michel KE. Hypomagnesemia and hypocalcemia associated with protein-losing enteropathy in Yorkshire terriers: five cases (1992–1998). J Am Vet Med Assoc 2000;217(5):703–6.

23. Kolbjørnsen O, Press CM, Landsverk T. Gastropathies in the Lundehund. I. Gastritis and gastric neoplasia associated with intestinal lymphangiectasia. APMIS 1994; 102(9):647–61.

24. Eckburg PB, Bik EM, Bernstein CN, et al. Diversity of the human intestinal microbial flora. Science 2005;308(5728):1635–8.
25. Craven M, Dogan B, Schukken A, et al. Antimicrobial resistance impacts clinical outcome of granulomatous colitis in boxer dogs. J Vet Intern Med 2010;24(4): 819–24.
26. Janeczko S, Atwater D, Bogel E, et al. The relationship of mucosal bacteria to duodenal histopathology, cytokine mRNA, and clinical disease activity in cats with inflammatory bowel disease. Vet Microbiol 2008;128(1–2):178–93.
27. Suchodolski JS, Xenoulis PG, Paddock CG, et al. Molecular analysis of the bacterial microbiota in duodenal biopsies from dogs with idiopathic inflammatory bowel disease. Vet Microbiol 2010;142(3–4):394–400.
28. Xenoulis PG, Palculict B, Allenspach K, et al. Molecular-phylogenetic characterization of microbial communities imbalances in the small intestine of dogs with inflammatory bowel disease. FEMS Microbiol Ecol 2008;66(3):579–89.
29. Suchodolski JS, Dowd SE, Westermarck E, et al. The effect of the macrolide antibiotic tylosin on microbial diversity in the canine small intestine as demonstrated by massive parallel 16S rRNA gene sequencing. BMC Microbiol 2009;9:210.
30. Mandigers PJ, Biourge V, Van Den Ingh TS, et al. A randomized, open-label, positively-controlled field trial of a hydrolyzed protein diet in dogs with chronic small bowel enteropathy. J Vet Intern Med 2010;24(6):1350–7.
31. Craven M, SE Dowd, S McDonough, et al. High throughput pyrosequencing reveals reduced bacterial diversity in the duodenal mucosa of dogs with IBD [abstract #158]. Proceedings of the 2009 ACVIM Congress in Montreal, Canada. J Vet Inter Med 2009;23(3):731.
32. Guilford WG, Jones BR, Markwell PJ, et al. Food sensitivity in cats with chronic idiopathic gastrointestinal problems. J Vet Intern Med 2001;15(1):7–13.
33. Marks SL, Laflamme D, McCandlish A. Dietary trial using a commercial hypoallergenic diet containing hydrolyzed protein for dogs with inflammatory bowel disease. Vet Ther 2002;3:109–18.
34. Bhattacharyya S, Dudeja PK, Tobacman JK. Tumor necrosis factor {alpha}-induced inflammation is increased and apoptosis is inhibited by common food additive carrageenan. J Biol Chem 2010;285(50):39511–22.
35. Jergens AE, Schreiner CA, Frank DE, et al. A scoring index for disease activity in canine inflammatory bowel disease. J Vet Intern Med 2003;7(3):291–7.
36. Allenspach K, Wieland B, Gröne A, et al. Chronic enteropathies in dogs: evaluation of risk factors for negative outcome. J Vet Intern Med 2007;21(4):700–8.
37. Craven M, Duhammel G, NB Sutter, et al. Absence of a bacterial association in Yorkshire terriers with protein-losing enteropathy and cystic intestinal crypts. Proceedings of the 2009 ACVIM Congress in Montreal, Canada. Vet Inter Med 2009;23(3):757.
38. Willard MD, Mansell J, Fosgate GT, et al. Effect of sample quality on the sensitivity of endoscopic biopsy for detecting gastric and duodenal lesions in dogs and cats. J Vet Intern Med 2008;22(5):1084–9.
39. Wiinberg B, Spohr A, Dietz HH, et al. Quantitative analysis of inflammatory and immune responses in dogs with gastritis and their relationship to Helicobacter spp. infection. J Vet Intern Med 2005;19(1):4–14.
40. Kleinschmidt S, Meneses F, Nolte I, et al. Characterization of mast cell numbers and subtypes in biopsies from the gastrointestinal tract of dogs with lymphocytic-plasmacytic or eosinophilic gastroenterocolitis. Vet Immunol Immunopathol 2007; 120(3–4):80–92.

41. Peterson PB, Willard MD. Protein-losing enteropathies. Vet Clin North Am Small Anim Pract 2003;33(5):1061–82.

42. Schreiner NM, Gaschen F, Gröne A, et al. Clinical signs, histology, and CD3-positive cells before and after treatment of dogs with chronic enteropathies. J Vet Intern Med 2008;22(5):1079–83.

43. Waly NE, Stokes CR, Gruffydd-Jones TJ, et al. Immune cell populations in the duodenal mucosa of cats with inflammatory bowel disease. J Vet Intern Med 2004;18(6):816–25.

44. Roth L, Walton AM, Leib MS, et al. A grading system for lymphocytic plasmacytic colitis in dogs. J Vet Diagn Invest 1990;2(4):257–62.

45. van der Gaag I. The histological appearance of large intestinal biopsies in dogs with clinical signs of large bowel disease. Can J Vet Res 1988;52(1):75–82.

46. Craven M, Simpson JW, Ridyard AE, et al. Canine inflammatory bowel disease: retrospective analysis of diagnosis and outcome in 80 cases (1995–2002). J Small Anim Pract 2004;45(7):336–42.

47. Willard MD, Zenger E, Mansell JL. Protein-losing enteropathy associated with cystic mucoid changes in the intestinal crypts of two dogs. J Am Anim Hosp Assoc 2003;39(2):187–91.

48. Willard MD, Jergens AE, Duncan RB, et al. Interobserver variation among histopathologic evaluations of intestinal tissues from dogs and cats. J Am Vet Med Assoc 2002;220(8):1177–82.

49. Day MJ, Bilzer T, Mansell J, et al. Histopathological standards for the diagnosis of gastrointestinal inflammation in endoscopic biopsy samples from the dog and cat: a report from the World Small Animal Veterinary Association Gastrointestinal Standardization Group. J Comp Pathol 2008;138(Suppl 1):S1–43.

50. Willard MD, Moore GE, Denton BD, et al. Effect of tissue processing on assessment of endoscopic intestinal biopsies in dogs and cats. J Vet Intern Med 2010;24(1):84–9.

51. Simpson KW. Small intestinal bacterial overgrowth. J Am Vet Med Assoc 1994; 205(3):405–7.

52. Allenspach K, Rüfenacht S, Sauter S, et al. Pharmacokinetics and clinical efficacy of cyclosporine treatment of dogs with steroid-refractory inflammatory bowel disease. J Vet Intern Med 2006;20(2):239–44.

53. Bush WW, Kimmel SE, Wosar MA, et al. Secondary hypoparathyroidism attributed to hypomagnesemia in a dog with protein-losing enteropathy. J Am Vet Med Assoc 2001;219(12):1732–4, 1708.

54. Mellanby RJ, Mellor PJ, Roulois A, et al. Hypocalcaemia associated with low serum vitamin D metabolite concentrations in two dogs with protein-losing enteropathies. J Small Anim Pract 2005;46(7):345–51.

55. Desai AP, Guvenc BH, Carachi R. Evidence for medium chain triglycerides in the treatment of primary intestinal lymphangiectasia. Eur J Pediatr Surg 2009;19(4): 241–5.

56. Dijkstra M, Kraus JS, Bosje JT, et al. Protein-losing enteropathy in Rottweilers. Tijdschr Diergeneeskd 2010;135(10):406–12 [in Dutch].

57. Lecoindre P, Chevallier M, Guerret S. Protein-losing enteropathy of non neoplastic origin in the dog: a retrospective study of 34 cases. Schweiz Arch Tierheilkd 2010;152(3):141–6 [in French].

58. Tanaka H, Nakayama M, Takase K. Histiocytic ulcerative colitis in a French bulldog. J Vet Med Sci 2003;65(3):431–3.

59. Gaschen L, Kircher P, Stüssi A, et al. Comparison of ultrasonographic findings with clinical activity index (CIBDAI) and diagnosis in dogs with chronic enteropathies. Vet Radiol Ultrasound 2008;49(1):56–64.

Protein-Losing Enteropathies in Dogs

Olivier Dossin, DVM, PhD*, Rachel Lavoué, DVM, MSc

KEYWORDS

- Intestine • Protein-losing enteropathy • Dogs
- Lymphangiectasia • Inflammatory bowel disease

Protein-losing enteropathy (PLE) is a syndrome associated with an abnormal loss of albumin through the gastrointestinal (GI) mucosa. PLE is identified when hypoalbuminemia occurs because the loss of albumin cannot be compensated by liver synthesis. PLE can be associated with various disease conditions, especially inflammatory bowel disease (IBD), intestinal lymphoma, and intestinal lymphangiectasia (IL) in small animal patients. PLE is more frequent in dogs than in cats and most of this review is related to canine PLE.

CLASSIFICATION

In human medicine, PLE is classified into three groups according to the main mucosal alteration causing albumin loss: (1) nonulcerated mucosal changes with abnormal permeability causing protein leakage in the intestinal lumen, (2) mucosal erosions or ulcerations with secondary exudation of proteins, and (3) lymphatic dysfunction with protein-rich lymph leakage in the gut (lymphangiectasia).[1,2] Apart from the conditions associated with intestinal epithelial erosion or IL and lacteal dilation/rupture, the mechanism of the protein loss is not clearly identified. It may involve mucosal edema and disruption of the intestinal epithelial barrier at the level of the complex protein network that connects enterocytes, such as tight and adherent junctions.[3] There is a wide spectrum of disease conditions associated with PLE in humans (**Box 1**). The vast majority of these conditions, however, have not yet been reported as causing PLE in dogs and cats.

The loss of protein in PLE is independent of the molecular weight and, therefore, panhypoproteinemia is theoretically expected. Several clinical studies in dogs, however, have reported that this is not always the case, and isolated albumin loss can also be observed.[5–7]

The authors have no conflict of interest to disclose.

Department of Clinical Sciences, National Veterinary School, 23 Chemin des Capelles, BP 87614, 31076 Toulouse cedex 3, France

* Corresponding author.

E-mail address: o.dossin@envt.fr

Vet Clin Small Anim 41 (2011) 399–418
doi:10.1016/j.cvsm.2011.02.002
0195-5616/11/$ – see front matter © 2011 Elsevier Inc. All rights reserved.

| Box 1 |
| Main causes of protein-losing enteropathy in human medicine |

Erosive GI diseases

    IBD[a] (Crohn's disease)

    Gastric and intestinal neoplasia[a] (carcinoma or lymphoma)

    Carcinoid syndrome

    Erosive gastritis or enteritis

    Helicobacter pylori gastritis

    Pseudomembranous enterocolitis

    Macroglobulinemia

Nonerosive GI disease

    Giant hypertrophic gastropathy[a] (Ménétrier disease)

    IBD[a]

    Intestinal parasites[a] (giardiasis or schistosomiasis)

    Celiac disease

    Small intestinal bacterial overgrowth

    Eosinophilic gastroenteritis[a]

    Cobalamin deficiency

    Systemic lupus erythematosus

    Whipple disease

Increased lymphatic pressure

    IL[a] (primary or secondary)

    Cardiac diseases (congestive heart failure, constrictive pericarditis, or congenital heart diseases)

    Neoplasia involving mesenteric lymph nodes or lymphatics

    IBD[a] (Crohn's disease)

    Portal hypertensive gastroenteropathy

    Sclerosing mesenteritis

    Mesenteric venous thrombosis

    Systemic lupus erythematosus

    Mesenteric tuberculosis and sarcoidosis

[a] Denotes conditions also reported in dogs as causing PLE.
Data from Refs.[1–4]

Lymphangiectasia

IL is a condition characterized by dilation of the lymphatic vessels and leakage of lymph from the villi or from deeper portions of the intestinal wall into the intestinal lumen (**Fig. 1**). The leakage of protein, lipid, and lymphocyte-rich lymph into the intestinal lumen is responsible for the protein loss and also the lymphopenia sometimes observed in IL.[2,6] Hypertension in the lymphatic vessels often induces edema of the submucosa or muscularis because of fluid accumulation in the surrounding tissues.

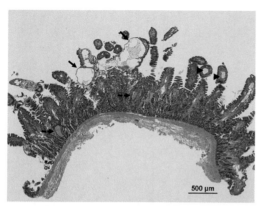

Fig. 1. Low-magnification (hematoxylin-eosin, ×40) photomicrograph of the jejunal mucosa of a dog with severe PLE and lymphangiectasia with crypt disease. Note the dilation of lacteals that ranges from moderate to severe. In moderately affected villi (*arrowheads*), the lacteals comprise greater than 25% to 50% of the villous width. Severe cystic lacteal dilation (*arrows*) is often observed and several ruptured villi are present. In addition, there are scattered markedly dilated crypts (*dashed arrows*), which are filled with a brightly eosinophilic proteinaceous material (see **Fig. 2** for higher magnification). Infiltrating the lamina propria throughout are normal numbers of lymphocytes and plasma cells. (*Courtesy of Luke Borst, DVM, PhD, North Carolina State University College of Veterinary Medicine, Raleigh, NC.*)

IL may be primary (idiopathic or congenital) or secondary to another disease condition that increases hydrostatic pressure in the lymphatic vessels of the digestive tract (eg, inflammatory mucosal infiltrates). The distinction between primary and secondary IL, however, is often challenging in dogs because leakage of lymph in the intestinal tissue may also induce secondary inflammation.

Approximately 50% of all Norwegian lundehunds living in North America are affected by PLE, which is thought to be due to primary (idiopathic) IL because of similarities with the disease in human patients.[8,9] Primary IL has also been reported in rottweilers, Yorkshire terriers, shar-peis, and Maltese.[6,10] Lymphangiectasia can affect lymphatic vessels at the villus level and also in the deeper parts of the intestinal wall, such as submucosa, muscularis, serosa, and in the mesentery.[6,11,12] Dilated intestinal crypts filled with mucin and cells (**Fig. 2**) are another common finding in lundehund enteropathy.[12] Granuloma formation (**Fig. 3**) due to leakage of lymph and ensuing inflammatory reaction around the lympathic vessels is observed in the mesentery of affected dogs.[6,13] The mechanism of primary lymphangiectasia in dogs is not clarified but an anomaly of the lymphatic vessels in the intestinal wall has been described in human medicine,[14] and dysregulation of lymphangiogenesis has been reported in people with primary lymphangiectasia.[15]

Secondary IL is associated with mucosal inflammation in IBD, intestinal neoplasia, or infectious diseases in dogs. It has also been described in humans in association with right-sided heart failure, constrictive pericarditis, and several other conditions (see **Box 1**).[1,2,4]

Inflammatory Bowel Disease

PLE is associated with IBD in dogs[5,6,16–19] and cats.[19–21] The magnitude of hypoalbuminemia is less severe in cats than in dogs; consequently, cats do not frequently present with ascites.[20,21] IBD-induced PLE is not always associated with IL.[5,17,19,22]

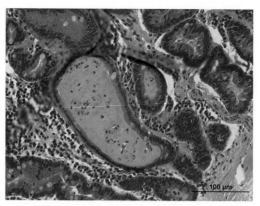

Fig. 2. High-magnification (hematoxylin-eosin, ×400) image of the jejunal crypts of the same dog as in **Fig. 1**. The crypts are multifocally, moderately to markedly dilated, and completely filled with a brightly eosinophilic hyaline material consistent with high protein content. Additionally, the fluid is punctuated by several degenerative and nondegenerative neutrophils mixed with fewer foamy macrophages and scant cellular and nuclear debris. The epithelium lining the dilated crypts is occasionally attenuated. (*Courtesy of* Luke Borst, DVM, PhD, North Carolina State University College of Veterinary Medicine, Raleigh, NC.)

It is likely that, as in human medicine, permeability changes associated with intestinal inflammation are responsible for the protein loss in these cases. Recent studies in transgenic rodent models and human epithelial cell lines revealed that heparan sulfate deficiency induces intestinal protein loss and inflammation associated with increased intestinal venous pressure.[23,24] Moreover, a nonanticoagulant heparin derivative prevented intestinal leakage in PLE-affected mice[24] and heparin has been used to successfully treat PLE secondary to surgical correction of a congenital cardiac

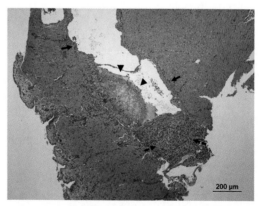

Fig. 3. High-magnification (hematoxylin-eosin, ×100) photomicrograph of the external muscular layers of the jejunum from the same dog as in **Fig. 1**. Pictured is a severely dilated lymphatic (*arrows*) that is partially filled with fibrillar strands of eosinophilic material (fibrin) (*arrowheads*), which entraps several degenerative neutrophils and moderate cellular debris. Adjacent to the dilated lymphatic is a focal accumulation of foamy macrophages (*dashed arrows*), which are interspersed with fewer lymphocytes and rare plasma cells (lipogranuloma). (*Courtesy of* Luke Borst, DVM, PhD, North Carolina State University College of Veterinary Medicine, Raleigh, NC.)

anomaly in humans.[25,26] Recently, colonic IBD in dogs has been associated with up-regulation of claudin, a protein associated with paracellular colonocytes junctions,[27] suggesting that alterations of paracellular intestinal permeability may occur in canine IBD. Because the intestinal biopsies performed in dogs affected with IBD are focal (surgical biopsies) or limited to only a superficial and small part of the duodenum and ileum (endoscopic biopsies), it is possible that IL may sometimes be missed because the lesions may only occur focally.[28]

Specific Forms of IBD Associated with PLE in Dogs

Basenji enteropathy is a rare immunoproliferative disease with intense intestinal inflammatory infiltration associated with gastric hypertrophy inducing PLE with severe hypoalbuminemia in some cases.[29–33] Hypergammaglobulinemia is reported in some cases.[30,34,35]

Giant hypertrophic gastritis resembling Ménétrier disease in humans has been reported in basenjis in association with immunoproliferative enteritis,[30,32,36] in a boxer,[37] an Old English sheepdog[38] and Drentse patrijshond dogs,[39] although hypo-albuminemia was not a consistent finding.

Soft-coated wheaten terriers are affected by a specific form of familial IBD associated with PLE. In approximately half of cases, PLE and protein-losing nephropathy occur simultaneously, which can render the diagnosis of PLE more challenging.[40] The intestinal histopathologic lesions reported in these dogs with PLE are IBD, lymphatic dilation, or combination of both and lymphangitis.[40] The lymphangitis is transmural and found mostly in the deeper layers of the intestinal wall.[40] Affected dogs exhibit sensitivity to different food allergens, including chicken, corn, milk, egg, soybean/tofu, cottage cheese, lamb, and wheat.[41] Exposure to food allergens is associated with a decrease in serum albumin concentration.[41]

Crypt Disease

Recently, PLE has been associated with crypt disease.[7,22,42] The hallmark of crypt disease (see **Figs. 1** and **2**) is a severe dilation of the intestinal crypts that are filled with mucus, sloughed epithelial cells, and sometimes inflammatory cells.[7] These lesions can be isolated and are not always associated with histologic signs of IBD or IL.[7,42] In some cases, the distribution of the lesions can be patchy or multifocal and separated by normal intestinal mucosa.[42] Crypt lesions could easily be missed during surgical biopsy because they are not visible to the surgeon.[42] Therefore, endo-scopic biopsy is probably preferable for diagnosing focal crypt disease. The lesions are located below the level of the villi (see **Fig. 2**), however, and can easily be missed if the biopsy is too superficial.[7,42] Crypt lesions seem to be especially prevalent in Yorkshire terriers and rottweilers.[7,22,42] The mechanism of crypt disease is unknown and a recent study did not show any association with intestinal bacteria and crypt disease in Yorkshire terriers with PLE.[43]

Regional Enteritis

Regional enteritis is characterized by focal transmural granulomatous infiltration mostly localized in the distal small intestine. It has been associated with hypoprotei-nemia in dogs.[44] Recently, idiopathic focal eosinophilic masses of the GI tract have been reported as a potential cause of hypoalbuminemia and panhypoproteinemia in dogs.[45] None of the 7 dogs reported in this study, however, had ascites.

Infectious Diseases Associated with PLE

GI tract infection by *Histoplasma capsulatum* can induce severe granulomatous intestinal infiltration and secondary PLE in dogs and cats.[46] Most of the time, GI histoplasmosis is associated with respiratory histoplasmosis, but isolated GI disease is possible in both species.[10,46] In patients with histoplasmosis, hypoalbuminemia is frequently associated with hyperglobulinemia,[46] as has also recently been described in canine pythiosis.[47] There is no definitive evidence, however, that the hypoalbuminemia is induced by GI loss in these diseases.

Parasitism

Severe intestinal parasitism, especially hookworm infestation, may induce PLE with ascites or edema. Positive response to a therapeutic trial is the only way to prove that the parasites were responsible for the PLE. It has been suggested that parasites may induce an inflammatory reaction that eventually leads to IBD.[18,48] In humans, giardiasis has been associated with PLE.[2,49]

Gastrointestinal Neoplasia

Mild to marked hypoalbuminemia is reported in dogs with alimentary lymphoma.[50–52] The prevalence seems high, with 11 of 18 dogs[51] and 24 of 30 dogs[50] affected in two different studies (range of hypoalbuminemia from 1.6 to 2.9 g/dL). In most of these cases, however, hypoalbuminemia is moderate and does not lead to formation of an abdominal transudate.[50–53] A case of large granular intestinal lymphoma and leukemia derived from natural killer cells and associated with PLE with concurrent hypoalbuminemia and hypoglobulinemia has been reported recently.[53] Mild hypoalbuminemia has been reported in 6 of 26 cats with intestinal lymphoma[54] but recently low-grade alimentary lymphoma in 15 cats has not been associated with hypoalbuminemia.[55] Other GI tumors, such as adenocarcinoma, can also induce hypoalbuminemia and PLE.[10]

Miscellaneous

Intestinal intussusception is sometimes associated with hypoproteinemia and hypoalbuminemia.[10] GI ulcers can also be associated with hypoalbuminemia because of the blood loss in the GI lumen. Fluid collection or edema is rare in such conditions, however. Severe GI albumin loss also occurs in parvoviral enteritis and can sometimes cause pitting edema. Primary bacterial overgrowth has been associated with PLE in humans,[56] and some dogs with PLE may improve with antibiotic treatment.

CLINICAL PRESENTATION

Some breeds, such as Yorkshire terriers, rottweilers, shar-peis, or German shepherds, are predisposed to PLE.[6,10,22] The classical clinical presentation of PLE is a combination of chronic relapsing digestive signs (mostly diarrhea and less frequently vomiting) with weight loss and edematous signs associated with chronic hypoalbuminemia (pitting edema of the limbs, scrotum or face, and ascites due to a pure transudate). Some affected dogs have concurrent abdominal and pleural effusion,[5–7,43] chylothorax,[57] or even isolated pleural effusion.[7] Pleural effusion is especially prevalent in Yorkshire terriers with PLE.[43,58] Care must be taken when a dog with PLE needs to be anesthetized for biopsy collection because a nondiagnosed pleural effusion may be fatal during anesthesia. Melena is rare in canine PLE.[6] Because these classical clinical findings are not always present, PLE should always be considered in hypoalbuminemic dogs, even in the absence of digestive signs. Other less frequent clinical signs are related to complications resulting from the protein loss.

COMPLICATIONS

A hypercoagulable state may occur in dogs with PLE. It has been associated with reduced antithrombin III (AT III) plasma concentration,[59] increased thrombin-antithrombin complexes,[60] or an abnormal thromboelastogram.[61] Even after clinical improvement, dogs with PLE remained hypercoagulable based on their thromboelastogram profiles. This suggests that intestinal loss of AT III is not the only mechanism inducing hypercoagulability in PLE.[61] Thromboembolic events are reported in 12% to 18% of soft-coated wheaten terriers with PLE.[40] In a report compiling several case series of PLE, clinically noticeable thromboembolic disease occurred in 7.5% of dogs.[10] PLE has been reported in cats with pulmonary thromboembolism[62] and in 4 dogs with aortic thrombosis (1 intestinal lymphoma and 3 idiopathic PLE).[63,64] Moreover, femoral artery thrombus was associated with intestinal lymphoma in one dog.[65] Sudden death with suspected pulmonary thromboembolism was reported in case series of dogs with crypt disease.[7,43] Some dogs with PLE, especially Yorkshire terriers,[43,58] also exhibit thrombocytosis. In a study of 16 dogs with PLE, a platelet/albumin (expressed in g/dL) ratio above 240,000 identified all the dogs with increased thrombin-antithrombin complexes, one of the markers for a hypercoagulable state.[60]

Hypocalcemia may occur in dogs with PLE, particularly in Yorkshire terriers, but also in several other breeds.[43,66–68] Hypocalcemia may be associated with hypomagnesemia[43,58,66,67] that may induce secondary hypoparathyroidism.[66] Hypocalcemia can be severe enough to induce twitching episodes[67] or even seizures in dogs with PLE.[69] These disturbances are probably due to a combination of poor intestinal absorption and increased leakage of calcium and magnesium in the GI lumen. Other causes of hypocalcemia in canine PLE include inappropriate PTH secretion,[66] calcitriol deficiency[68] due to reduced intestinal absorption of lipid soluble vitamins (A, D, E, and K), and decreased 1α-hydroxylation by the kidney.[67]

Granulomatous lymphangitis is reported in 35% of soft-coated wheaten terriers with PLE, with a transmural distribution of lesions typically predominating in the submucosa, muscularis, and serosa (see **Fig. 3**).[40] In other breeds, lymphangitis can also be found in the mesentery.[13] Granulomas surrounding lymphatic vessels[8,13] and intestinal lymphangitis[6] can further impair intestinal lymphatic drainage and worsen the intestinal loss of protein.

Gut wall edema is thought to be another possible complication of canine PLE, which may further aggravate protein loss.[10] It is probably due to a combination of decreased oncotic pressure and leakage of lymph in the intestinal wall. Complications of segmental intestinal ileus have been reported in humans and related to intestinal wall edema inducing dysfunction in motility.[70]

DIAGNOSIS

The first step when facing a pet with presumptive PLE is to rule out other conditions associated with hypoalbuminemia, such as protein-losing nephropathy, liver failure, and third spacing associated with severe pleuritis or peritonitis. Therefore, the work-up should include a urinalysis with a urine protein-to-creatinine ratio; a liver function test, such as preprandial and postprandial serum bile acid concentration; and a search for inflammatory fluid accumulation in the thorax or abdomen.

Identifying the Origin of the Protein Loss

Unfortunately, protein loss through the GI tract is not easily confirmed in clinical practice. The only available test is the measurement of fecal α_1-proteinase inhibitor (α_1-PI) at the Gastrointestinal Laboratory at Texas A&M University (www.vetmed.tamu.edu/

gilab). α_1-PI is a protease inhibitor of similar size to albumin and is also synthesized in the liver. α_1-PI is neither actively absorbed nor secreted in the normal gut.[1] It can leak with other protein through the gut. Because of its antiproteolytic activity, it is resistant to hydrolysis in the GI tract and can be recovered unchanged in the feces.[71,72] The measurement is performed on samples of freshly voided feces from 3 consecutive days (no intrarectal collection). The feces are collected with special preweighed collecting tubes, immediately frozen, and shipped frozen overnight. This test can be useful to confirm enteric protein loss in animals that exhibit concurrent protein-losing nephropathy or liver disease. Fecal α_1-PI is increased in dogs with chronic GI signs but does not correlate with plasma albumin.[73] Fecal α_1-PI measurement could also be used to screen dogs prone to PLE, such as lundehund, and in dogs with poorly responsive IBD to document PLE before the animals become overtly hypoalbuminemic.

Hypoalbuminemia is the hallmark of PLE, and concurrent hypocholesterolemia, hypoglobulinemia, and lymphopenia are frequently observed, although these changes are not always present.[6,8,17] It is particularly important not to rule out PLE in hypoalbuminemic dogs that are not hypoglobulinemic.[6] Some dogs with PLE may be hyperglobulinemic.[6,17] Hyperglobulinemia should prompt a search for inflammatory (especially fungal diseases) or neoplastic diseases that may underlie the PLE. Fecal parasite screening with flotation and, if indicated, antigen test for giardia using 3 different fecal samples should be performed. A coagulation panel, including prothrombin time, activated partial thromboplastin time, AT III, and D-dimers is recommended to evaluate patients for hypercoagulability and thrombosis.[59,61,74]

Low serum cobalamin and low serum albumin may occur concurrently in dogs with chronic enteropathies.[5] Therefore, serum cobalamin concentration should be measured in all PLE patients to assess the need for cobalamin supplementation. Similarly, hypocalcemia and hypomagnesemia should be documented. Evaluation of ionized calcium is the most accurate method to diagnose hypocalcemia.[75]

Perinuclear antineutrophil cytoplasmic autoantibodies (pANCAs) are early markers of PLE in soft-coated wheaten terriers.[76] Serum pANCAs are positive in affected dogs on average 2.4 years before the onset of hypoalbuminemia[76] but unfortunately this test is not routinely available.

Diagnostic Imaging

Abdominal imaging is essential in most cases of PLE. Abdominal ultrasound is a prerequisite to select the biopsy method. Identification of focal or patchy lesions that cannot be reached by an endoscope provides a good indication for surgical biopsy. Specific findings, such as hyperechoic mucosal striations, can be suggestive of PLE.[77,78] In a recent study of ultrasonographic findings in dogs with chronic enteropathies, 8 of 8 dogs with PLE had changes in the jejunal mucosa and 6 of 8 had changes in the duodenal mucosa.[77] When compared with dogs with chronic enteropathies that did not result in protein loss, hyperechoic mucosal striations had a sensitivity of 75% and a specificity of 96% for PLE in dogs with PLE, of which 7 of 8 had secondary IL in duodenal biopsies.[77] Fine-needle aspiration of any abnormal organ should always be performed because it can help with diagnosis of lymphoma or histoplasmosis. In endemic areas and in cases of suggestive clinical presentation, cytologic examination of a rectal scraping or a urinary antigen test for histoplasmosis should be performed. Finally, the thoracic cavity should be screened for the presence of pleural fluid.

In cases of negative findings, the next step in the diagnosis of PLE is a biopsy of the stomach and small intestinal walls. Systematic treatment of intestinal parasites is recommended, however, before performing invasive procedures. Fenbendazole, administered daily (50 mg/kg orally) for 5 days, eliminates most intestinal nematodes as well as giardia.

Obtaining Small Intestinal Biopsies

The selection of the biopsy method is a matter of debate. Bidirectional (combination of upper and lower GI) endoscopy, including gastric, duodenal, and ileal biopsies, is the authors' preferred method because histologic diagnosis can be different between duodenal and ileal samples in up to 73% of the cases of canine IBD,[79] and lymphangiectasia may only be found on ileal biopsies in some cases. In a case series of 13 dogs with IBD and full-thickness biopsy from the authors' practice, lymphangiectasia was found exclusively in the ileum in 4 of 13 dogs and was more severe in the ileum than in the duodenum in 3 of 13 dogs. When the jejunum was affected, however, equally severe or worse lesions were also observed either in the duodenum or in the ileum.[80] In certain cases, passing the endoscope through the ileocolic valve may be difficult. In such instances, the biopsy forceps can be pushed blindly through the ileocolic valve to perform blinded biopsies or to serve as a guide for passage of the endoscope through the valve. Endoscopic mucosal biopsies may sometimes be too superficial to diagnose IL. The canine GI lymphatic system has a complex architecture and exhibits vessels and plexuses in all the layers of the intestinal wall.[81] Therefore, IL may affect different levels of this complex system, including the deeper layers.[6,22,40] Deeper lesions, especially those located in the muscularis or serosa, may not always be associated with more superficial changes in the mucosa and may not appear in endoscopic biopsies. For the same reason, diagnosis of crypt disease requires good endoscopic biopsies that include sufficient numbers of intestinal crypts.[7,22,42,82,83] Endoscopic findings in PLE range from normal aspect of the intestinal mucosa to severe changes, such as increase granularity and uperficial erosions or ulcers. The endoscopic presentation of IL ranges from normal appearance to more classically described features, such as multiple scattered pinpoint villi (Movie 1), diffuse prominent villi with white-discolored tips (rice grain aspect), or focal whitish macules or nodules,[10,22,42,84] as described in humans. A recent study in rottweilers with PLE suggested that the rice grain aspect is more likely associated with focal and moderate IL and the multiple scattered pinpoint aspect more associated with severe IL.[22] Foamy whitish lipid discharge or chylous fluid in the duodenal lumen may also be observed, especially after the biopsy (see Movie 1). Providing a liquid fat source, such as cream or corn oil orally 2 to 4 hours before the endoscopy can accentuate the abnormal appearance of severely lipid-laden villi in the postabsorptive stage of dogs with IL. The lipid-rich meal can also accentuate microscopic lesions of lacteal dilation on the biopsy.[10]

Coeliotomy or laparoscopy with full-thickness biopsy offers the advantage of a thorough inspection of the abdomen, including a search for lipogranulomas and biopsy from all three segments of the small intestine. Because lesion distribution may be patchy (in particular crypt lesions),[7] they can be missed if only one single biopsy is sampled from each segment. Although hypoalbuminemia has traditionally been considered a risk factor for intestinal suture dehiscence, two independent studies did not show a significant additional risk of dehiscence in hypoalbuminemic dogs.[85,86] Especially in the presence of severe gut wall edema, serosal patching is recommended to optimize wound healing when performing full-thickness intestinal biopsies in dogs with PLE.[10]

Histopathologic Evaluation

Consistency in the definition of histopathologic intestinal lesions on endoscopic biopsies has been recently greatly improved by the publication of standards with templates for dogs and cats.[87] The World Small Animal Veterinary Association template (**Fig. 4**) should be used to warrant consistency in histopathologic interpretation of the severity of IL. Using this template, the severity of hypoalbuminemia could be related to the histologic grade of IL in dogs.[83] The pathologist should always evaluate the quality of the endoscopic biopsies before interpretation because the chances of diagnosing IL decrease if the samples are inadequate.[82] Even with biopsy samples of adequate quality from dogs with IL, lesions are only found in 56% of the submitted specimen.[82] A crush artifact squeezing the dilated lymphatic vessels may induce a false-negative diagnosis of LE, particularly when small endoscopic biopsy forceps are used and also when surgical biopsies are not correctly handled.

PROGNOSIS

The prognosis is always guarded in PLE because the response to treatment is unpredictable and relapses may occur. Therefore, continuous or intermittent lifelong

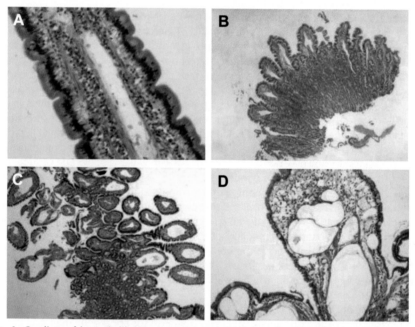

Fig. 4. Grading of lacteal dilation in endoscopic biopsies of canine duodenal mucosa. (*A*) Normal mucosa. Central lacteal represents up to approximately 25% of width of the villous lamina propria when sectioned longitudinally (hematoxylin-eosin). (*B*) Mild lacteal dilation. Central lacteal represents up to approximately 50% of width of the villous lamina propria when sectioned longitudinally. Villi are generally wider than normal (hematoxylin-eosin). (*C*) Moderate lacteal dilation. Central lacteal represents up to approximately 75% of width of the villous lamina propria when sectioned longitudinally. Affected villi are wider than normal (hematoxylin-eosin). (*D*) Marked lacteal dilation. Central lacteal dilated to occupy up to 100% of width of the villous lamina propria. Surrounding lamina propria is oedematous. Villi are markedly distended-particularly at tips, giving a "club-shapped"appearance (hematoxylin-eosin). (*From* Day MJ, Bilzer T, Mansell J, et al. Histopathological standards for the diagnosis of gastrointestinal inflammation in endoscopic biopsy samples from the dog and cat: a report from the World Small Animal Veterinary Association Gastrointestinal Standardization Group. J Comp Pathol 2008;138(Suppl 1):S1–43; with permission.)

treatment is frequently required. Hypoalbuminemia was not a strong predictive factor of euthanasia because of refractoriness to treatment in one study that included dogs with chronic enteropathies[5] but has been associated with a lack of response to treatment and euthanasia due to treatment failure in another study that included IBD dogs.[17] Recently, a new canine chronic enteropathy clinical activity index (CCECAI) (**Table 1**) has been proposed for dogs with various forms of chronic intestinal diseases, including PLE.[5] Receiver operating characteristic curve analysis of this index as a predictor of refractoriness to treatment and euthanasia within 3 years after the diagnosis revealed a sensitivity and specificity of 91% and 82%, respectively, for a cutoff value of CCECAI equal to 12 (see **Table 1**). Recent studies have also suggested that the prognosis of PLE is guarded in rottweilers[88] and Yorkshire terriers.[43,58]

TREATMENT

The treatment of PLE is focused on the primary disease causing the protein loss. It is beyond the scope of this review to discuss the treatment of infectious diseases or neoplasia associated with PLE. The nonspecific treatment has four main goals: to provide adequate nutritional support, to provide oncotic support, to address complications, and to treat intestinal lesions.

Providing Nutritional Support

Dogs with PLE are usually in severe negative energetic and protein balance. The goal of the nutritional support is to provide a high-energy density (above 3.5 kcal/g) with a combined low-fat and high-carbohydrate content. Current recommendations for dogs with PLE are below 10% to 15% of fat, above 25% to 30% of protein, less than 5% of crude fibers (on a dry matter basis), and above 87% and 90% digestibility for the protein and fat/carbohydrate sources, respectively.[89] High-fiber diets are not recommended because fibers inhibit digestion and absorption of protein and also provide a bulk of nondigestible content. A novel protein diet is also recommended in these patients because IBD is frequently associated with PLE. The fat content of the currently available dry novel protein diets ranges from 9% up to 24% on a dry matter basis; care should be taken during selection of a particular diet. Hydrolyzed protein diets are a good source of highly digestible protein. Royal Canin/Medi-Cal Gastro Intestinal Low Fat (7% fat on a dry matter basis with chicken as protein source) is a diet with one of the lowest fat content currently available. Medium chain triglycerides have been suggested as an alternative source of energy from fat. In dogs, however, medium chain triglycerides are absorbed via the lymphatic system and, therefore, provide a stimulus for intestinal lymph flow that should be avoided in PLE.[90,91] Therefore, the clinical utility of these expensive and poorly palatable products is questionable. Supplementation with cooked egg whites is an option to provide additional highly digestible proteins (1 or 2 cooked large egg whites/10 kg body weight as needed to maintain serum albumin above 2 g/dL).[89] Finally, because of the severe digestive impairment and the concurrent high-energy/protein requirements of the affected dogs, frequent and small meals are initially necessary.

Oligomeric or elemental diets providing small peptides or amino acids are a useful alternative in the most severe or nonresponsive cases to provide readily available sources for protein synthesis.[10,92] Tolerex and Vivonex or Peptamen products provide free amino acids or oligopeptides, respectively. Their fat contents range from 1.3% for Tolerex to 3% to 6% for Vivonex and to 33% to 36% for Peptamen. These products are available online (www.nestle-nutrition.com/Public/Default.aspx) and are usually supplemented with additional amino acids solutions.[10] They are thought to hasten

Table 1
Clinical scoring for dogs with PLE

Criteria	Scoring Chart	Results
Attitude/activity	0 Normal 1 Slightly decreased 2 Moderately decreased 3 Severely decreased	
Appetite	0 Normal 1 Slightly decreased 2 Moderately decreased 3 Severely decreased	
Weight loss	0 None 1 Mild (<5%) 2 Moderate (5%–10%) 3 Severe (>10%)	
Vomiting	0 None 1 Mild (1/wk) 2 Moderate (2–3/wk) 3 Severe (>3/wk)	
Stool consistency	0 Normal 1 Slightly soft feces 2 Very soft feces 3 Watery diarrhea	
Stool frequency	0 Normal 1 Slightly increased (2–3/d) or fecal blood mucus or both 2 Moderately increased (4–5/d) 3 Severely increased (>5/d)	
Serum albumin (lowest concentration at any time during the follow-up)	0 Serum albumin >2.0 g/dL 1 Serum albumin 1.5–1.9 g/dL 2 Serum albumin 1.2–1.4 g/dL 3 Serum albumin <1.2 g/dL	
Ascites/edema	0 None 1 Mild ascites or peripheral edema 2 Moderate ascites or peripheral edema 3 Severe ascites, pleural effusion and peripheral edema	
Pruritus	0 None 1 Occasional episodes of itching 2 Regular episode of itching but stops when the dog is asleep 3 Dog regularly wakes up because of itching	
Cobalamin (optional)	0 Normal range 1 Below normal range	
Total	<4 Insignificant disease <6 Mild disease <9 Moderate disease <12 Severe disease >12 Very severe disease	

Adapted from Allenspach K, Wieland B, Grone A, et al. Chronic enteropathies in dogs: evaluation of risk factors for negative outcome. J Vet Intern Med 2007;21(4):700–8; with permission.

clinical recovery in some cases.[7,10,42] In the most severely affected cases, total parenteral nutrition can be beneficial at least initially.[10,93] The daily cost and the risk of complications, however, are high.

Parenteral fat-soluble vitamin supplementation might be necessary in severe long-standing cases of fat malabsorption and steatorrhea (intramuscular injection of an adequate vitamin supplement solution with 300 IU of vitamin E; 100,000 IU of vitamin A; and 10,000 IU of vitamin D_3 should be sufficient for 3 months in dogs).[89]

Providing Oncotic Support

There is no efficient way to provide long-term oncotic support in dogs with PLE if the continuous leakage of protein in the GI lumen is not treated. In critical cases, it might be useful to give intravenous oncotic support at the beginning of the treatment or before performing intestinal biopsies. Hydroxyethyl starches are used at a maximal dosage rate of 20 to 30 mL/kg/d, although they provide short-term oncotic support only. Additionally, higher dosage may impair coagulation.[94] Aggressive oncotic support is also advocated in cases of PLE associated with severe gut edema that may further worsen GI protein loss.[10] Albumin can be provided through plasma transfusion. A large volume of plasma, however, is required to increase a patient's serum albumin concentration, and this raises the concern of hypervolemia. Concentrated human albumin solutions (25%) are an alternative option, but these solutions have been associated with severe and sometimes fatal adverse reactions in dogs.[95–98] Moreover, the increase in plasma albumin concentration in dogs with PLE is short-lived until the ongoing intestinal losses can be halted.[99] Therefore, this approach should be limited to the most critical cases and synthetic colloid support is preferred by the authors in dogs with PLE. Recently, the use of 5% human albumin solution has been evaluated in dogs.[100] None of the dogs developed severe hypersensitivity reaction, such as anaphylaxis, urticaria, or angioedema. Transient diarrhea, hyperthermia, tremors, or perivascular inflammation at catheter site, however, were observed in 43.5% of the dogs.[100] Canine purified albumin has recently become available in 5-g vials (www.abrint.net) and might be a good option to benefit from the colloid support while avoiding allergic reaction to human albumin.

Addressing Complications

Coagulation should be monitored in patients with PLE because hypercoagulability and thrombosis have been reported. When antithrombin is severely reduced, supplementation with fresh frozen plasma transfusion may be beneficial. In cases of suspected thrombosis, heparin treatment combined with low dosage of aspirin (0.5 mg/kg/d orally in dogs) is recommended. The authors use standard heparin (at a dose of 200 to 250 IU/kg subcutaneously 3 times a day) with concurrent monitoring of clotting times every day during hospitalization. If plasma AT III concentration is decreased, fresh frozen plasma complemented with 10 IU/kg of standard heparin should be administered before starting heparin therapy. Vitamin K is a fat-soluble vitamin whose absorption may be decreased in dogs with PLE. Vitamin K deficiency may play a role in coagulopathies associated with PLE, and parenteral supplementation may be useful in some cases.

Hypocobalaminemia is frequent in PLE dogs. Serum concentrations of cobalamin and albumin seem to be correlated in dogs with PLE.[5] Cobalamin supplementation is recommended and can be started early while the test results for serum cobalamin are pending (500 to 1500 µg/dog depending on the size).

Abdominal and thoracic transudates should not be drained unless they induce respiratory impairment. Diuretics are usually not useful in PLE because edema and fluid collections are secondary to decreased oncotic pressure.[4] Spironolactone may help limit fluid collection in some cases but the effect is usually minimal. Furosemide is not recommended because it may induce dehydration and further activate the renin-aldosterone axis in PLE.

Intravenous supplementation with calcium and magnesium salts is required in cases of hypocalcemia and/or hypomagnesemia. If hypocalcemia relapses after intravenous calcium boluses, parenteral vitamin D supplementation should be attempted because some affected dogs may experience vitamin D deficiency due to poor intestinal absorption.[68] Sometimes, long-term oral supplementation with calcium and magnesium is required.

Treating Intestinal Lesions

Because PLE is frequently secondary to IBD, using immune-suppressive treatment is recommended. Granuloma formation secondary to lymph leakage may occur and further impair lymphatic circulation in the GI tract. This may worsen the lymph leakage through the intestinal wall and, therefore, aggressive treatment of these inflammatory reactions is recommended.[13] Standard treatments include steroids at immune-suppressive dosages or azathioprine. A recent study demonstrated the efficacy of cyclosporine (5 mg/kg/d) orally in dogs with steroid-refractory PLE.[16] For this reason, in severe cases of PLE, the authors now recommend starting cyclosporine and steroid at the same time. Also, the authors prefer starting with injectable steroids because intestinal absorption may be impaired in dogs with severe PLE. Recently, a dog with PLE associated with lymphocytic plasmacytic enteritis that failed to respond to a combination of prednisolone and cyclosporine was treated successfully with methotrexate (0.6 mg/kg intramuscularly once a week for 5 weeks). The dog was subsequently maintained on a combination of prednisolone and azathrioprine administered on alternate days.[101] Sodium chromoglycate has been recommended in soft-coated wheaten terriers with PLE. The reported dosage is 100 mg/dog 3 or 4 times daily orally; however, efficacy and safety still have to be evaluated.[102]

The authors have observed rare cases of PLE that are antibiotic responsive. It is possible that bacterial overgrowth is associated with PLE either as a cause or as a complication, as it is the case in human medicine.[56] Therefore, an antibiotic trial with metronidazole or tylosin is probably a reasonable option when starting treatment of PLE.

Follow-up of dogs with PLE is based on clinical response and normalization of albumin concentration. Serum albumin concentration should be measured on a regular basis even if the dog is stable. Decreased serum albumin may be used as an early marker of relapse. In combination with clinical assessment, it is computed to obtain a disease activity score (see **Table 1**) and decide if aggressive treatment of PLE should be resumed.

SUMMARY

PLE is a complex syndrome characterized by intestinal loss of albumin and secondary hypoalbuminemia. In dogs, it is most frequently associated with IBD or lymphoma but can also be observed with histoplasmosis. The diagnosis requires elimination of other causes of hypoalbuminemia, such as liver failure or renal disease. Possible life-threatening complications include extreme denutrition, thromboembolic disease, and hypocalcemia or hypomagnesemia. Identification of intestinal lesions is necessary to differentiate between inflammatory, infectious, and neoplastic conditions and initiate appropriate treatment. Abdominal ultrasonography is necessary to help choose the most appropriate approach for intestinal biopsy (endoscopy vs surgery). The nonspecific treatment is mostly based on dietary changes (high digestibility, intense energy support, and relative fat restriction) and immune suppressive medications. Complications, such as thomboembolism, hypocalcemia, and hypomagnesemia, should be addressed and monitored during follow-up.

SUPPLEMENTARY DATA

Supplementary data related to this article available at doi: 10.1016/j.cvsm.2011.02. 002.

The following is the Supplementary data related to this article: Movie 1 Endoscopy of a dog with PLE and moderate lymphangiectasia on proximal duodenal biopsies. Note diffuse pinpoint aspect of the villi and reflux of greenish foamy material that was especially marked after the biopsy.

REFERENCES

1. Kim KE. Protein-losing gastroenteropathy. In: Feldman M, Friedman LS, Sleisenger MH, editors. Sleisenger and Fordtran's gastrointestinal and liver disease—pathophysiology, diagnosis and management, vol. 1. 7th edition. Philadelphia: Saunders; 2002. p. 446–52.

2. Levin MS. Miscellaneous diseases of the small intestine. In: Yamada T, Alpers DA, Kaplowitz N, et al, editors. Textbook of gastroenterology, vol. 1. 4th edition. Philadelphia: Lippincott, Williams and Wilkins; 2003. p. 1663–83.

3. Groschwitz KR, Hogan SP. Intestinal barrier function: molecular regulation and disease pathogenesis. J Allergy Clin Immunol 2009;124(1):3–20 [quiz: 21–2].

4. Umar SB, DiBaise JK. Protein-losing enteropathy: case illustrations and clinical review. Am J Gastroenterol 2010;105(1):43–9 [quiz: 50].

5. Allenspach K, Wieland B, Grone A, et al. Chronic enteropathies in dogs: evaluation of risk factors for negative outcome. J Vet Intern Med 2007;21(4): 700–8.

6. Kull PA, Hess RS, Craig LE, et al. Clinical, clinicopathologic, radiographic, and ultrasonographic characteristics of intestinal lymphangiectasia in dogs: 17 cases (1996–1998). J Am Vet Med Assoc 2001;219(2):197–202.

7. Willard MD, Helman G, Fradkin JM, et al. Intestinal crypt lesions associated with protein-losing enteropathy in the dog. J Vet Intern Med 2000;14(3):298–307.

8. Berghoff N, Ruaux CG, Steiner JM, et al. Gastroenteropathy in Norwegian Lundehunds. Compend Contin Educ Vet 2007;29(8):456–65, 468–70 [quiz: 470–1].

9. Berghoff N, Steiner JM, Ruaux CG, et al. Prevalence of enteropathy in the North American population of the Norvegian Lundehund [abstract]. J Vet Intern Med 2004;18:435.

10. Peterson PB, Willard MD. Protein-losing enteropathies. Vet Clin North Am Small Anim Pract 2003;33(5):1061–82.

11. Flesja K, Yri T. Protein-losing enteropathy in the Lundehund. J Small Anim Pract 1977;18(1):11–23.

12. Landsverk T, Gamlem H. Intestinal lymphangiectasia in the Lundehund. Scanning electron microscopy of intestinal mucosa. Acta Pathol Microbiol Immunol Scand A 1984;92(5):353–62.

13. Van Kruiningen HJ, Lees GE, Hayden DW, et al. Lipogranulomatous lymphangitis in canine intestinal lymphangiectasia. Vet Pathol 1984;21(4):377–83.

14. Liu NF, Lu Q, Wang CG, et al. Magnetic resonance imaging as a new method to diagnose protein losing enteropathy. Lymphology 2008;41(3):111–5.

15. Hokari R, Kitagawa N, Watanabe C, et al. Changes in regulatory molecules for lymphangiogenesis in intestinal lymphangiectasia with enteric protein loss. J Gastroenterol Hepatol 2008;23(7 Pt 2):e88–95.

16. Allenspach K, Rufenacht S, Sauter S, et al. Pharmacokinetics and clinical efficacy of cyclosporine treatment of dogs with steroid-refractory inflammatory bowel disease. J Vet Intern Med 2006;20(2):239–44.

17. Craven M, Simpson JW, Ridyard AE, et al. Canine inflammatory bowel disease: retrospective analysis of diagnosis and outcome in 80 cases (1995–2002). J Small Anim Pract 2004;45(7):336–42.

18. Jacobs G, Collins-Kelly L, Lappin M, et al. Lymphocytic-plasmacytic enteritis in 24 dogs. J Vet Intern Med 1990;4(2):45–53.

19. Jergens AE, Moore FM, Haynes JS, et al. Idiopathic inflammatory bowel disease in dogs and cats: 84 cases (1987–1990). J Am Vet Med Assoc 1992;201(10): 1603–8.

20. Baez JL, Hendrick MJ, Walker LM, et al. Radiographic, ultrasonographic, and endoscopic findings in cats with inflammatory bowel disease of the stomach and small intestine: 33 cases (1990–1997). J Am Vet Med Assoc 1999;215(3): 349–54.

21. Bailey S, Benigni L, Eastwood J, et al. Comparisons between cats with normal and increased fPLI concentrations in cats diagnosed with inflammatory bowel disease. J Small Anim Pract 2010;51(9):484–9.

22. Lecoindre P, Chevallier M, Guerret S. Protein-losing enteropathy of non neoplastic origin in the dog: a retrospective study of 34 cases. Schweiz Arch Tierheilkd 2010;152(3):141–6 [in French].

23. Bode L, Freeze HH. Applied glycoproteomics—approaches to study genetic-environmental collisions causing protein-losing enteropathy. Biochim Biophys Acta 2006;1760(4):547–59.

24. Bode L, Salvestrini C, Park PW, et al. Heparan sulfate and syndecan-1 are essential in maintaining murine and human intestinal epithelial barrier function. J Clin Invest 2008;118(1):229–38.

25. Bendayan I, Casaldaliga J, Castello F, et al. Heparin therapy and reversal of protein-losing enteropathy in a case with congenital heart disease. Pediatr Cardiol 2000;21(3):267–8.

26. Kelly AM, Feldt RH, Driscoll DJ, et al. Use of heparin in the treatment of protein-losing enteropathy after fontan operation for complex congenital heart disease. Mayo Clin Proc 1998;73(8):777–9.

27. Ridyard AE, Brown JK, Rhind SM, et al. Apical junction complex protein expression in the canine colon: differential expression of claudin-2 in the colonic mucosa in dogs with idiopathic colitis. J Histochem Cytochem 2007;55(10):1049–58.

28. Louvet A, Denis B. Ultrasonographic diagnosis—small bowel lymphangiectasia in a dog. Vet Radiol Ultrasound 2004;45(6):565–7.

29. Barta O, Breitschwerdt EB, Shaffer LM, et al. Lymphocyte transformation and humoral immune factors in Basenji dogs with immunoproliferative small intestinal disease. Am J Vet Res 1983;44(10):1954–9.

30. Breitschwerdt EB, Waltman C, Hagstad HV, et al. Clinical and epidemiologic characterization of a diarrheal syndrome in Basenji dogs. J Am Vet Med Assoc 1982;180(8):914–20.

31. De Buysscher EV, Breitschwerdt EB, MacLachlan NJ. Elevated serum IgA associated with immunoproliferative enteropathy of Basenji dogs: lack of evidence for alpha heavy-chain disease or enhanced intestinal IgA secretion. Vet Immunol Immunopathol 1988;20(1):41–52.

32. MacLachlan NJ, Breitschwerdt EB, Chambers JM, et al. Gastroenteritis of basenji dogs. Vet Pathol 1988;25(1):36–41.

33. Ochoa R, Breitschwerdt EB, Lincoln KL. Immunoproliferative small intestinal disease in Basenji dogs: morphologic observations. Am J Vet Res 1984;45(3): 482–90.

34. Breitschwerdt EB, Barta O, Waltman C, et al. Serum proteins in healthy Basenjis and Basenjis with chronic diarrhea. Am J Vet Res 1983;44(2):326–8.

35. Breitschwerdt EB, Ochoa R, Barta M, et al. Clinical and laboratory characterization of Basenjis with immunoproliferative small intestinal disease. Am J Vet Res 1984;45(2):267–73.

36. Kruiningen HJ. Giant hypertrophic gastritis of Basenji dogs. Vet Pathol 1977; 14(1):19–28.

37. van der Gaag I, Happe RP, Wolvekamp WT. A boxer dog with chronic hypertrophic gastritis resembling Menetrier's disease in man. Vet Pathol 1976;13(3): 172–85.

38. Rallis TS, Patsikas MN, Mylonakis ME, et al. Giant hypertrophic gastritis (Menetrier's-like disease) in an Old English sheepdog. J Am Anim Hosp Assoc 2007; 43(2):122–7.

39. Slappendel RJ, Vandergaag I, Vannes JJ, et al. Familial Stomatocytosis Hypertrophic Gastritis (Fshg), a newly recognized disease in the Dog (Drentse Patrijshond). Vet Q 1991;13(1):30–40.

40. Littman MP, Dambach DM, Vaden SL, et al. Familial protein-losing enteropathy and protein-losing nephropathy in Soft Coated Wheaten Terriers: 222 cases (1983–1997). J Vet Intern Med 2000;14(1):68–80.

41. Vaden SL, Hammerberg B, Davenport DJ, et al. Food hypersensitivity reactions in Soft Coated Wheaten Terriers with protein-losing enteropathy or protein-losing nephropathy or both: gastroscopic food sensitivity testing, dietary provocation, and fecal immunoglobulin E. J Vet Intern Med 2000;14(1):60–7.

42. Willard MD, Zenger E, Mansell JL. Protein-losing enteropathy associated with cystic mucoid changes in the intestinal crypts of two dogs. J Am Anim Hosp Assoc 2003;39(2):187–91.

43. Craven M, Duhamel GE, Sutter NB, et al. Absence of bacterial association in Yorkshire terriers with protein-losing enteropathy and cystic intestinal crypts [abstract]. J Vet Intern Med 2009;23:757.

44. Lecoindre P, Gouni V, Chevallier M. Regional granulomatous enteritis in 8 dogs. Paper presented at: Proceedings of the 17th ECVIM -CA congress. Budapest, September 2007.

45. Lyles SE, Panciera DL, Saunders GK, et al. Idiopathic eosinophilic masses of the gastrointestinal tract in dogs. J Vet Intern Med 2009;23(4):818–23.

46. Bromel C, Sykes JE. Histoplasmosis in dogs and cats. Clin Tech Small Anim Pract 2005;20(4):227–32.

47. Berryessa NA, Marks SL, Pesavento PA, et al. Gastrointestinal pythiosis in 10 dogs from California. J Vet Intern Med 2008;22(4):1065–9.

48. Jergens AE. Inflammatory bowel disease. Current perspectives. Vet Clin North Am Small Anim Pract 1999;29(2):501–21, vii.

49. Korman SH, Bar-Oz B, Mandelberg A, et al. Giardiasis with protein-losing enteropathy: diagnosis by fecal alpha 1-antitrypsin determination. J Pediatr Gastroenterol Nutr 1990;10(2):249–52.

50. Frank JD, Reimer SB, Kass PH, et al. Clinical outcomes of 30 cases (1997–2004) of canine gastrointestinal lymphoma. J Am Anim Hosp Assoc 2007;43(6): 313–21.

51. Rassnick KM, Moore AS, Collister KE, et al. Efficacy of combination chemotherapy for treatment of gastrointestinal lymphoma in dogs. J Vet Intern Med 2009;23(2):317–22.

52. Steinberg H, Dubielzig RR, Thomson J, et al. Primary gastrointestinal lymphosarcoma with epitheliotropism in three Shar-pei and one boxer dog. Vet Pathol 1995;32(4):423–6.

53. Snead EC. Large granular intestinal lymphosarcoma and leukemia in a dog. Can Vet J 2007;48(8):848–51.

54. Mahony OM, Moore AS, Cotter SM, et al. Alimentary lymphoma in cats: 28 cases (1988–1993). J Am Vet Med Assoc 1995;207(12):1593–8.

55. Lingard AE, Briscoe K, Beatty JA, et al. Low-grade alimentary lymphoma: clinicopathological findings and response to treatment in 17 cases. J Feline Med Surg 2009;11(8):692–700.

56. Su J, Smith MB, Rerknimitr R, et al. Small intestine bacterial overgrowth presenting as protein-losing enteropathy. Dig Dis Sci 1998;43(3):679–81.

57. Fossum TW, Sherding RG, Zack PM, et al. Intestinal lymphangiectasia associated with chylothorax in two dogs. J Am Vet Med Assoc 1987;190(1):61–4.

58. Simmerson SM, Wunschmann A, Crews L, et al. Description of protein-losing enteropathy in Yorkshire terriers using the W.S.A.V.A. gastrointestinal classification system [abstract]. J Vet Intern Med 2009;23:732.

59. Brownlee L, Sellon RK. Antithrombin and plasminogen activities are decreased and fibrinogen levels are increased in dogs with protein-losing enteropathy [abstract]. J Vet Intern Med 2002;16:348.

60. Lahmers SM, Sellon RK, Peterson PB. Dogs with protein losing enteropathy are in a hypercoagulable state [abstract]. J Vet Intern Med 2006;20:790.

61. Goodwin LV, Goggs R, Chan DL, et al. Evaluation of hypercoagulability using thromboelastography in dogs with protein losing enteropathy [abstract]. J Vet Intern Med 2010;24:723–4.

62. Norris CR, Griffey SM, Samii VF. Pulmonary thromboembolism in cats: 29 cases (1987–1997). J Am Vet Med Assoc 1999;215(11):1650–4.

63. Clare AC, Kraje BJ. Use of recombinant tissue-plasminogen activator for aortic thrombolysis in a hypoproteinemic dog. J Am Vet Med Assoc 1998;212(4):539–43.

64. Goncalves R, Penderis J, Chang YP, et al. Clinical and neurological characteristics of aortic thromboembolism in dogs. J Small Anim Pract 2008;49(4):178–84.

65. Ihle SL, Baldwin CJ, Pifer SM. Probable recurrent femoral artery thrombosis in a dog with intestinal lymphosarcoma. J Am Vet Med Assoc 1996;208(2):240–2.

66. Bush WW, Kimmel SE, Wosar MA, et al. Secondary hypoparathyroidism attributed to hypomagnesemia in a dog with protein-losing enteropathy. J Am Vet Med Assoc 2001;219(12):1732–4, 1708.

67. Kimmel SE, Waddell LS, Michel KE. Hypomagnesemia and hypocalcemia associated with protein-losing enteropathy in Yorkshire terriers: five cases (1992–1998). J Am Vet Med Assoc 2000;217(5):703–6.

68. Mellanby RJ, Mellor PJ, Roulois A, et al. Hypocalcaemia associated with low serum vitamin D metabolite concentrations in two dogs with protein-losing enteropathies. J Small Anim Pract 2005;46(7):345–51.

69. Brauer C, Jambroszyk M, Tipold A. Metabolic and toxic causes of canine seizure disorders: a retrospective study of 96 cases. Vet J 2011;187(2):272–5.

70. Vignes S, Bellanger J. Primary intestinal lymphangiectasia (Waldmann's disease). Orphanet J Rare Dis 2008;3:5.
71. Melgarejo T, Williams DA, Asem EK. Enzyme-linked immunosorbent assay for canine alpha 1-protease inhibitor. Am J Vet Res 1998;59(2):127–30.
72. Melgarejo T, Williams DA, Griffith G. Isolation and characterization of alpha 1-protease inhibitor from canine plasma. Am J Vet Res 1996;57(3):258–63.
73. Murphy KF, German AJ, Ruaux CG, et al. Fecal alpha1-proteinase inhibitor concentration in dogs with chronic gastrointestinal disease. Vet Clin Pathol 2003;32(2):67–72.
74. Kuzi S, Segev G, Haruvi E, et al. Plasma antithrombin activity as a diagnostic and prognostic indicator in dogs: a retrospective study of 149 dogs. J Vet Intern Med 2010;24(3):587–96.
75. Schenck PA, Chew DJ. Prediction of serum ionized calcium concentration by use of serum total calcium concentration in dogs. Am J Vet Res 2005;66(8): 1330–6.
76. Allenspach K, Lomas B, Wieland B, et al. Evaluation of perinuclear anti-neutrophilic cytoplasmic autoantibodies as an early marker of protein-losing enteropathy and protein-losing nephropathy in Soft Coated Wheaten Terriers. Am J Vet Res 2008;69(10):1301–4.
77. Gaschen L, Kircher P, Stussi A, et al. Comparison of ultrasonographic findings with clinical activity index (CIBDAI) and diagnosis in dogs with chronic enteropathies. Vet Radiol Ultrasound 2008;49(1):56–64.
78. Sutherland-Smith J, Penninck DG, Keating JH, et al. Ultrasonographic intestinal hyperechoic mucosal striations in dogs are associated with lacteal dilation. Vet Radiol Ultrasound 2007;48(1):51–7.
79. Casamian-Sorrosal D, Willard MD, Murray JK, et al. Comparison of histopathologic findings in biopsies from the duodenum and ileum of dogs with enteropathy. J Vet Intern Med 2010;24(1):80–3.
80. Dossin O, Tesseydre J-F, Concordet D, et al. Is duodenal mucosa representative of other small intestinal pats in inflammatory bowel disease affected dogs? [abstract]. J Vet Intern Med 2007;22(3):613.
81. Yamanaka Y, Araki K, Ogata T. Three-dimensional organization of lymphatics in the dog small intestine: a scanning electron microscopic study on corrosion casts. Arch Histol Cytol 1995;58(4):465–74.
82. Willard MD, Mansell J, Fosgate GT, et al. Effect of sample quality on the sensitivity of endoscopic biopsy for detecting gastric and duodenal lesions in dogs and cats. J Vet Intern Med 2008;22(5):1084–9.
83. Willard MD, Moore GE, Denton BD, et al. Effect of tissue processing on assessment of endoscopic intestinal biopsies in dogs and cats. J Vet Intern Med 2010; 24(1):84–9.
84. Kim JH, Bak YT, Kim JS, et al. Clinical significance of duodenal lymphangiectasia incidentally found during routine upper gastrointestinal endoscopy. Endoscopy 2009;41(6):510–5.
85. Harvey HJ. Complications of small intestinal biopsy in hypoalbuminemic dogs. Vet Surg 1990;19(4):289–92.
86. Shales CJ, Warren J, Anderson DM, et al. Complications following full-thickness small intestinal biopsy in 66 dogs: a retrospective study. J Small Anim Pract 2005;46(7):317–21.
87. Day MJ, Bilzer T, Mansell J, et al. Histopathological standards for the diagnosis of gastrointestinal inflammation in endoscopic biopsy samples from the dog and

cat: a report from the World Small Animal Veterinary Association Gastrointestinal Standardization Group. J Comp Pathol 2008;138(Suppl 1):S1–43.

88. Dijkstra M, Kraus JS, Bosje JT, et al. Protein-losing enteropathy in Rottweilers. Tijdschr Diergeneeskd 2010;135(10):406–12.

89. Davenport DJ, Jergens AE, Remillard RL. Protein-losing enteropathy. In: Hand MS, Thatcher GD, Remillard RL, et al, editors. Small animal clinical nutrition. 5th edition. Topeka (KS): Mark Morris Institute; 2010. p. 1077–83.

90. Jensen GL, McGarvey N, Taraszewski R, et al. Lymphatic absorption of enterally fed structured triacylglycerol vs physical mix in a canine model. Am J Clin Nutr 1994;60(4):518–24.

91. Newton JD, McLoughlin MA, Birchard SJ, et al. Transport pathways of enterally administered medium-chain triglycerides in dogs. Paper presented at: Proceedings of the Iams Nutritional Symposium: Recent advances in canine and feline nutrition. San Francisco, 2000.

92. Moore LE. Protein-losing enteropathies. In: Bonagura JD, Twedt DC, editors, Kirk's current veterinary therapy XIV, vol. 14. St Louis (MO): Saunders Elsevier; 2009. p. 512–5.

93. Lane IF, Miller E, Twedt DC. Parenteral nutrition in the management of a dog with lymphocytic-plasmacytic enteritis and severe protein-losing enteropathy. Can Vet J 1999;40(10):721–4.

94. Chan DL. Colloids: current recommendations. Vet Clin North Am Small Anim Pract 2008;38(3):587–93, xi.

95. Cohn LA, Kerl ME, Lenox CE, et al. Response of healthy dogs to infusions of human serum albumin. Am J Vet Res 2007;68(6):657–63.

96. Martin LG, Luther TY, Alperin DC, et al. Serum antibodies against human albumin in critically ill and healthy dogs. J Am Vet Med Assoc 2008;232(7):1004–9.

97. Mathews KA. The therapeutic use of 25% human serum albumin in critically ill dogs and cats. Vet Clin North Am Small Anim Pract 2008;38(3):595–605, xi–xii.

98. Trow AV, Rozanski EA, Delaforcade AM, et al. Evaluation of use of human albumin in critically ill dogs: 73 cases (2003–2006). J Am Vet Med Assoc 2008;233(4):607–12.

99. Mathews KA, Barry M. The use of 25% human serum albumin: outcome and efficacy in raising serum albumin and systemic blood pressure in critically ill dogs and cats. J Vet Emerg Crit Care (San Antonio) 2005;15:110–8.

100. Vigano F, Perissinotto L, Bosco VR. Administration of 5% human serum albumin in critically ill small animal patients with hypoalbuminemia: 418 dogs and 170 cats (1994–2008). J Vet Emerg Crit Care (San Antonio) 2010;20(2):237–43.

101. Yuki M, Sugimoto N, Takahashi K, et al. A case of protein-losing enteropathy treated with methotrexate in a dog. J Vet Med Sci 2006;68(4):397–9.

102. Vaden SL. Protein-losing enteropathies. In: Steiner JM, editor. Small animal gastroenterology. Hannover (Germany): Schlütersche; 2008. p. 207–10.

Alimentary Lymphoma in Cats and Dogs

Tracy Gieger, DVM

KEYWORDS

- Lymphoma • Lymphosarcoma • Chemotherapy • Cancer
- Lymphoid neoplasia • Gastrointestinal neoplasia

FELINE ALIMENTARY LYMPHOMA

Lymphoma is the most common feline malignancy, and the gastrointestinal (GI) tract is the most common location for this disease.[1] Alimentary lymphoma may affect the upper or lower GI tract, liver, or pancreas, and is characterized by infiltration with neoplastic lymphocytes with or without mesenteric lymph node involvement. Lymphoma can be divided histopathologically into small cell (lymphocytic [LL]; low grade; well differentiated) or large cell (lymphoblastic [LBL]; high grade) types. At one institution, feline GI lymphoma was equally divided among those types,[2] but in another study LL occurred 3 times more often than LBL.[3] Large granular lymphoma (LGL) is a subtype that is characterized by the presence of natural killer T lymphocytes that have characteristic intracytoplasmic granules.[4,5] Clinically these types of lymphoma are distinct entities with different clinical presentations, therapies, and outcomes.

Etiology and Pathogenesis

Although infection with feline leukemia virus (FeLV) and feline immunodeficiency virus (FIV) are major risk factors for the development of lymphoma, cats with GI lymphoma are usually negative for both viruses.[1,2] *Helicobacter* infection may play a role in the development of feline GI lymphoma.[6] In one study, gastric biopsy samples from 16 of 24 cats with lymphoma were positive for *Helicobacter heilmannii*. The potential importance of this infection is that eradication of the bacteria with antibiotics may resolve or hinder the progression of the underlying neoplasm. Exposure to cigarette smoke is another risk factor for development of lymphoma in cats. Cats living in households with any exposure to cigarette smoke have a 2.4-fold increased risk of developing lymphoma than cats from nonsmoking households, and the amount and duration of exposure is linearly correlated with increasing risk of lymphoma development.[7]

Department of Veterinary Clinical Sciences, Louisiana State University School of Veterinary Medicine, Skip Bertman Drive, Baton Rouge, LA 70803, USA
E-mail address: tgieger@vetmed.lsu.edu

Vet Clin Small Anim 41 (2011) 419–432
doi:10.1016/j.cvsm.2011.02.001
0195-5616/11/$ – see front matter © 2011 Elsevier Inc. All rights reserved.
vetsmall.theclinics.com

Signalment, History, and Physical Examination

Alimentary lymphoma has been reported in cats ranging in age from 1 to 20 years (median 13 years), with most cats being middle-aged to older.[1]

Lymphocytic lymphoma is typically a slowly progressive disease with a protracted history (**Table 1**). In one study, the median duration of clinical signs of illness before diagnosis was 6 months.[8] Clinical signs included weight loss, vomiting, diarrhea, anorexia or hyporexia, and lethargy.[2] Physical examination findings in cats with LL may be unremarkable or can reveal diffusely thickened intestinal loops, a mass lesion consisting of mesenteric lymph nodes, and/or an intramural intestinal mass.[2]

Lymphoblastic lymphoma is most often characterized by an acute onset of weight loss, vomiting, diarrhea, anorexia or hyporexia, and icterus if concurrent liver involvement is present (see **Table 1**). The physical examination often reveals dehydration,

Table 1 Lymphocytic versus lymphoblastic lymphoma		
Clinical signs of illness	Gradual weight loss, vomiting, diarrhea, decreased appetite	Rapid weight loss, anorexia, vomiting, diarrhea, icterus
Duration of clinical signs	Typically prolonged (weeks to months)	Typically acute (days to weeks)
Physical examination findings	May be normal; thickened bowel loops; palpable masses uncommon	Palpable mass lesions common; hepatomegaly; icterus
Diagnostic workup	Rule out non-GI causes of weight loss; endoscopy versus full-thickness surgical biopsy required for definitive diagnosis	Aspiration cytology of mass lesions, mesenteric lymph nodes or abnormal liver usually diagnostic
Pitfalls of diagnostic testing and therapy	False negatives common when enlarged mesenteric lymph nodes are aspirated; histopathology to differentiate from inflammatory bowel disease can be challenging	Hepatic lipidosis and pancreatitis may be concurrent diseases
Surgical intervention	Useful to obtain samples for diagnosis	Therapeutic if obstructing mass lesions are present
Therapy	Oral chemotherapy: prednisone and chlorambucil; radiation therapy may be useful to prolong survival	Injectable chemotherapy: CHOP (cyclophosphamide, doxorubicin, vincristine, prednisone ± L-asparaginase ± methotrexate), CCNU (lomustine), MOPP (mustargen, vincristine, prednisone, procarbazine); radiation therapy may be useful to prolong survival
Response to therapy	75%–90% response rate	50%–60% response rate
Outcome	Most cats live >2 years and are managed long term with chemotherapy	Median survival 6–7 months; if complete response to therapy 40% chance of living a year or longer

hepatomegaly, an abdominal mass consisting of mesenteric lymph nodes or an intramural mass, and/or diffusely thickened intestinal loops.[3]

Diagnosis of Lymphoma

Lymphoma should be suspected in cats with thickened intestinal loops, mesenteric lymphadenopathy, intestinal masses, or multicentric organ infiltration. For cats with a history of gastrointestinal illness, weight loss, or hyporexia/anorexia, a thorough workup to identify primary and concurrent diseases is indicated. Baseline bloodwork including a complete blood count (CBC), chemistry panel, thyroid function testing, and urinalysis is essential. Testing for FeLV and FIV is generally indicated in any sick cat. For cats with suspected neoplasia, 3-view (ventrodorsal or dorsoventral, right and left lateral views) thoracic radiographs should be obtained to rule out gross metastatic disease. Abdominal radiography can be helpful to evaluate cats for the presence of abdominal masses, GI outflow tract obstruction, organomegaly, and constipation. Abdominal ultrasonography is indicated to evaluate intestinal wall thickness, to document the presence of GI outflow tract obstructions, to identify mass lesions and changes in liver/spleen parenchyma, and to evaluate mesenteric lymph nodes.

CBC abnormalities in cats with GI lymphoma may include anemia (usually nonregenerative anemia of chronic disease or regenerative anemia secondary to intestinal blood loss) and neutrophilia (secondary to inflammation, neoplasia, or stress). Biochemical abnormalities may include hypoalbuminemia and/or panhypoproteinemia secondary to intestinal loss; in one study, 49% of cats with LL and 50% of cats with LBL were hypoalbuminemic.[3] Increased liver enzymes may indicate hepatic lymphoma or concurrent liver disease (hepatic lipidosis, cholangiohepatitis). Bone marrow aspiration and cytology is recommended as part of systemic staging for lymphoma in cats that are FeLV positive or in cats with cytopenias or circulating malignant lymphocytes. Polymerase chain reaction (PCR) of the bone marrow for detection of FeLV should be considered if a bone marrow aspirate is obtained.

Because the ileum is the sole site of cobalamin (vitamin B12) absorption, low serum cobalamin concentrations support a diagnosis of primary intestinal disease in cats with normal exocrine pancreatic function. In addition, determination of serum feline pancreatic lipase immunoreactivity may be useful, as the clinical signs of feline pancreatitis may be difficult to distinguish from those of GI lymphoma.

Ultrasound findings in cats with LL are usually indistinguishable from those with inflammatory bowel disease (IBD), and consist of normal or increased intestinal wall thickness with preservation of intestinal layers.[2,9] Mesenteric lymphadenopathy, intestinal intussusceptions, or distinct intramural mass lesions may also be noted. In a recent study evaluating differences in ultrasound findings between cats with LL versus IBD, thickening of the muscularis propria was present in 12.5% of normal cats, 4.2% of cats with IBD, and 48.4% of cats with LL.[10] Cats with lymphoma were 18 times more likely to have a thickened muscularis layer than were cats with IBD (**Figs. 1** and **2**). Mesenteric lymphadenopathy was present in 47% of cats with LL and 17% of cats with IBD. Of the cats with lymphoma, 26% had both muscularis thickening and lymphadenopathy, whereas only 1 of 24 cats with IBD had this combination of findings. In another study of 16 cats with LL, mesenteric lymphadenopathy was present on ultrasonography in 12 cats, diffuse small intestinal wall thickening in 9, and a focal intestinal mass in 1.[2] The diagnostic value of cytologic evaluation of an ultrasound-guided aspiration of enlarged mesenteric lymph nodes for confirmation of LL was reported to be questionable: benign lymphoid hyperplasia was diagnosed in 9 of 12 cats with LL and abdominal lymphadenopathy. However, when surgical

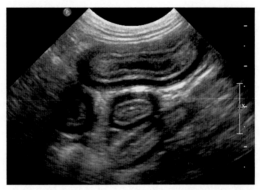

Fig. 1. Abdominal ultrasonogram of a cat with lymphocytic lymphoma (LL). The hypoechoic small intestinal muscularis layer is diffusely thickened. Although this change is not specific, it has been reported to occur more frequently in cats with LL as well as in cats with IBD. (*Courtesy of* Dr L. Gaschen, Louisiana State University.)

biopsies were obtained of the affected lymph nodes, lymphoma was confirmed in 8 of 9 cases.[2]

Ultrasound findings in cats with LBL may include transmural intestinal thickening, disruption of normal wall layering, reduced wall echogenicity, localized hypomotility, abdominal lymphadenomegaly, and mass lesions (**Fig. 3**).[10] Concurrent liver involvement may also be present, as evidenced by a hyperechoic or hypoechoic liver. Pancreatic and splenic involvement may also be noticed. The presence of diffuse echogenicity changes and/or nodular lesions in these organs supports possible infiltration with lymphoma.[10]

The optimal approach to definitively diagnosing feline GI lymphoma varies among clinicians. Fine-needle aspiration and cytology of intestinal masses, enlarged mesenteric lymph nodes, or the liver may be diagnostic for lymphoma, and are relatively noninvasive and rapid diagnostic methods. However, the presence of inflammation and/or lymphoid reactivity may hinder a definitive diagnosis, and histopathology of

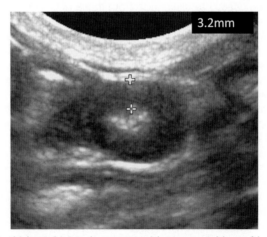

Fig. 2. Moderately thickened jejunal segment with transmural loss of layering in an older cat with lymphocytic lymphoma. (*Courtesy of* Dr L. Gaschen, Louisiana State University.)

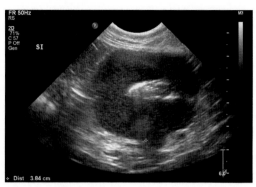

Fig. 3. Large jejunal mass of 3.84 cm diameter with transmural loss of layering in a vomiting cat with lymphoblastic lymphoma. (*Courtesy of* Dr L. Gaschen, Louisiana State University.)

tissue biopsies may be necessary to confirm the diagnosis of lymphoma. Controversy exists regarding whether endoscopically or surgically obtained intestinal biopsies are most helpful to differentiate feline IBD from GI lymphoma.

Surgically versus endoscopically obtained intestinal biopsies

The obvious advantage of surgically obtained biopsies is that they are transmural and therefore include all of the layers of the GI tract, allowing the pathologist to evaluate the disease process thoroughly. In addition, the clinician can obtain biopsies of the mesenteric lymph nodes, liver, and pancreas during the laparotomy. Disadvantages of surgery include longer anesthesia time and a more invasive procedure followed by a period of wound healing in an often debilitated cat. In a recent study of 43 cats with chronic signs of illness related to the GI tract, full-thickness biopsies were obtained.[11] Twenty-three percent of cats were diagnosed with LL; the majority of cats had IBD (46.5%), and fewer cats had fibrosis (9.3%), gastritis (7%), lymphangiectasia (7%), and mast cell tumors (4.7%).

In a study of 17 cats with LL diagnosed via full-thickness GI biopsies, lymphoma was detected in the stomach (33%), duodenum (83%), jejunum (100%), ileum (93%), mesenteric lymph nodes (59%), liver (27%), colon (20%), and pancreas (7%); however, not all sites were biopsied in all cats.[2] All but one cat had lymphoma present in multiple biopsied sites and in 4 cats, IBD was present in other parts of the intestinal tract. Concurrent GI tract diseases including chronic pancreatitis (n = 1), neutrophilic cholangitis (n = 1), and hepatic lipidosis (n = 1) were also diagnosed.

The advantage of endoscopic biopsy is that it is a less invasive, shorter procedure that is often better suited to a critically ill feline than is exploratory laparotomy. Furthermore, it allows visualization of the mucosa, which helps to identify the best sites for collection of biopsies. The skills and persistence of the endoscopist are critical in obtaining diagnostic samples. In a recent study,[12] "marginal" duodenal biopsy samples were defined as samples with the presence of at least one villus plus subvillous lamina propria, and "adequate" samples had at least 3 villi and subvillous lamina propria that extended to the muscularis mucosa. If 6 marginal or adequate samples of the feline stomach or duodenum were obtained, the correct histologic diagnosis was very likely to be achieved. Once endoscopic biopsies are obtained, sample handling to properly orient the samples for the pathologist is critical for optimal interpretation.

The disadvantage of endoscopy is that biopsies are limited to the gastric, duodenal, ileal, and colonic mucosa. In addition, detection of lymphoma in deeper tissues (submucosal/muscularis/serosal layers) is often difficult because of the limited depth of the biopsy specimen. A study of 22 cats (12 with IBD and 10 with LL) examined differences in histopathology results between endoscopic biopsy samples that had been collected immediately before exploratory laparotomy and full-thickness GI biopsy specimens collected during the surgical procedure.[13] Of the 10 cats diagnosed with LL, full-thickness surgical biopsies revealed jejunal and ileal involvement, and 9 of 10 had duodenal involvement. Lymphoma was also detected in the mesenteric lymph nodes, the liver, or both. Evaluation of gastric biopsies revealed no significant difference in the ability to diagnose lymphoma between full-thickness and endoscopically obtained biopsies. Because the pylorus could not be passed in 8 of 22 cats because of the large size of the endoscope (chosen in an attempt to obtain large biopsy specimens), one-third of the duodenal biopsies had to be obtained blindly (with collection of only 3 samples per cat). When comparing the method used to obtain duodenal samples, 9 cats were diagnosed with LL via full-thickness biopsies and only 1 was definitively diagnosed via endoscopy. The study clearly demonstrates that the suboptimal endoscopic technique has a significant impact on the diagnostic accuracy of the method; however, it does not evaluate the diagnostic value of a thorough duodenoscopy with sampling of adequate numbers of good-quality samples. Overall, it underscores the fact that the quality of the endoscopist's work significantly influences the diagnostic value of upper GI endoscopy.

In some veterinary clinics, the use of laparoscopy has largely replaced the need for laparotomy.[14] This less invasive technique has many of the advantages of laparotomy, with a significantly shorter recovery period.

Histopathologic evaluation of biopsy specimens

Histologically, IBD is characterized by a diffuse infiltration of various proportions of lymphocytes, plasma cells, eosinophils, neutrophils, and/or macrophages that are primarily found in the mucosal layer of the intestine. Lymphoma causes mucosal infiltration by neoplastic lymphocytes that are often irregularly distributed between and among intestinal villi, with frequent progression to submucosal and transmural infiltration (**Fig. 4**).[11,15] Lymphoma is not associated with mucosal edema or inflammation that typically occurs with IBD.[2,3] LL and LGL typically consist of T cells, and LBL

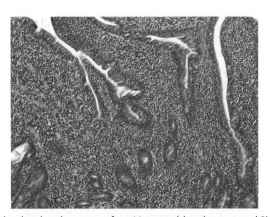

Fig. 4. Section of the duodenal mucosa of an 11-year-old male neutered Siamese cat with an 8-month history of chronic diarrhea and intermittent vomiting. There is villus blunting, and the lamina propria is expanded by small neoplastic lymphocytes (hematoxylin-eosin stain, original magnification ×100). (*Courtesy of* Dr N. Wakamatsu, Louisiana State University.)

consists of B cells.[2,8] Epitheliotropic intestinal lymphoma (EIL) is a subset of LL that is characterized by infiltration of malignant T cells into the mucosal epithelium of the intestinal tract.[9] In one study,[2] evidence of concurrent IBD was diagnosed in 3 of 19 cats diagnosed with LL.

The use of immunohistochemistry (IHC) for B-cell and T-cell markers may help to distinguish IBD from LL because cats with lymphoma should have a monoclonal population of B or T lymphocytes (**Fig. 5**). In one study, of 32 cats diagnosed with LL based on routine hematoxylin-eosin stains, 16% of cases were reclassified as having IBD, based on a mixed population of B and T cells and plasma cells after IHC was performed.[15] Immunohistochemistry results may be difficult to interpret because staining techniques and the antibodies used vary among laboratories, and there is often inconsistent stain uptake in cells of an individual tumor and between tumors from the same species. Also, the presence of T lymphocytes alone is not diagnostic for lymphoma because of MALT (mucosal-associated lymphoid tissue), which consists primarily of T cells and is expanded in cases of intestinal inflammation.

The use of PCR may be useful to confirm the diagnosis of GI lymphoma, because detection of a clonal expansion of either B or T lymphocytes would be diagnostic for lymphoma, while a mixed population of lymphoid cells supports a diagnosis of IBD. In a study of intestinal biopsies from 28 cats with intestinal T-cell lymphoma diagnosed by light microscopy and IHC, 22 had clonal rearrangements of their T-cell receptor gamma genes; this is in contrast to a polyclonal arrangement of receptors in 9 cats with IBD.[16]

Treatment Options and Prognosis for Cats with Lymphoma

Surgery for cats with obstructing GI masses is indicated to relieve the obstruction and discomfort associated with the mass. Complete resection may not be possible in some cases, however, and dehiscence of the anastomosis site must be considered as a possible complication. Surgical excision of intestinal masses should be followed by biopsy of other parts of the GI tract, liver, pancreas, and mesenteric lymph nodes, because it is rare to have a solitary mass of lymphoma with no concurrent organ involvement. Postoperative chemotherapy is indicated because lymphoma is almost always considered a multicentric disease, but a gold-standard protocol does not exist. Selection of a chemotherapy protocol depends on the type of lymphoma (lymphocytic

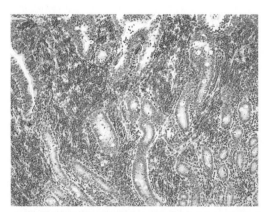

Fig. 5. Same biopsy as in **Fig. 4**. The majority of neoplastic cells stain positive for CD3. Diagnosis: T-cell lymphoma, LL (CD3 immunohistochemistry, original magnification ×100). (*Courtesy of* Dr N. Wakamatsu, Louisiana State University.)

vs lymphoblastic), as well as patient-associated factors including concurrent disease and owner-associated factors such as finances, ability to medicate the cat, and ability to return for rechecks. In general, cats with LL have better responses to therapy and longer survival times than those with LBL. In one study of cats with alimentary lymphoma treated with various chemotherapy protocols, 50 cats with LL had a complete response (CR) rate of 69% and a median survival time (MST) of 17 months as compared with an 18% CR rate and an MST of 3 months for 17 cats with LBL.[3]

Lymphocytic lymphoma is typically a slowly progressive disease, and chlorambucil, a chemotherapeutic agent that targets slowly dividing lymphocytes, is used along with steroids such as prednisone or prednisolone (**Table 2**). There is some debate about whether chlorambucil should be administered as a bolus dose (a single large dose every 3 weeks) or every other day continuous dosing. Because cats will potentially be treated with chlorambucil for several months to year(s), the clinician must determine a therapeutic plan that is suitable for both the cat and the client. The potential advantages of the bolus-dosing regimen include (1) less owner exposure to chemotherapy and (2) less continuous exposure of the cat to chemotherapy.[17]

In one study of 42 cats with LL treated with prednisone (5–10 mg orally [PO] every 24 h) and chlorambucil (2 mg PO every 48–72 h), there was an overall response rate of 95% with a 56% CR rate (ie, 100% resolution of clinical signs and detectable tumor) and 39% partial response (PR) rate (ie, >50% but <100% decrease in the amount of measurable disease).[8] For cats achieving a CR to therapy, the median remission duration was 897 days as compared with 428 days for cats achieving a PR. Twelve cats died of lymphoma during the study period (median follow-up time of 476 days). Overall, the MST of affected cats was 704 days. In another study of 17 cats with LL treated with either prednisone (1–2 mg/kg PO every 24–48 hours) and chlorambucil (15 mg/m^2 PO every 24 hours for 4 consecutive days every 3 weeks) or a multidrug injectable chemotherapy protocol (including vincristine, cyclophosphamide, doxorubicin, and L-asparaginase), the CR rate was 76% with a median remission duration of 19 months (range, 3.5–73 months).[2]

In one study of 28 cats with LL (24 were diagnosed via full-thickness biopsy) treated with prednisone and chlorambucil, the clinical response rate was 96%.[17] In this study, IHC confirmed that 94% of cases were of T-cell origin. Rescue therapy with cyclophosphamide was successful in 7 of 9 cats that developed recurrence of clinical signs of their of their disease during treatment with chlorambucil (complete restaging was not always performed). The median duration of clinical remission was 786 days. Of interest, 4 of 28 cats developed a second, unrelated malignancy.

There are few studies that address rescue chemotherapy for cats with LL, because many cats do not develop clinical relapse and survival times are typically long (**Table 3**). Cyclophosphamide has been used as a rescue therapy, with good responses.[17] Other drugs typically used to treat LBL including (but not limited to) vincristine, vinblastine, doxorubicin, and L-asparaginase could be used to attempt reinduction of clinical remission. Additional considerations for cats with recurrent clinical signs include repeat staging (ultrasonography, endoscopy) to look for new concurrent diseases and/or the progression of LL to the lymphoblastic form; this has not been well described, however.

Because cats with LBL are often severely ill at the time of diagnosis, intensive supportive care in addition to chemotherapy is warranted. This treatment may include intravenous (IV) fluid therapy, blood products, IV antibiotics, and enteral or parenteral nutrition. For cats with LBL, multidrug protocols are the most widely studied, and COP (cyclophosphamide, vincristine, prednisone) or CHOP (cyclophosphamide, doxorubicin, vincristine, prednisone ± L-asparaginase ± methotrexate) based protocols

Table 2
Chlorambucil + prednisone chemotherapy protocols for cats with lymphocytic lymphoma

Chlorambucil Dose (PO)	Prednisone Dose (PO)	Response Rate	Median Response Duration (months)	Median Survival Time (months)	Comments	References
2 mg every 48–72 h	5 or 10 mg/cat/d	56% CR 39% PR	30 mo if CR 14 mo if PR	n/a		8
15 mg/m² every 24 h × 4 d every 3 wk	3 mg/kg every 24 h then 1–2 mg/kg when remission is achieved	76% CR	19 mo	19 mo if CR; 4 mo if not CR		2
15 mg/m² every 24 h × 4 d every 3 wk	3 mg/kg every 24 h then 1–2 mg/kg when remission is achieved	69% CR	16 mo	17 mo overall; 23 mo if CR		3
20 mg/m² every 2 wk (round to nearest 2 mg tablet size)	Variable	96% CR	26 mo		Good response to cyclophosphamide when clinical relapse occurred	17

Abbreviations: CR, complete response (100% of clinically evident disease resolved); n/a, no data available; PO, by mouth; PR, partial response (>50% but <100% of clinically evident disease resolved).

Table 3
Chemotherapy protocols for cats with lymphoblastic lymphoma

Drugs	Response Rate	Median Response Duration (months)	Median Survival Time (months)	Comments	References
CHOP	18% CR	n/a	2.7 mo	Part of a larger study comparing lymphocytic and lymphoblastic alimentary lymphoma	3
COP	75% CR	8 mo	9 mo	If CR, 51% clinical remission rate at 1 y and 38% at 2 y; cats that did not achieve CR usually did not live 1 y	26,a,b
COP	32% CR	7 mo if CR	n/a	n/a	32,a
COP or COP then doxorubicin	n/a	3 mo if COP; 9 mo if COP then doxorubicin	n/a	Study comparing COP to doxorubicin maintenance therapy	18,a,b
CVM	52%	4 mo	n/a	Addition of prednisone and L-asparaginase did not improve results	24,a,b
CVM-L	62% CR 20% PR		7 mo if CR; 2.5 mo if PR	Cats with minimal response to therapy: MST 1.5 mo; FeLV + worse prognosis; cats with stages I and II lymphoma had a better prognosis	23,a,b
Doxorubicin	42%	Median 2 mo; 3 mo if CR		Cats with CR to therapy and FeLV-negative cats have a better prognosis	19,a,b
Doxorubicin	22% response	n/a	n/a	Doxorubicin used as a rescue therapy; small cell lymphoma and cats receiving drugs in addition to doxorubicin were more likely to respond to therapy; not thought to be an effective rescue therapy	33,a,b
CHOP-L-M	47% CR 37% PR	22 mo if CR 4 mo if PR	22 mo if CR 4 mo if PR		27,a,b
CHOP-L-M	n/a	5 mo	10 mo	Longer duration of first remission resulted in longer survival time	25,a
CHOP-L-M	74% CR 14% PR	9 mo if CR	10 mo if CR	6-mo clinical remission rate 75%; 1-y clinical remission rate 50%	21,a,b

Abbreviations: C, cyclophosphamide; CR, complete response (100% of clinically evident disease resolved); FeLV, feline leukemia virus; H, hydroxydaunorubicin, doxorubicin; L, L-asparaginase; M, methotrexate; MST, median survival time; O, vincristine; P, prednisone or prednisolone; PR, partial response (>50% but <100% of clinically evident disease resolved); V, vincristine.

a A diagnosis of lymphoma was confirmed in these studies; however, it was not documented whether it was lymphocytic or lymphoblastic.
b Not all cats in these studies had alimentary lymphoma.

have been shown to have better efficacy than single-agent protocols and steroids alone.[18,19] Recently, CCNU (lomustine) used as a single agent or in combination with steroids has been shown to be effective in the treatment of feline lymphoma, and appears to be a reasonable treatment option for many cats.[20] In general, cats are less responsive to chemotherapy than dogs when they are treated for LBL. Most studies document response rates for cats with LBL at approximately 50% to 75% with an MST of 7 to 9 months.[21–28] One of the few consistent prognostic indicators in cats treated for LBL is response to therapy; several studies have documented that cats that have a CR to therapy have longer survival times than those that only have a PR to therapy.[23,25] Other possible indicators of prognosis include the World Health Organization stage of disease. Cats with stage 1 (single extranodal or lymphoid site) and stage 2 (regional lymphadenopathy or resectable GI mass) lymphoma have longer survival times than other stages.[23] Finally, a positive FeLV antigen test is considered a negative prognostic factor, because cats infected with this virus typically die of viral-associated syndromes even if therapy for lymphoma is effective.[21]

LGL is an uncommon form of feline alimentary lymphoma that has a poor prognosis.[5] In a study of 45 cats with LGL, all cats tested negative for retroviruses. Twenty-three cats were treated with chemotherapy. Thirty percent responded, and the MST was 57 days (range, 0–267 days). Prognostic factors for improved survival were not detected.

In general, cats tolerate chemotherapy very well and clinically significant neutropenia is uncommon.[22] In a recently published survey of 31 owners whose cats were undergoing COP chemotherapy, 83% of owners were happy that they treated their cats and 87% stated they would treat another cat.[22]

Dietary modifications should be considered as part of the treatment protocol for cats with lymphoma. Diets should be highly digestible and palatable. For cats with concurrent IBD, hypoallergenic diets should be considered. For cats that are anorexic or hyporexic, enteral nutritional support should be provided by means of an esophageal or gastric feeding tube. Appetite stimulants such as cyproheptadine and mirtazapine may also be helpful. For many cats, once chemotherapy (including steroids) is initiated, the appetite improves and the tube can be removed.

Parenteral cobalamin supplementation should be considered even if serum concentrations are not measured, because the prevalence of hypocobalaminemia in cats with GI lymphoma was reported to be 78% in one study.[8] In another study of cats with a history of clinical signs related to the GI tract and confirmed severe hypocobalaminemia (<100 ng/L), the serum cobalamin concentrations and mean body weight increased, and signs of GI disease improved in the majority of animals after 4 weeks of administration of cobalamin at a dose of 250 μg subcutaneously once weekly.[26] Limitations of this study included that the cats did not have biopsy-confirmed diagnoses of GI disease and that the majority of cats were receiving other therapy (steroids, antibiotics) concurrently with vitamin B12 supplementation.

Radiation therapy for alimentary lymphoma may be an underutilized treatment modality in cats, because lymphoma is generally a radiation-responsive disease. Radiotherapy is used successfully for the treatment of solitary site lymphomas, including nasal and spinal lymphoma. In a pilot study of 8 cats with LBL treated with 6 weeks of standard multidrug chemotherapy followed by 10 daily 1.5-Gy fractions of radiation, 5 of 8 cats had long-term (>266 days) progression-free survival.[29] Radiation therapy was well tolerated. Further studies are warranted that will hopefully result in prolongation of survival times in cats with alimentary lymphoma.

CANINE ALIMENTARY LYMPHOMA

Alimentary lymphoma is less common in dogs than in cats, representing only 7% of all canine lymphomas. Alimentary lymphoma in dogs may be part of the syndrome of multicentric lymphoma (ie, peripheral lymph nodes ± other organ systems), but most commonly, it is confined to the GI tract.[30] In one study of 18 dogs with alimentary LBL, 13 (72%) had lymphoma confined to the intestinal tract, and lymphoma was part of multicentric disease in the remaining 5 (28%). Unlike in cats, lymphocytic lymphoma of the alimentary tract is rare. The majority of dogs have rapidly progressive clinical signs associated with lymphoblastic lymphoma, including (in decreasing order of frequency) vomiting, diarrhea, weight loss, anorexia, and lethargy.[31] Physical examination findings in dogs with LBL may include ascites, poor body condition, a palpable abdominal mass, abdominal pain, and thickened intestinal loops. Staging tests are similar to those for feline lymphoma. The most common biochemical abnormality is hypoalbuminemia (which occurs in 61%–80% of dogs); and hypercalcemia is uncommon. The majority of alimentary lymphomas in dogs are of T-cell origin.[30,31]

Chemotherapy and supportive care are the mainstays of the treatment of alimentary lymphoma in dogs. The overall response rate to treatment with a multidrug chemotherapy protocol (vincristine, L-asparaginase, cyclophosphamide, doxorubicin, prednisone, lomustine, procarbazine, mustargen) was 56% in the largest published study of dogs with alimentary lymphoma.[30] For the responders, the overall median first remission duration was 86 days and the MST was 117 days. Dogs that did not respond to treatment were euthanized a median of 10 days after initiation of therapy. Dogs with diarrhea as a presenting complaint had a worse prognosis, with 13 diarrheic dogs having an MST of 70 days versus 700 days for 5 dogs without diarrhea. Similar to cats with alimentary LBL, intensive fluid therapy and nutritional support (enteral or parenteral) is indicated concurrently with chemotherapy in clinically ill dogs with alimentary lymphoma.

SUMMARY

This article presents a review of feline and canine alimentary GI lymphoma. Gastrointestinal lymphoma should be suspected in animals with an acute or prolonged history of clinical signs of disease related to the GI tract. Systemic staging tests (CBC/chemistry/urinalysis/thyroxin levels/thoracic radiographs) are used to identify concurrent disease. Abdominal ultrasonography is useful for the documentation of intestinal wall thickening, mass lesions, concurrent organ involvement, lymphadenopathy, and abdominal lymphadenopathy. The ultrasonographic findings can be used to decide whether the next diagnostic test should be laparotomy, laparoscopy, or endoscopy, with the goal of obtaining diagnostic histologic specimens. Histopathologically, lymphoma may be lymphoblastic or lymphocytic; these diseases have different therapies and prognosis. Chemotherapy, including steroids and nutritional support, are essential in the management of alimentary lymphoma.

REFERENCES

1. Louwerens M, London CL, Pedersen NC, et al. Feline lymphoma in the post-feline leukemia virus era. J Vet Intern Med 2005;19:329–35.
2. Lingard AE, Briscoe K, Beatty JA, et al. Low-grade alimentary lymphoma (LGAL): clinicopathological findings and response to treatment in 17 cases. J Feline Med Surg 2009;11:692–700.

3. Fondacaro JV, Richter KP, Carpenter JL, et al. Feline gastrointestinal lymphoma: 67 cases. Eur J Comp Gastroenterol 1999;4(2):69–74.

4. Wellman ML, Hammer AS, DiBartola SP, et al. Lymphoma involving large granular lymphocytes in cats: 11 cases. J Am Vet Med Assoc 1992;201(8):1265–9.

5. Krick EL, Little L, Shofer FS, et al. Description of clinical and pathological findings, treatment and outcome of feline large granular lymphocyte lymphoma. Vet Comp Oncol 2008;6(2):102–10.

6. Bridgeford EC, Marini RP, Feng Y, et al. Gastric *Helicobacter* species as a cause of feline gastric lymphoma. Vet Immunol Immunopathol 2008;123:106–13.

7. Bertone ER, Snyder LA, Moore AS. Environmental tobacco smoke and risk of malignant lymphoma in pet cats. Am J Epidemiol 2002;156(3):268–73.

8. Kiselow MA, Rassnick KM, McDonough SP, et al. Outcome of cats with low-grade lymphocytic lymphoma: 41 cases. J Am Vet Med Assoc 2008;232(3):405–10.

9. Carreras JK, Goldschmidt M, Lamb M, et al. Feline epitheliotropic intestinal malignant lymphoma: 10 cases. J Vet Intern Med 2003;17:326–31.

10. Zwingenberger AL, Marks SL, Baker TW, et al. Ultrasonographic evaluation of the muscularis propria in cats with diffuse small intestinal lymphoma or inflammatory bowel disease. J Vet Intern Med 2010;24:289–92.

11. Kleinschmidt S, Harder J, Nolte I, et al. Chronic inflammatory and noninflammatory diseases of the gastrointestinal tract in cats: diagnostic advantages of full-thickness intestinal and extraintestinal biopsies. J Feline Med Surg 2010;12:97–103.

12. Willard MD, Mansell J, Fosgate GT, et al. Effect of sample quality on the sensitivity of endoscopic biopsy for detecting gastric and duodenal lesions in dogs and cats. J Vet Intern Med 2008;22:1084–9.

13. Evans SE, Bonczynski JJ, Broussard JD, et al. Comparison of endoscopic and full-thickness biopsy specimens for diagnosis of inflammatory bowel disease and alimentary tract lymphoma in cats. J Am Vet Med Assoc 2006;229(9):1447–50.

14. Webb CB. Feline laparoscopy for intestinal disease. Top Companion Anim Med 2008;23:193–9.

15. Waly NE, Gruffydd-Jones TJ, Stokes CR, et al. Immunohistochemical diagnosis of alimentary lymphomas and severe intestinal inflammation in cats. J Comp Pathol 2005;133:253–60.

16. Moore PF, Woo JC, Vernau W, et al. Characterization of feline T cell receptor gamma variable region genes for the molecular diagnosis of feline intestinal T cell lymphoma. Vet Immunol Immunopathol 2005;106:167–78.

17. Stein TJ, Pellin M, Steinberg H, et al. Treatment of feline gastrointestinal small-cell lymphoma with chlorambucil and glucocorticoids. J Am Anim Hosp Assoc 2010;46:413–7.

18. Moore AS, Cotter SM, Frimberger AE, et al. A comparison of doxorubicin and COP for maintenance of remission in cats with lymphoma. J Vet Intern Med 1996;10(6):372–5.

19. Kristal O, Lana SE, Ogilvie GK, et al. Single agent chemotherapy with doxorubicin for feline lymphoma: a retrospective study of 19 cases. J Vet Intern Med 2001;15:125–30.

20. Rassnick KM, Gieger TL, Williams LE, et al. Phase I evaluation of CCNU (lomustine) in tumor-bearing cats. J Vet Intern Med 2001;15:196–9.

21. Simon D, Eberle N, Laacke-Singer L, et al. Combination chemotherapy in feline lymphoma: treatment outcome, tolerability, and duration in 23 cats. J Vet Intern Med 2008;22:394–400.

22. Tzannes S, Hammond MF, Murphy S, et al. Owners' perception of their cats' quality of life during COP chemotherapy for lymphoma. J Feline Med Surg 2008;10:73–81.
23. Mooney SC, Hayes AA, MacEwen EG, et al. Treatment and prognostic factors in lymphoma in cats: 103 cases. J Am Vet Med Assoc 1989;194(5):696–9.
24. Jeglum KA, Whereat A, Young K. Chemotherapy of lymphoma in 75 cats. J Am Vet Med Assoc 1987;190(2):174–8.
25. Zwahlen CH, Lucroy MD, Kraegel SA, et al. Results of chemotherapy for cats with alimentary malignant lymphoma: 21 cases. J Am Vet Med Assoc 1998;213(8): 1144–9.
26. Teske E, vanStraten G, van Noort R, et al. Chemotherapy with cyclophosphamide, vincristine, and prednisolone. J Vet Intern Med 2002;16:179–86.
27. Milner RJ, Peyton J, Cooke K, et al. Response rates and survival times for cats with lymphoma treated with UWM chemotherapy protocol: 38 cases. J Am Vet Med Assoc 2005;227:1118–22.
28. Ruaux CG, Steiner JM, Williams DA. Early biochemical and clinical responses to cobalamin supplementation in cats with signs of gastrointestinal disease and severe hypocobalaminemia. J Vet Intern Med 2005;19:155–60.
29. Williams LE, Pruitt AF, Thrall DE. Chemotherapy followed by abdominal cavity irradiation for feline lymphoblastic lymphoma. Vet Radiol Ultrasound 2010;51(6): 681–7.
30. Rassnick KM, Moore AS, Collister KE, et al. Efficacy of combination chemotherapy for treatment of gastrointestinal lymphoma in dogs. J Vet Intern Med 2009;23:317–22.
31. Frank JD, Reimer SB, Kass PH, et al. Clinical outcomes of 30 cases of canine gastrointestinal lymphoma. J Am Anim Hosp Assoc 2007;43:313–21.
32. Mahoney OM, Moore AS, Cotter SM, et al. Alimentary lymphoma in cats: 28 cases. J Am Vet Med Assoc 1995;207(12):1593–7.
33. Oberthaler KT, Mauldin E, McManus P, et al. Rescue therapy with doxorubicin-based chemotherapy for relapsing or refractory feline lymphoma: a retrospective study of 23 cases. J Feline Med Surg 2009;11:259–65.

Granulomatous Colitis of Boxer Dogs

Melanie Craven, BVetMed, PhD, MRCVS[a],*,
Caroline S. Mansfield, BVMS, MVM[b],
Kenneth W. Simpson, BVM&S, PhD[a]

KEYWORDS

• Histiocytic ulcerative colitis • *E coli* • Enrofloxacin • IBD • AIEC

Granulomatous colitis (GC) is an uncommon type of inflammatory bowel disease (IBD), predominant in Boxer dogs younger than 4 years.[1–4] There are sporadic reports of GC in other dog breeds, particularly young French bulldogs,[5,6] and in the authors' observation. Affected dogs typically present with signs of colitis, hematochezia, and weight loss, progressing to cachexia in severe cases (**Fig. 1**).[1,7–9] GC was first reported in the United States in 1965[1] and later emerged in Australia, Japan, and Europe, becoming better known as histiocytic ulcerative colitis. However, the authors subscribe to the original name as described by Van Kruiningen and colleagues[1] for several reasons. First, this name more accurately reflects the histopathologic appearance of the inflammatory response, that is, a mix of macrophages, lymphocytes and neutrophils, almost invariably reported by pathologists as granulomatous inflammation (**Fig. 2**).[2,3,9–13] Second, a histiocyte is a fixed tissue macrophage, whereas the mucosa in GC is transiently packed with recruited macrophages that egress with successful treatment.[14]

The cytoplasm of macrophages in GC stains positive with periodic acid–Schiff (PAS) (see **Fig. 2**, inset), a unique and pathognomonic feature that is strikingly similar to that of Whipple disease in humans.[1] Whipple disease is a rare, systemic bacterial infection primarily affecting the small intestine. It is caused by *Tropheryma whipplei* and diagnosed by the presence of PAS-positive macrophages in intestinal biopsies.[15,16] Because of this similarity and following the occurrence of GC in 9 Boxer dogs from the same kennel, 6 of which responded to chloramphenicol treatment,[1] an infectious cause has long been suspected in GC. Thus, initial studies focused on searching for a GC-associated pathogen. Electron microscopic imaging of colon mucosa revealed occasional bacteria in 4 of 13 affected dogs and abundant coccobacillary structures resembling *Chlamydia* within the macrophages of 5 dogs.[17] In a later report of GC, the

The authors have nothing to disclose.
[a] Department of Veterinary Clinical Sciences, Cornell University, Tower Road, Ithaca, NY 14853–6401, USA
[b] University of Melbourne, 250 Princes Highway, Werribee, Victoria 3030, Australia
* Corresponding author. Department of Veterinary Clinical Sciences, VMC 2013, College of Veterinary Medicine, Cornell University, Tower Road, Ithaca, NY 14853–6401.
E-mail address: mdc57@cornell.edu

Vet Clin Small Anim 41 (2011) 433–445
doi:10.1016/j.cvsm.2011.01.003
0195-5616/11/$ – see front matter © 2011 Elsevier Inc. All rights reserved.

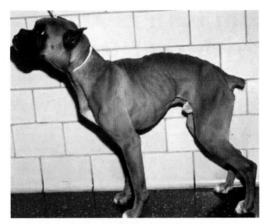

Fig. 1. Cachexia in a young Boxer dog with severe GC.

isolation of *Mycoplasma* spp from the colon of 4 of 11 dogs and the draining lymph nodes of 3 of 11 dogs raised the possibility of *Mycoplasma* as a causative agent. However, experimental inoculation of 8-week-old Boxer puppies with the isolated *Mycoplasma* spp did not induce GC.[18]

With no definitive evidence for a specific pathogen, other investigators suggested that the scant bacteria visualized within the superficial mucosa were opportune invaders of an inflamed and ulcerated mucosa.[7,19] A primary immune-mediated pathogenesis was presumed, and the mucosal immune response in GC was evaluated using immunohistochemistry.[7,19] This evaluation revealed increased numbers of IgG+ plasma cells, CD3+ T cells, L1 cells, and major histocompatibility complex class II cells, analogous to ulcerative colitis in humans.[20] Until 2004, the mainstay of treatment of GC involved immunosuppression with agents such as corticosteroids and azathioprine in combination with antibiotic therapy and dietary change.[3] Responses to treatment were generally poor, frequently resulting in euthanasia. GC became considered an incurable immune-mediated disease.[4–7,19]

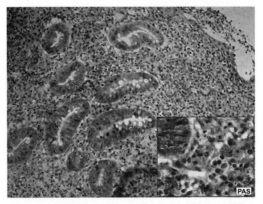

Fig. 2. GC-affected colon mucosa showing mucosal ulceration; goblet cell loss; and dense cellular infiltration with macrophages, lymphocytes, plasma cells, and eosinophils (hematoxylin-eosin, original magnification × 40). Inset: oamy macrophages positive on periodic acid–Schiff (PAS) staining, pathognomonic for GC (original magnification × 200).

RECENT DISCOVERIES
GC and Invasive Escherichia coli

The search for an infectious cause of GC was reignited by reports of long-term remission in dogs treated with enrofloxacin.[3,21–23] The application of culture-independent molecular methods, namely, immunohistochemistry and fluorescence in situ hybridization (FISH), enabled the identification of mucosally invasive E coli. Using a polyclonal E coli antibody, immunoreactivity was documented in the lamina propria macrophages and the regional lymph nodes of 10 affected dogs.[22] Also, immunostaining of colonic mucosa gave positive results with antibodies against Salmonella, Campylobacter, and Lawsonia intracellularis. Concurrent work using advanced molecular methods demonstrated the presence of metabolically active invasive E coli packed within colonic macrophages.[23] This finding was accomplished using FISH, a technique that uses fluorescent molecules attached to oligonucleotide probes that hybridize to bacterial 16S ribosomal DNA (rDNA). Fluorescent labeling enables clear visualization of bacterial morphology and spatial localization, even against a busy background of severe inflammation. In this study, FISH analysis was done in 13 dogs with GC with a eubacterial 16S rDNA library construction generated from GC mucosa. In all dogs evaluated, the authors discovered intramucosal and macrophage invasion exclusively by E coli (**Fig. 3**).[23] GC-associated E coli were shown to lack genes associated with virulence present in diarrheagenic E coli and were able to invade epithelial cells and persist within macrophages.[23] This pathogen-like behavior is similar to that of a newly identified E coli pathotype, the adherent and invasive E coli (AIEC) that is increasingly associated with Crohn's disease (CD) in humans.[24,25]

A direct causal role for E coli in GC pathogenesis is supported by the correlation between clinical remission of the disease and eradication of invasive E coli using enrofloxacin.[14,23] A series of 7 dogs with histologically confirmed GC and intramucosal E coli invasion confirmed by FISH were treated with enrofloxacin (7 ± 3 mg/kg/d for 9.5 ± 4 weeks) and reevaluated by repeat histology and FISH (**Fig. 4**).[14] Long-term clinical remission coincided with the eradication of invasive E coli in 4 dogs. In a relapsing case, the E coli were enrofloxacin resistant and the animal was euthanized because of refractory disease. The result of PAS staining in this study remained positive for more than 6 months despite remission of clinical signs and eradication of the

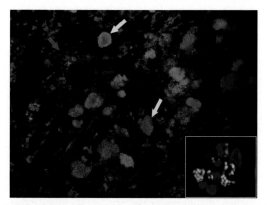

Fig. 3. FISH image (original magnification × 40) of GC colon mucosa showing typical clusters of E coli within the mucosa (*red arrow*) and intracellularly with macrophages (*yellow arrows*). Inset: invasive E coli within a macrophage. E coli-Cy3 probe (*red*) with non-EUB3386FAM (*green*) and 4′,6-diamidino-2-phenylindole (4′-6-diamidino-2-phenylindole [DAPI]) (nuclei in *blue*).

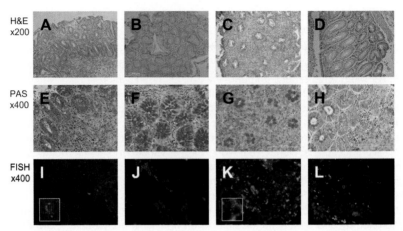

Fig. 4. Colon mucosa from 2 dogs with GC before and after enrofloxacin treatment. Pretreatment sections: histologically, (*A, C*) there is severe loss of glandular structure and cellular infiltration in both cases. Mucosal infiltration with macrophages that show positive with PAS (*E, G*) is a dominant feature. FISH (*I, K*) shows invasive *E coli* (*Insets I* and *K*, magnified *E coli* ×100). Posttreatment sections: 10 weeks after initial diagnosis in dog 1, inflammation is resolving, but mild PAS staining persists (*B, F*) and the result of FISH is negative for bacterial invasion (*J*). In dog 2, enrofloxacin resistance developed, and after 3 months of enrofloxacin treatment, severe inflammation and positive staining with PAS persist (*D, H*). Result of FISH remains positive for *E coli* invasion (*L*). (*A–D*) Hematoxylin-eosin, original magnification × 60; (*E–H*) PAS, original magnification × 60; and (*I–L*) FISH, original magnification × 60.

invasive *E coli*. The reasons for this positivity are not clear, but it is important to note that the complete histologic remission of disease seems to lag behind clinical improvement, a feature also reported in Whipple disease (see **Fig. 4**).[26]

The importance of appropriate antimicrobial selection in the treatment of GC was recently demonstrated in a prospective study of 14 GC cases.[27] In this study, the *E coli* isolates from 6 of 6 complete responders were enrofloxacin sensitive, whereas those from 4 of 4 nonresponders and 2 of 4 partial responders were enrofloxacin resistant. Clinical response was directly influenced by susceptibility of *E coli* to enrofloxacin (*P*<.01).

Taken as a whole, this evidence indicates a 1:1 correlation between GC and invasive *E coli* in 32 cases collectively evaluated by FISH to date.[14,23,27] This discovery has transformed the diagnostic approach, therapy, and prognosis of GC.

Genetics

Because GC is breed specific and rare, it is suspected to be an autosomal recessive genetic defect involving the immune system that confers susceptibility to *E coli* invasion. Research is currently being undertaken to identify the genetic basis of GC, and a genome-wide association scan (GWAS) is underway.[28,29] The principle of a GWAS is to observe the frequency with which certain alleles are present in affected and control groups in order to identify disease associations in candidate genes. The Broad Institute Dog Genome Project identified more than 2.5 million single nucleotide polymorphisms (SNPs) in the Boxer dog and 10 additional dog breeds and developed a custom canine SNP array the GeneChip Canine Genome 2.0 Array in collaboration with Affymetrix Inc, Santa Clara, CA, USA.[30,31] This array relies on the hybridization of fluorescently labeled fragments of SNP-containing DNA to complementary DNA olig-omers that are tiled on a silicon wafer. The SNP genotype calls are made using the integration of fluorescent signal intensities at each location.

The GWAS of GC has revealed GC-associated SNPs in the gene encoding neutrophil cytosolic factor (NCF) 2.[28,29] This gene encodes a cytosolic subunit, p67[phox], of the multiprotein complex NADPH oxidase.[32,33] Within phagocytes, NADPH oxidase plays a crucial role in innate immunity by reducing molecular oxygen to superoxide, gener-ating numerous toxic reactive oxygen species (ROS). ROS are used as microbicidal agents against pathogens in the respiratory burst generated by phagocytic cells.[34,35] An ineffective respiratory burst results in a compromised ability to eliminate intracellular pathogens, particularly catalase-producing bacteria and fungi.[36] Mutations in NCF2 in humans are known to cause chronic granulomatous disease (CGD), a disease complex comprising immunodeficiency disorders and predisposition to chronic infections.[36,37] Patients with CGD can develop colitis with striking histologic similarities to GC, including macrophages that stain positive with PAS.[37–39] The initial screening test for CGD in humans is the evaluation of the neutrophil respiratory burst in peripheral blood. The authors have recently evaluated a flow cytometric method of assessing the neutro-phil respiratory burst in dogs and have demonstrated marked reductions in the neutro-phil oxidative burst in 2 dogs with GC compared with healthy controls.[29] It is notable that a recent GWAS in human IBD has identified CD-associated SNPs in the gene encoding another NADPH oxidase complex subunit, NCF4.[40]

To summarize, a GWAS of GC has identified NCF2 (a gene associated with CGD in humans) as a candidate gene, and further disease mapping and phenotypic charac-terization by neutrophil function testing are ongoing. The bacteria involved in the gastrointestinal manifestations of CGD are poorly characterized, but their striking simi-larities with those involved in GC suggest a potential role for *E coli*. The identification of NCF2 in GC suggests that the Boxer dog may prove to be a useful model for CGD, but further work is required to confirm NCF2 gene involvement.

AIEC in Crohn's Disease

The association of AIEC with GC is similar to findings in humans with IBD, especially ileal CD, one of the most prevalent forms of IBD occurring in humans. CD is a hetero-geneous group of disorders resulting from the convergence of multiple factors such as genetically determined susceptibility, altered immune tolerance of the enteric bacteria, and environmental triggers. The role of the resident microflora in CD pathogenesis was initially thought to arise from a lack of immunologic tolerance and an overly aggressive T-cell response to microbial components in individuals with genetic susceptibility (eg, nucleotide-binding oligomerization domain containing 2 [NOD2] mutation).[41] More recent work shows that CD is in fact associated with specific alterations in the status quo of the intestinal microbial ecosystem that can develop independent of genetic susceptibility.[42–44] This phenomenon termed dysbiosis refers to an altered balance of "aggressive" species (eg, *Bacteroidetes*, *Proteobacteria*) versus "protective" species (eg, *Firmicutes*). Specific pathogens, such as *Mycobacterium tuberculosis*, *Salmonella*, *Helicobacter*, and *Listeria*, are frequently cited in CD pathogenesis but cause and effect have never been convincingly demonstrated. New evidence for a specific pathogen in CD lies in the ability of AIEC to invade and persist intracellularly in intestinal epithelial cells and macrophages and to induce granulomatous lesions in vitro.[24,25,41,45–50]

This unique group of *E coli* was first associated with IBD when recovered from 100% of the biopsy specimens of early ileal CD lesions and 65% of chronically inflamed ileal resections, compared with 3.7% of colonic biopsies from the same patients, and 6%

of healthy control ileal biopsies.[25] Numerous subsequent studies have confirmed these observations,[45,46,51] but the precise role of AIEC in CD, that is, whether it is a secondary invader or a primary pathogen, remains the subject of much debate. These commensal flora are, however, increasingly cited as emerging pathogens in CD because the number of E coli in CD have been shown to be strongly correlated with the severity of disease ($P<.001$) and in a FISH-based study, invasive E coli were found only in inflamed mucosa.[45]

AIEC are unique in that they do not possess any of the known virulence genes for invasion used by enteroinvasive or enteropathogenic E coli, or Shigella strains.[45,46,52] They are similar to extraintestinal avian and uropathic E coli strains in phylogeny and virulence gene profile.[45,53] A functional change in the resident E coli, characterized by proliferation and upregulation of virulence genes, has been suggested to account for the ability of AIEC to invade and persist in the epithelial cells and macrophages of patients with CD.[24,25,45] There is emerging evidence that AIEC use specific mechanisms to facilitate cellular invasion and survival, such as flagellin,[48] type I pili,[54] cell adhesion molecule CEACAM6, which acts as a receptor for AIEC,[51] the stress response protein Gp96,[55] and long polar fimbriae.[25,42,45]

A role for AIEC in CGD has not yet been appreciated but is implied by our understanding not only of the GC pathogenesis but also of the pathophysiologic similarities between CD and CGD that culminate in defective bacterial killing, which includes phagocyte dysfunction because of defective NADPH oxidase[36,40] and polymorphisms of genes regulating clearance of intracellular pathogens.[56–58] The most well-recognized CD-associated polymorphism involves NOD2, which encodes an intracellular sensor for a bacterial wall peptidoglycan, and facilitates a nuclear factor-κ B–mediated proinflammatory and antibacterial response.[57] More recently, GWAS in patients with CD has shown disease-associated polymorphisms in autophagy pathway components, which also play important roles in eliminating intracellular microbes, autophagy-related 16-like protein 1, and immunity-related GTPase family, M.[40,59] Evidently, an increasingly emerging theme in the pathophysiology of IBD involves the abnormal interfacing of host immunity with resident intestinal microbes, which has major implications for disease management.

DIAGNOSIS
Clinical Features

GC typically affects Boxer dogs younger than 4 years with no sex predilection, and some reports describe clinical signs in animals as young as 6 weeks.[2,7,14] Clinical signs are typical of colitis, that is, frequent small-volume diarrhea, hematochezia, mucoid feces, and tenesmus. The degree of hematochezia is often significantly greater than for other types of colitis, and affected dogs may fail to thrive or may lose weight. Affected dogs are usually clinically well and afebrile but may be lethargic with severe disease. Differential diagnoses aside from GC include idiopathic IBD, enteric parasites, and infectious agents (whipworms, hookworms, Giardia, Cryptosporidium, Salmonella, Campylobacter, fungal infections, pathogen causing protothecosis), neoplasia, rectoanal polyps, chronic intussusceptions, and rectal stricture. It is not uncommon in the authors' experience for there to have been a recent episode of suspected infectious gastroenteritis (eg, caused by Salmonella or Campylobacter) that may act as a trigger for GC.

Traditional Diagnostics

Routine clinicopathologic testing is usually unremarkable but may detect mild to moderate anemia. This diagnosis could reflect anemia of chronic disease, or hemorrhage if hematochezia is severe. The degree and chronicity of blood loss can be sufficient in rare cases to cause iron deficiency anemia, characterized by red cell microcytosis and hypochromia. Hypoalbuminemia may also occur in some affected dogs because of hemorrhage, protein exudation via diffusely ulcerated mucosa, anorexia, and inflammation (albumin is a negative acute phase protein). Parasitologic analysis of feces is usually unrewarding but is required to exclude other causes of clinical signs. Imaging studies (radiographs, ultrasound) are largely unremarkable but may be useful to detect other causes of large-bowel signs (eg, partial intestinal obstruction, abdominal masses, chronic intussusceptions, prostatomegaly). Definitive diagnosis is achieved by ruling out other causes of clinical signs and histologic confirmation on colonic mucosal biopsies. Mucosal pinch biopsies obtained via endoscopy are adequate for diagnosis, but a patchy distribution of disease and PAS staining is not uncommon; hence the authors suggest obtaining a minimum of 10 endoscopic biopsies. Grossly, the colonic mucosa may be reddened, cobblestoned, and ulcerated. The histologic appearance of GC is unique relative to other types of colitis in dogs because of the severe mucosal ulceration and infiltration of the submucosa and lamina propria with macrophages that stain positive with PAS (see **Fig. 2**).[7,9,14,60] Additional histologic features include mucosal ulceration, loss of goblet cells, and cellular infiltration with granulocytes and lymphocytes.[1,17] Enlargement of draining lymph nodes, or more rarely, generalized lymphadenopathy, can develop as a result of lymphoid hyperplasia and macrophage infiltration.[17,18]

FISH Analysis

Demonstration of invasive *E coli* in GC is now integral to disease diagnosis and management and is best accomplished using FISH (see **Fig. 3**). The advantage of FISH over other methods such as Gram staining is that it uses fluorescent probes that bind with high specificity to bacterial rDNA and increase the likelihood of visualizing bacteria in tissues with a busy inflammatory background. The degree of cellular infiltration and the foamy appearance of macrophages in GC make it difficult to differentiate bacteria from cytoplasmic contents, granules, and inflammatory debris using routine stains. Poor visualization is likely the reason why the association with *E coli* was not uncovered in earlier studies because cultures positive for *E coli* were actually obtained from the colic lymph nodes of 7 affected Boxer dogs in 1966, but the *E coli* were considered to be secondary invaders.[60]

FISH is performed on formalin-fixed paraffin-embedded colonic mucosal biopsy specimens. An *E coli*–specific probe is colocalized with a eubacterial probe and slides spotted with other bacteria are used to control probe specificity, such as *Salmonella, Proteus, Klebsiella, Enterococcus, Staphylococcus, Streptococcus,* and genera of Clostridiales. A negative FISH result does not completely exclude *E coli* invasion because a patchy distribution of invasion can occur. Thus, a minimum of 10 mucosal biopsies is recommended. Other reasons for false-negative results include the presence of dead or dying bacteria during biopsy sampling, low bacterial numbers, overfixation, and sulfasalazine treatment. False-positive results on FISH are also possible but unlikely, given the additional probes used as positive and negative controls. FISH for GC is currently performed by the Simpson Laboratory at Cornell University, and additional information is available online at www.vet.cornell.edu/labs/simpson.

Antimicrobial Susceptibility Testing

Although FISH analysis may identify the presence, and sometimes specific species of bacteria, it is only moderately helpful for antimicrobial selection because it does not reveal antimicrobial resistance genes or intracellular versus extracellular bacterial location. It is also necessary to culture colonic mucosa, particularly (but not only) when invasive *E coli* are documented, in order to determine antimicrobial susceptibility. It is of course impossible to be certain that the *E coli* strain isolated is in fact the invasive strain and not just a surface colonizer. However, in the authors' experience (M. C. and K. W. S.), only 1 or 2 *E coli* strains are usually cultivable from 1 to 2 colon biopsies because the invading pathotype is likely to predominate, having outcompeted other strains. Collection of 2 to 3 mucosal biopsies into Luria-Bertani broth for gram-negative enrichment and antimicrobial sensitivities of all isolated *E coli* strains is recommended (further information and sampling kits for FISH and culture are available at www.vet.cornell.edu/labs/simpson).

Future Directions

Pending further evaluation of the genetic basis of GC, it is possible that a genetic screening test may become available in the near future. Initial screening of patients with CGD is accomplished by simple tests of neutrophil function, and this may also become a useful diagnostic tool in GC, if NCF2 gene involvement is confirmed.

TREATMENT

Before recent developments, treatment with standard recommended protocols for idiopathic colitis, namely dietary modification and therapy with metronidazole/tylosin, sulfasalazine, prednisolone, and azathioprine, failed to produce satisfactory clinical results.[5,7,10,11] The administration of enrofloxacin alone, 5 mg/kg once daily for a total of 6 to 8 weeks, has been associated with long-term remission.[3,14,23,27] It is now apparent that a successful response to treatment hinges on the successful eradication of invasive *E coli*. Thus the antimicrobial used must not only be able to kill *E coli* but also achieve an adequate intracellular concentration.

In order to optimize antimicrobial selection against GC-associated *E coli*, a recent study analyzed antimicrobial sensitivity profiles in 14 GC cases and discovered enrofloxacin resistance in 43% (**Table 1**). The resistant *E coli* strains were uniformly resistant to all fluoroquinolones tested (ciprofloxacin, marbofloxacin, enrofloxacin, danofloxacin) and tended to harbor resistance to other macrophage-penetrating antimicrobials, such as chloramphenicol, florfenicol, rifampin, trimethoprim-sulfa (TMPS),

Table 1
Prevalence of antimicrobial resistance in *E coli* strains isolated from 14 GC-affected Boxer dogs versus 17 healthy dogs

Antimicrobial	Resistant Strains (%)		Resistant Dogs (%)	
	GC	Healthy	GC	Healthy
Amoxicillin-clavulanate	35*	8	57*	12
Ampicillin	49**	15	64**	18
Cefoxitin	30***	0	50***	0
Tetracycline	48*	18	64*	24
Trimethoprim-sulfa	44***	6	57**	7
Ciprofloxacin	35***	0	43**	0
Gentamicin	13	18	14	36
Chloramphenicol	17*	0	21	0

GC significantly different from healthy using Fisher exact test: *P<.05, **P<.01,***P<.001.
Data from Craven M, Dogan B, Schukken A, et al. Antimicrobial resistance impacts clinical outcome of granulomatous colitis in boxer dogs. J Vet Intern Med 2010;24(4):819–24.

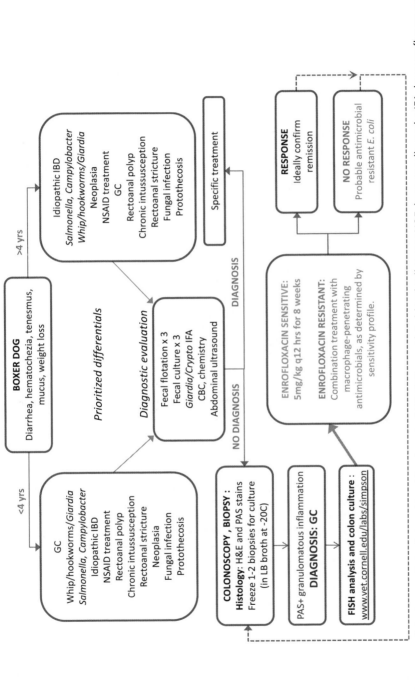

Fig. 5. Summary of the approach to diagnosis and treatment of GC. CBC, complete blood cell count; H&E, hematoxylin-eosin; IFA, immunofluorescence assay; NSAID, nonsteroidal antiinflammatory drug.

tetracyclines, and clarithromycin. Empirical treatment with enrofloxacin before performing colon biopsy was associated with the isolation of resistant E coli (P<.01), perhaps associated with inadequate duration of treatment.[27] In skeletally immature dogs, damage to developing cartilage is a potential adverse effect of enrofloxacin treatment and practitioners may be understandably reluctant to prescribe the drug for extended periods. However, it is important in GC that a sufficient duration of enrofloxacin is given, even if significant clinical improvement is noted within 1 to 2 weeks. Cartilage defects are rarely appreciated and are perhaps the lesser of the 2 evils because resistance to enrofloxacin in GC is significantly associated with a poor outcome.[27] Currently, the suggested treatment regimen for cases with enrofloxacin-sensitive E coli is 5 to 10 mg/kg every 24 hours for a minimum of 6 weeks. The authors suggest enrofloxacin specifically because it has been proved to induce remission. Other fluoroquinolones such as ciprofloxacin and marbofloxacin may also be effective but have not been evaluated. Posttreatment colonoscopy and biopsy are advisable to demonstrate remission of disease and successful eradication of E coli invasion. The role of other medications such as mesalamine or sulfasalazine as adjunctive treatment in GC is unknown. Mesalamine has been shown to downregulate cytokine production in response to AIEC in vitro[61] and may have synergistic effects alongside antimicrobials in the treatment of GC, but this drug has yet to be critically evaluated.

A poor response to treatment is usually associated with development of enrofloxacin resistance. Repeat colonoscopic biopsy for FISH and culture is required to guide further treatment. Potential reasons for development of enrofloxacin resistance in GC include treatment with an inadequate dosage and duration of enrofloxacin and the acquisition of resistance plasmids.[62,63] In enrofloxacin-resistant cases, the antimicrobial selection should be determined by susceptibility testing. Aside from the spectrum of activity, it is of critical importance that the antimicrobial used is capable of penetrating macrophages. Agents likely to do so include chloramphenicol, florfenicol, TMPS, tetracyclines, clarithromycin, and rifampicin.[63] When a multidrug-resistant strain of E coli is present, the authors recommend considering the use of a combination antimicrobial protocol, to include a fluoroquinolone and several other of these macrophage-penetrating agents (eg, chloramphenicol, TMPS). Even though the E coli may be resistant to these agents individually, they may have synergistic effects when the drugs are administered together over an extended period (the authors suggest at least 1 month beyond the resolution of clinical signs). This perhaps heavy-handed approach seems to be justified when considering that refractory cases are usually euthanized. No obvious universal alternative was identified as the next-best antimicrobial to enrofloxacin in the aforementioned case series, but of note is that 100% of the GC-associated E coli strains were sensitive to the aminoglycoside amikacin. However, the molecular properties of amikacin result in a poor ability to penetrate mammalian cells, precluding its clinical application for the treatment of intracellular infections. Additional therapies for GC are clearly needed, and future directions include intracellular targeting of amikacin, E coli vaccination, and gene transfer therapy. **Fig. 5** provides a summary of the diagnosis and management of GC.

REFERENCES

1. Van Kruiningen HJ, Montali RJ, Strandberg JD, et al. A granulomatous colitis of dogs with histologic resemblance to Whipple's disease. Pathol Vet 1965;2(6): 521–44.
2. Churcher RK, Watson AD. Canine histiocytic ulcerative colitis. Aust Vet J 1997; 75(10):710–3.

3. Hostutler RA, Luria BJ, Johnson SE, et al. Antibiotic-responsive histiocytic ulcerative colitis in 9 dogs. J Vet Intern Med 2004;18(4):499–504.
4. Van Kruiningen HJ. Granulomatous colitis of boxer dogs: comparative aspects. Gastroenterology 1967;53(1):114–22.
5. Stokes JE, Kruger JM, Mullaney T, et al. Histiocytic ulcerative colitis in three non-boxer dogs. J Am Anim Hosp Assoc 2001;37(5):461–5.
6. Tanaka H, Nakayama M, Takase K. Histiocytic ulcerative colitis in a French bulldog. J Vet Med Sci 2003;65(3):431–3.
7. Hall EJ, Tennant BJ, Payne-Johnson CE, et al. Boxer colitis. Vet Rec 1992; 130(7):148.
8. Fletcher WD. Advanced granulomatous colitis in a Siberian Husky (a case report). Vet Med Small Anim Clin 1978;73(11):1409.
9. Kennedy PC, Cello RM. Colitis of boxer dogs. Gastroenterology 1966;51(5): 926–31.
10. Hill FW, Sullivan ND. Histiocytic ulcerative colitis in a Boxer dog. Aust Vet J 1978; 54(9):447–9.
11. Lindberg R, Segall T. Histiocytic ulcerative colitis in a boxer. A case report. Nord Vet Med 1977;29(12):552–5.
12. Arai K, Sudo M, Saeki Y, et al. Granulomatous colitis in a Boxer dog. Journal of the Japan Veterinary Medical Association 1983;36:29–33.
13. van der Gaag I, Happe RP, Wolvekamp WT. A boxer dog with chronic hypertrophic gastritis resembling Menetrier's disease in man. Vet Pathol 1976;13(3):172–85.
14. Mansfield CS, James FE, Craven M, et al. Remission of histiocytic ulcerative colitis in Boxer dogs correlates with eradication of invasive intramucosal Escherichia coli. J Vet Intern Med 2009;23(5):964–9.
15. Afshar P, Redfield DC, Higginbottom PA. Whipple's disease: a rare disease revisited. Curr Gastroenterol Rep 2010;12(4):263–9.
16. Desnues B, Al Moussawi K, Fenollar F. New insights into Whipple's disease and Tropheryma whipplei infections. Microbes Infect 2010;12(14–15):1102–10.
17. Van Kruiningen HJ. The ultrastructure of macrophages in granulomatous colitis of Boxer dogs. Vet Pathol 1975;12(5–6):446–59.
18. Bowe PS, Van Kruiningen HJ, Rosendal S. Attempts to produce granulomatous colitis in Boxer dogs with a mycoplasma. Can J Comp Med 1982; 46(4):430–3.
19. German AJ, Hall EJ, Kelly DF, et al. An immunohistochemical study of histiocytic ulcerative colitis in boxer dogs. J Comp Pathol 2000;122(2–3):163–75.
20. Hanauer SB. Inflammatory bowel disease: epidemiology, pathogenesis, and therapeutic opportunities. Inflamm Bowel Dis 2006;12(Suppl 1):S3–9.
21. Davies DR, O'Hara AJ, Irwin PJ, et al. Successful management of histiocytic ulcerative colitis with enrofloxacin in two Boxer dogs. Aust Vet J 2004;82(1–2):58–61.
22. Van Kruiningen HJ, Civco IC, Cartun RW. The comparative importance of E. coli antigen in granulomatous colitis of Boxer dogs. APMIS 2005;113(6):420–5.
23. Simpson KW, Dogan B, Rishniw M, et al. Adherent and invasive Escherichia coli is associated with granulomatous colitis in boxer dogs. Infect Immun 2006;74(8): 4778–92.
24. Darfeuille-Michaud A, Neut C, Barnich N, et al. Presence of adherent Escherichia coli strains in ileal mucosa of patients with Crohn's disease. Gastroenterology 1998;115(6):1405–13.
25. Darfeuille-Michaud A, Boudeau J, Bulois P, et al. High prevalence of adherent-invasive Escherichia coli associated with ileal mucosa in Crohn's disease. Gastroenterology 2004;127(2):412–21.

26. Schneider T, Moos V, Loddenkemper C, et al. Whipple's disease: new aspects of pathogenesis and treatment. Lancet Infect Dis 2008;8(3):179–90.

27. Craven M, Dogan B, Schukken A, et al. Antimicrobial resistance impacts clinical outcome of granulomatous colitis in Boxer dogs. J Vet Intern Med 2010;24(4): 819–24.

28. Craven M, Acland G, Mezey J, et al. Genome-wide association scan reveals polymorphisms in the P67phox subunit (NCF2) In Boxer dogs with E.coli-associated granulomatous colitis: a potential model of chronic granulomatous disease [abstract]. In: Digestive Disease Week. New Orleans (Louisiana), 2010.

29. Craven M, Gao C, Acland G, et al. Genome-wide analysis of granuomatous colitis in the Boxer dog. Research report. Forum of the ACVIM 2010.

30. Karlsson EK, Baranowska I, Wade CM, et al. Efficient mapping of mendelian traits in dogs through genome-wide association. Nat Genet 2007;39(11):1321–8.

31. Salmon Hillbertz NH, Isaksson M, Karlsson EK, et al. Duplication of FGF3, FGF4, FGF19 and ORAOV1 causes hair ridge and predisposition to dermoid sinus in Ridgeback dogs. Nat Genet 2007;39(11):1318–20.

32. von Rosenvinge EC, O'Donnell TG, Holland SM, et al. Chronic granulomatous disease. Inflamm Bowel Dis 2010;16(1):9.

33. Holland SM. Update on phagocytic defects. Pediatr Infect Dis J 2003;22(1):87–8.

34. Mizuki K, Kadomatsu K, Hata K, et al. Functional modules and expression of mouse p40(phox) and p67(phox), SH3-domain-containing proteins involved in the phagocyte NADPH oxidase complex. Eur J Biochem 1998;251(3):573–82.

35. Han CH, Freeman JL, Lee T, et al. Regulation of the neutrophil respiratory burst oxidase. Identification of an activation domain in p67(phox). J Biol Chem 1998; 273(27):16663–8.

36. Holland SM. Chronic granulomatous disease. Clin Rev Allergy Immunol 2010; 38(1):3–10.

37. Marciano BE, Rosenzweig SD, Kleiner DE, et al. Gastrointestinal involvement in chronic granulomatous disease. Pediatrics 2004;114(2):462–8.

38. Schappi MG, Smith VV, Goldblatt D, et al. Colitis in chronic granulomatous disease. Arch Dis Child 2001;84(2):147–51.

39. Schappi MG, Klein NJ, Lindley KJ, et al. The nature of colitis in chronic granulomatous disease. J Pediatr Gastroenterol Nutr 2003;36(5):623–31.

40. Roberts RL, Hollis-Moffatt JE, Gearry RB, et al. Confirmation of association of IRGM and NCF4 with ileal Crohn's disease in a population-based cohort. Genes Immun 2008;9(6):561–5.

41. Sartor RB. Microbial influences in inflammatory bowel diseases. Gastroenterology 2008;134(2):577–94.

42. Sartor RB. Targeting enteric bacteria in treatment of inflammatory bowel diseases: why, how, and when. Curr Opin Gastroenterol 2003;19(4):358–65.

43. Sartor RB, Muehlbauer M. Microbial host interactions in IBD: implications for pathogenesis and therapy. Curr Gastroenterol Rep 2007;9(6):497–507.

44. Willing B, Halfvarson J, Dicksved J, et al. Twin studies reveal specific imbalances in the mucosa-associated microbiota of patients with ileal Crohn's disease. Inflamm Bowel Dis 2009;15(5):653–60.

45. Baumgart M, Dogan B, Rishniw M, et al. Culture independent analysis of ileal mucosa reveals a selective increase in invasive Escherichia coli of novel phylogeny relative to depletion of Clostridiales in Crohn's disease involving the ileum. ISME J 2007;1(5):403–18.

46. Barnich N, Darfeuille-Michaud A. Adherent-invasive Escherichia coli and Crohn's disease. Curr Opin Gastroenterol 2007;23(1):16–20.

47. Bringer MA, Glasser AL, Tung CH, et al. The Crohn's disease-associated adherent-invasive Escherichia coli strain LF82 replicates in mature phagolysosomes within J774 macrophages. Cell Microbiol 2006;8(3):471–84.

48. Eaves-Pyles T, Allen CA, Taormina J, et al. Escherichia coli isolated from a Crohn's disease patient adheres, invades, and induces inflammatory responses in polarized intestinal epithelial cells. Int J Med Microbiol 2008;298(5–6):397–409.

49. Glasser AL, Boudeau J, Barnich N, et al. Adherent invasive Escherichia coli strains from patients with Crohn's disease survive and replicate within macrophages without inducing host cell death. Infect Immun 2001;69(9): 5529–37.

50. Meconi S, Vercellone A, Levillain F, et al. Adherent-invasive Escherichia coli isolated from Crohn's disease patients induce granulomas in vitro. Cell Microbiol 2007;9(5):1252–61.

51. Barnich N, Carvalho FA, Glasser AL, et al. CEACAM6 acts as a receptor for adherent-invasive E. coli, supporting ileal mucosa colonization in Crohn disease. J Clin Invest 2007;117(6):1566–74.

52. Packey CD, Sartor RB. Interplay of commensal and pathogenic bacteria, genetic mutations, and immunoregulatory defects in the pathogenesis of inflammatory bowel diseases. J Intern Med 2008;263(6):597–606.

53. Martinez-Medina M, Aldeguer X, Lopez-Siles M, et al. Molecular diversity of Escherichia coli in the human gut: new ecological evidence supporting the role of adherent-invasive E. coli (AIEC) in Crohn's disease. Inflamm Bowel Dis 2009; 15(6):872–82.

54. Ryan P, Kelly RG, Lee G, et al. Bacterial DNA within granulomas of patients with Crohn's disease–detection by laser capture microdissection and PCR. Am J Gastroenterol 2004;99(8):1539–43.

55. Rolhion N, Barnich N, Bringer MA, et al. Abnormally expressed ER stress response chaperone Gp96 in CD favours adherent-invasive Escherichia coli invasion. Gut 2010;59(10):1355–62.

56. Barrett JC, Hansoul S, Nicolae DL, et al. Genome-wide association defines more than 30 distinct susceptibility loci for Crohn's disease. Nat Genet 2008;40(8): 955–62.

57. Eckmann L, Karin M. NOD2 and Crohn's disease: loss or gain of function? Immunity 2005;22(6):661–7.

58. Homer CR, Richmond AL, Rebert NA, et al. ATG16L1 and NOD2 interact in an autophagy-dependent, anti-bacterial pathway implicated in Crohn's disease pathogenesis. Gastroenterology 2010;139(5):1630–41.

59. Massey DC, Parkes M. Genome-wide association scanning highlights two autophagy genes, ATG16L1 and IRGM, as being significantly associated with Crohn's disease. Autophagy 2007;3(6):649–51.

60. van Kruiningen HJ. Granulomatous colitis of Boxer dogs [PhD thesis]. New York: State Veterinary College, Cornell University; 1966.

61. Subramanian S, Rhodes JM, Hart CA, et al. Characterization of epithelial IL-8 response to inflammatory bowel disease mucosal E. coli and its inhibition by mesalamine. Inflamm Bowel Dis 2008;14(2):162–75.

62. Warren A, Townsend K, King T, et al. Multi-drug resistant escherichia coli with extended-spectrum beta-lactamase activity and fluoroquinolone resistance isolated from clinical infections in dogs. Aust Vet J 2001;79(9):621–3.

63. Subramanian S, Roberts CL, Hart CA, et al. Replication of colonic Crohn's disease mucosal Escherichia coli isolates within macrophages and their susceptibility to antibiotics. Antimicrob Agents Chemother 2008;52(2):427–34.

Chronic Idiopathic Large Bowel Diarrhea in the Dog

Patrick Lecoindre, Dr med vet[a],*,
Frédéric P. Gaschen, Dr med vet, Dr habil[b]

KEYWORDS

• Colon • Dietary fiber • Large bowel diarrhea • Behavior • Dog

In dogs, large bowel diarrhea is usually characterized by small amounts of feces often admixed with mucous and/or fresh blood (hematochezia), frequent defecation with urgency, and tenesmus. These signs reflect colonic dysfunction with decreased water reabsorption and decreased fecal storage capacity, as well as mucosal damage (hematochezia) and response to inflammation (excessive mucous).[1,2] Acute colitis is most commonly associated with whipworm infestation (*Trichuris vulpis*), dietary indiscretion, and *Clostridium perfringens* or *Clostridium difficile* infections.[1,2] Differential diagnoses for chronic and chronic-recurring canine colitis include whipworm infestation, clostridial infections (see the article by J. Scott Weese elsewhere in this issue for further exploration of this issue), infections with mucosa adherent-invasive *Escherichia coli* in specific breeds (eg, Boxer, English Bulldog, and similar breeds) and resulting granulomatous colitis (see the article by Craven and colleagues elsewhere in this issue for further exploration of this topic), diet-responsive colitis,[3,4] idiopathic inflammatory bowel disease (IBD),[2] neoplasia,[5] and functional disorders.[4–8]

Large bowel diarrhea may also occur in dogs without any evidence of inflammation. In the only case series of canine chronic idiopathic large bowel diarrhea (CILBD) published to date, 37 dogs were reported that responded well to treatment with a highly digestible diet added with psyllium, a source of soluble fibers.[5] Two groups of canine patients with CILBD have been defined: the fiber-responsive group and the group with suspect stress-associated large bowel diarrhea.[7,8]

This article briefly reviews functional intestinal disorders in people and summarizes the data published on CILBD with addition of a case series from the practice of one of the authors. Current recommendations for diagnostic approach and management of CILBD are also reviewed.

The authors have nothing to disclose.
[a] Clinique vétérinaire des Cerisioz, 5 Route Street, Symphorien d'Ozon, 69800 St Priest, France
[b] Department of Veterinary Clinical Sciences, School of Veterinary Medicine, Louisiana State University, Baton Rouge, LA 70803, USA
* Corresponding author.
E-mail address: patrick.lecoindre@wanadoo.fr

FUNCTIONAL INTESTINAL DISORDERS IN PEOPLE

Irritable bowel syndrome (IBS) is a chronic functional disorder of the gastrointestinal (GI) tract associated with abdominal pain and altered bowel activity in the absence of any pathologic organic change.[1,9,10] The prevalence of IBS in the general population is estimated to be between 2.5% and 22% in reports from multiple countries,[9,10] even though many patients with IBS may not search for medical help and are not included in the epidemiologic data.[10] Three forms have been described: one associated with diarrhea (IBS-D), another characterized by constipation (IBS-C), and a mixed form with both episodes of diarrhea and constipation (IBS-M).[9,10]

Clinical Presentation and Diagnosis of IBS in People

The predominating symptoms are recurring nonspecific abdominal pain or discomfort and altered bowel habits (ie, diarrhea or constipation). Eating worsens the pain, while defecation alleviates it.[9,10] Other symptoms include urgency, straining, bloating, a sensation of incomplete evacuation, and mucus in the stool.[1,10] Slow onset of IBS over weeks to months shows a strong correlation with stress disorders such as depression and anxiety, which are relatively frequent.[9] The differentiation between organic diseases and IBS is difficult based on the clinical phenotype only. Alarm features such as late onset of symptoms after age 50 years, unintentional weight loss, nocturnal diarrhea, anemia and bloody stools, and a family history of colon cancer are red flags that should prompt the physician to consider alternative diagnoses such as IBD or colon cancer.[10] A more comprehensive diagnostic work-up is indicated for patients with suspected IBS who show one or more alarm feature. Interestingly, IBS may also occur after an intestinal infection post-infectious IBS (PI-IBS) in a subset of patients.[10]

Pathogenesis of IBS

The pathogenesis of gut–brain axis dysfunction in IBS is multifactorial, but not fully understood. Several phenomena are known to contribute to symptom genesis. They include abnormal bowel motility (spasms), visceral hypersensitivity, altered cerebral processing of gut events, environmental stressors, and intrinsic psychopathology.[11] GI motility is affected differently in the various forms of IBS; generally GI transit is slowed in IBS-C and accelerated in IBS-D.[12] In patients with IBS-D, high-amplitude propagating contractions are of higher amplitude, and more likely to be associated with a sensation of pain.[12,13] Visceral hypersensitivity appears to be a hallmark of IBS, and IBS patients have enhanced perception of visceral events such as contractions and gas throughout their GI tract.[12]

Possible pathomechanisms for IBS have been explored and include stress,[14,15] diet, and microbiota,[11] as well as inflammation and neuroimmune interactions.[16] Stress is defined as an external disturbance or threat from the environment that disturbs homeostasis.[14] The response to stress triggers coordinated changes in behavior and autonomic and neuroendocrine responses that allow the organism to adapt to the new environment.[14,15] The hypothalamic-pituitary-adrenal axis is activated with secretion of corticotropin-releasing factor (CRF). However, severe or chronic stress may exceed the adaptive capacity of the organism and lead to the development of disease.[14,15] Various stressors such as early life stress (eg, childhood psychological trauma) and sustained stressful life events may significantly impact intestinal physiology.[10,14,15] Stress has been implicated in the pathogenesis of IBS in people and has been associated with exacerbations of clinical signs in patients with organic intestinal diseases such as IBD.[14,15] In rodent models, chronic stress results in epithelial barrier dysfunction, inflammation, and metabolic abnormalities in both small and large intestines.[14,15] Food ingestion commonly triggers the onset of symptoms in IBS patients.[9–11] Food intake initiates postprandial patterns of GI motility and associated abnormal events in IBS. Moreover, specific foods that are poorly absorbed and highly fermentable may potentiate IBS symptoms such as bloating and diarrhea. Finally, the enteric flora is also thought to play a role in the pathogenesis of IBS.[11] Some IBS patients have been found to have abnormal immune system function. The intestinal permeability may be increased; higher numbers of activated mucosal mast cells are present, and increased density of sensory mucosal nerve endings is observed in some IBS patients.[16] Mast cells located in the vicinity of nerve endings may contribute to the clinical disease.[16]

Management of IBS

The management of IBS in people is multifaceted. Depending on the severity of symptoms, education and dietary adjustment may suffice, or behavior modification with psychopharmacologic agents may be required.[9,10] Treatment options for IBS-D include motility-modifying agents such as loperamide (which acts on mu receptors of the myenteric plexus) and diphenoxylate, alosetron, a $5-HT_3$-antagonist that inhibits GI motility and reduces visceral sensitivity and abdominal pain, but may cause ischemic colitis, or rifaximin, a very poorly absorbed antibiotic with broad-spectrum activity against gram-negative aerobes and anaerobes.[9,10] Antispasmodics are used in the treatment of abdominal pain. Tricyclic antidepressants, serotonin reuptake inhibitors, and psychological and behavioral therapy are recommended in some patients.[10,14] Probiotics have been reported to cause modest improvement.[9]

CHRONIC IDIOPATHIC LARGE BOWEL DIARRHEA

The name canine idiopathic large bowel diarrhea (CILBD) was coined by Leib[7] in 2000. Although it is purely descriptive, it is more appropriate than IBS or spastic colon and should be preferred since studies of GI motility and visceral sensitivity in affected dogs are lacking to date.[7,8]

Colonic Motility in Dogs

The canine colon exhibits three types of contractions. While the individual phasic contractions and the migrating and nonmigrating motor complexes produce extensive mixing and kneading of fecal material and slow net distal propulsion, the giant motor complexes produce mass movements and expel feces during defecation.[17] Changes in colonic motility have been described in dogs with colitis and include decreased nonpropulsive motility and increased giant migrating contractions, resulting in frequent defecation and tenesmus.[18] The decreased nonpropulsive motility may be associated with disturbances in muscarinic receptors of circular colonic smooth muscle cells associated with inflammation.[19] No motility studies have been performed to date in dogs with noninflammatory colonic disorders such as CILBD.

Published Studies of CILBD

There is a paucity of published studies about CILBD in dogs. Many reports describing IBS or irritable or spastic colon were part of book chapters[6,20] or conference proceedings.[8] However, the prevalence of CILBD in dogs presented to referral hospitals for complete evaluation of chronic large bowel diarrhea appears to be significant. A study from Belgium reports that 7 of 40 dogs (17.5%) with chronic large bowel diarrhea evaluated with colonoscopy and histopathology had no evidence of organic disease.[21] In another study from the United States, 19 of 74 dogs (26%) undergoing colonoscopy were diagnosed with idiopathic large bowel diarrhea.[22] This contrasts with data from New Zealand, where fewer than 1 in 20 (5%) patients with large bowel diarrhea was diagnosed with IBS.[6] Leib[7] described a cohort of 37 dogs with CILBD that responded to a highly digestible diet and soluble fiber (psyllium). The clinical data from this cohort are summarized in **Table 1**. Even though no detailed behavioral evaluation was performed in these dogs, it is noteworthy that almost 40% had either environmental changes that coincided with the occurrence of clinical signs (visitors in household, travel, moving, house construction, or other events) or abnormal personality traits (separation anxiety, submissive urination, noise sensitivity, aggression, or nervousness).

Own Study

Selection criteria for CILBD

The medical records of dogs that underwent colonoscopy with collection of colonic mucosal biopsies at one of the authors' hospital (PL) were reviewed. Selection criteria for CILBD were history of chronic recurrent large bowel diarrhea, negative fecal examination, unremarkable complete blood cell (CBC) count and serum

Table 1
Summary of presentation and response to treatment in 2 case series of dogs with Chronic idiopathic large bowel diarrhea

	Leib[7] 2000	Authors' Cohort
Number of dogs	37	19
Female-to-male ratio	1.31	1.37
Median age in years (range)	6 (0.5–14)	6.3 (2–12)
Duration of signs before presentation/referral	1–65 mo	3–24 mo
Average number of daily defecations	3.5 (18 dogs)	N/A
Excessive mucus in feces	34 (92%)	19 (100%)
Tenesmus	22 (59%)	19 (100%)
Stool consistency	Median fecal score 2 out of 5 (mostly unformed, loose stool)	Liquid in 8 dogs (42%)
Hematochezia	29 (78%)	9 (47%)
Vomiting	23 (62%), frequent in 2 dogs	8 (42%)
Weight loss	3 (8%)	None
Decreased appetite during episodes of diarrhea	10 (27%)	8 (42%)
Abdominal pain during episodes of diarrhea	5 (13%)	6 (32%)
Anal pruritus	N/A	6 (32%)
Abnormal personality traits, environmental stress factors	14 (38%)	8 (42%)
Positive long-term response to fiber supplementation alone	26/27 (96%)	12 (63%)
Positive response to behavior modifying drugs	N/A	4 (21%)
No response to treatment	1 (4%)	3 (16%)

biochemistry, and absence of abnormalities on colonoscopy and histopathology. The initial treatment consisted of a broad-spectrum anthelmintic (fenbendazole 50 mg/kg by mouth daily for 5 days) and feeding a highly digestible diet with low fat content (Gastrointestinal Low Fat, Royal Canin, Aimargues, France). No consistent improvement was observed over a 3-week period.

The dogs diagnosed with CILBD using the previously mentioned criteria underwent a behavioral assessment based on a scoring system designed to assess emotional and cognitive disorders in dogs.[19,23] The system evaluates behavior associated with food and water intake, as well as sleep, somesthesis, exploration of environment, aggression, and learning abilities with weighted criteria. The various categories are graded and a final score is obtained.[23]

Following diagnosis, all dogs with CILBD were prescribed 1 of 2 commercial high fiber diets. They either received diet 1 (Canine Fiber Response FR 23, Royal Canin), containing 20.5% total dietary fiber from a specific blend consisting mostly of insoluble vegetable fiber associated with moderately soluble beet pulp fibers, fructooligosaccharides (FOS), and psyllium husk, or diet 2 (WD, Hills Pet Nutrition, Sophia-Antipolis, France), containing 29.5% total dietary fiber with 28.4% insoluble fiber and 1.1% soluble fiber. Additional medical treatment consisting of antimicrobials, motility-modifying agents, and antispasmodics was given depending on the animals' clinical signs.

Owners were called after 1 month of treatment and answered a questionnaire that included fecal scoring, evaluation of clinical signs (vomiting, tenesmus, appetite changes, flatulence, and hematochezia).

Results

Eighty-four dogs with large bowel diarrhea were referred to the author's hospital (PL) for colonoscopy over a 2-year period (Jan. 1, 2008 to Dec. 31, 2009). Of those, 19 (22.6%) satisfied the criteria listed previously. The 19 dogs consisted of 8 females, of which 3 were spayed, and 11 intact males, mean age 6.3 years old (range: 2–12), 13 small breed dogs less than 15 kg and 6 middle-sized to large breed dogs. Specifically, the breeds represented were 4 toy Poodles, 2 Yorkshire terriers, 1 Cairn terrier, 1 Beagle, 1 Bichon frisé, 1 Springer spaniel, 3 small mixed breed dogs (Poodle, Bichon), 3 Labradors, 1 Siberian Husky, 1 Akita Inu, 1 German Shepherd dog.

All dogs had chronic large bowel diarrhea with tenesmus and passed mucoid stool that was of liquid consistency in 8 dogs. Defecation frequency was increased in 16 dogs; 9 dogs had hematochezia (3 of them with abnormal behavior scores), and 8 dogs had decreased appetite, particularly at the onset of diarrhea episodes. No weight loss or other systemic changes were noted in these dogs. Intermittent vomiting was present in 8 animals. Five dogs had signs of anal pruritus, and 6 dogs showed abdominal pain during diarrhea episodes. Clinical signs had been present for 3 to 24 months (mean duration of 6 months), and owners frequently reported a disease course characterized by acute episodes of diarrhea followed by remission periods with normal stool or sometimes constipation.

Six small breed dogs had moderately increased behavioral scores and were diagnosed with anxiety disorders (2 Toy Poodles, 2 Yorkshire Terriers, 1 Cairn Terrier, and 1 Bichon frisé). Two large breed dogs (Akita Inu and Siberian Husky) had severely abnormal scores and were diagnosed with depressive disorders, one of them with aggressivity.

Thirteen dogs were fed diet 1, and 6 were fed diet 2. Eleven dogs were administered oral antimicrobials (combination of metronidazole 10–15 mg/kg twice daily by mouth and marbofloxacin 2 mg/kg by mouth once daily for several days) due to severe diarrhea or presence of hematochezia. Four dogs received loperamide, and 2 dogs were administered sulfasalazine (30 mg/kg by mouth three times daily) because of persistent tenesmus. Musculotropic antispasmodics such as mebeverine (3 dogs) and pinaverium (2 dogs) were also administered for various amounts of time as part of the long-term treatment (see posology in **Table 2**).

Table 2
Treatment modalities for chronic idiopathic large bowel diarrhea in dogs

Class	Name	Dose	Comment
Fiber	Psyllium	Daily dose: 0.5 T for toy breeds 1T for small breed dogs 2T for medium breed dogs 3T for large breed dogs	Median dose was 1.3 g/kg day in one study[9]
	Special diets supplemented with fiber		Available from reputable pet food manufacturers
Motility modifying agents	Loperamide	0.1 mg/kg PO q 6–8 h	
	Diphenoxylate	0.1 mg/kg PO q 6–8 h	Most formulation combine diphenoxylate and atropine sulfate
Antispasmodics (neurotropic)	Chlordiazepoxide (5 mg) and clidinium bromide (2.5 mg)	0.1–0.25 mg/kg clidinium PO q 8–12 h for a few days	Librax®. Give at time of onset of clinical signs, or when stressful situations are anticipated for a few days only
	Propantheline	0.25 mg/kg PO TID	Do not use longer than 48 to 72 h.
	Hyoscyamine	0.003–0.006 mg/kg PO BID to TID	Use during paroxysms, not for prolonged use
	Dicyclomine	0.15 mg/kg BID to TID	
Antispasmodics (musculotropic)	Mebeverine Pinaverium Trimebutine	2.5–5 mg/kg PO BID 1 mg/kg PO BID 0.33 mg/kg PO TID	
Behavior-modifying agents	Selegiline	Starting dose 0.5 mg/kg PO once daily	Dopamine agonist. Dose can be increased up to 2 mg/kg once daily if no response after 2 months
	Clomipramine	Starting dose 1mg/kg PO BID	Tricyclic antidepressant. Increase gradually up to 3 mg/kg PO BID if necessary after 14 days
	Tryptic hydrolysate of alpha casein	15 mg/kg PO once daily	

Twelve of 19 dogs responded very well to dietary modification, and medical treatment could be rapidly discontinued. Four dogs had behavioral changes that required specific treatment (selegiline [Selgian, CEVA Santé Animale, Libourne, France], clomipramine [Clomicalm, Novartis Santé Animale, Rueil-Malmaison, France], tryptic hydrolysate of alpha casein [Zylkène, Vétoquinol, Lure, France]). Antispasmodics were not helpful in these 4 dogs. Three dogs did not respond to dietary and medical treatment in the long term, and developed further paroxysms of diarrhea and abdominal pain. One of those dogs had a severely increased high behavioral score, while the other 2 had normal behavioral assessments.

Practical Relevance

In dogs referred for large bowel diarrhea, CILBD is a common problem (22% in the author's case series). The clinical signs displayed by dogs with CILBD are indicative of a large bowel disorder, but are in no way pathognomonic (**Box 1**). Unlike what had been reported earlier,[20] hematochezia occurs in a large proportion of dogs with CILBD, even in those with behavior disorders. Therefore, CILBD is a diagnosis that can only be made by exclusion of all other causes of large bowel diarrhea. In one study, colonoscopy revealed minimal mucosal changes in slightly less than half of dogs, which included very slight focal increases in friability, granularity or hyperemia; decreased or increased numbers of lymphoid follicles; decreased visualization of submucosal blood vessels; localized colonic spasm; and localized small superficial erosions.[7] No such lesions were appreciated in the author's cohort. It is noteworthy that many dogs with CILBD occasionally vomit, have a decreased appetite, and show abdominal pain during episodes of diarrhea (see **Table 1**). These additional signs suggest that the whole GI tract may be affected to some extent by the disease, much like is the case in human patients with IBS.

Based on the cases reported in the author's study, most dogs with CILBD appear to respond to a high fiber diet. Alternatively, supplementation with soluble fibers can also be successful based on the cases reported by Leib.[7] The beneficial effects of fiber supplementation for the canine colon have been previously documented and reviewed.[24,25] Nonsoluble fibers bind water and noxious agents in the colon and regulate colonic motility, while soluble fibers modulate colonic microbiota, increase production of short chain fatty acids, acidify colonic content, and stimulate of colonic cellular proliferation. These effects justify use of fiber supplementation as part of an

---

Box 1
Diagnostic criteria for Chronic idiopathic large bowel diarrhea

Chronic or chronic recurring diarrhea for at least 4 weeks

Diarrhea of large bowel origin with increased frequency, excess mucus, tenesmus, and hematochezia

No abnormal findings on physical examination, CBC, biochemical profile, and urinalysis or if minor changes observed on physical examination, CBC count, chemistry panel, urinalysis, absence of a severe systemic disorder

No identifiable cause for large bowel diarrhea

No or only minimal changes observed during colonoscopy

Histopathologic evaluation of colonic mucosal biopsies unremarkable

Data from Leib MS. Irritable bowel syndrome in dogs: fact or fiction? Compend Contin Educ Pract Vet 2009;31(2):14.

early treatment trial in dogs with various causes of large bowel diarrhea, and it is possible that fiber-responsive dogs with large bowel diarrhea may escape further scrutiny, causing CILBD to be underdiagnosed.

In the absence of control groups, both the author's study and the Leib[7] study could not rule out that other properties of the new diet fed to the dogs may have played a role in the improvement of clinical signs, such as optimized n3:n6 fatty acid ratio or higher bioavailability of nutrients. Moreover, it is also possible that some of the dogs included in the study may have had inflammatory bowel disease that could not be confirmed at the time of colonoscopy. This could have been due performing colonoscopy during quiescent phase, or not obtaining biopsies from the areas with histopathologic lesions. Like has been reported in a high proportion of dogs with chronic enteropathies, some dogs could have responded to an elimination diet consisting of novel proteins[3,4] or hydrolyzed peptides.[25] However, all precautions were taken in both case series to include only dogs that had undergone an adequate work-up to exclude the presence of other known colonic diseases.

Among all dogs with CILBD, some respond to fiber supplementation, while others do not and may require behavioral therapy. In the latter group, it is tempting to make a diagnosis of IBS, or irritable or spastic colon; however data are currently lacking to clearly document the existence of these diseases in the dog. In the cases reported by Leib,[7] almost 40% had evidence of abnormal personality traits or environmental stress factors, and they all responded to psyllium supplementation. In the author's case series, 8 dogs had increased behavioral scores; 4 responded to a switch to a high-fiber diet, while 4 required medical treatment of the behavior disorder (see **Table 2**). Fiber supplementation is therefore recommended in all dogs with CILBD, even in the presence of behavior disorders. Lack of response to treatment justifies the use of behavior-modifying drugs. Initial doses of psyllium can be found in **Table 2**. Motility-modifying agents and antispasmodics (see **Table 2**) have been recommended in severe acute paroxysms of CILBD and are associated with mixed success in the authors' experience.

One of the authors (PL) has observed CILBD occurring as a sequel of inflammatory disease. For instance, Boxers that recovered from granulomatous colitis with persistently soft feces benefited from dietary fiber supplementation. Onset of functional GI disorders after inflammatory intestinal diseases has been well documented in people (PI-IBS).[10]

Prognosis of CILBD is good, particularly for dogs that respond to fiber supplementation. Response to long-term treatment with soluble fiber (median 15 months) was deemed excellent in 63%, very good in 22%, good in 11%, and poor in 4% of dogs.[7] In the author's series, 63% of dogs responded to a high fiber diet and 21% to behavior-modifying drugs, while 16% did not respond to treatment. When the owners attempted to decrease fiber supplementation, diarrhea returned in 6 of 11 dogs with soluble fiber-responsive disease in the study by Leib.[7] While 7 dogs were switched back to a grocery store diet, only 2 experienced a recurrence of clinical signs.[7] It is therefore important to sensitize owners that recurrence is possible, and that long-term fiber supplementation may be required.

SUMMARY

CILBD is a diagnosis made by exclusion that describes dogs with chronic large bowel diarrhea in the absence of any other identifiable disorder. Most dogs respond to dietary fiber supplementation, and the prognosis is usually good. Even though CILBD appears to be quite common, at least among dogs referred for GI work-up, there are very few reports available in the literature. There is a great need for well-designed prospective studies to further define the clinical phenotype and evaluate possible treatment modalities.

REFERENCES

1. Leib MS. Large intestine. In: Steiner JM, editor. Small animal gastroenterology. Hannover (Germany): Schluetersche; 2008. p. 217–30.
2. Allenspach K. Diseases of the large intestine. In: Ettinger SJ, Feldman EC, editors. Textbook of veterinary internal medicine, vol. 2. 7th edition. St Louis (MO): Saunders Elsevier; 2010. p. 1573–94.
3. Allenspach K, Wieland B, Grone A, et al. Chronic enteropathies in dogs: evaluation of risk factors for negative outcome. J Vet Intern Med 2007;21(4):700–8.
4. Simpson JW, Maskell IE, Markwell PJ. Use of a restricted antigen diet in the management of idiopathic canine colitis. J Small Anim Pract 1994;35:234–8.
5. Henry CJ. Neoplastic diseases of the large intestine. In: Steiner JM, editor. Small animal gastroenterology. Hannover (Germany): Schluetersche; 2008. p. 236–40.
6. Guilford WG. Motility disorders of the bowel. In: Guilford WG, Center SA, Strombeck DR, et al, editors. Strombeck's small animal gastroenterology. 3rd edition. Philadelphia: W.B. Saunders; 1996. p. 532–9.
7. Leib MS. Treatment of chronic idiopathic large-bowel diarrhea in dogs with a highly digestible diet and soluble fiber: a retrospective review of 37 cases. J Vet Intern Med 2000;14(1):27–32.
8. Leib MS. Irritable bowel syndrome in dogs: fact or fiction? Compend Contin Educ Pract Vet 2009;31(2 Suppl A):13–6.
9. Grundmann O, Yoon SL. Irritable bowel syndrome: epidemiology, diagnosis and treatment: an update for health care practitioners. J Gastroenterol Hepatol 2010; 25(4):691–9.
10. Khan S, Chang L. Diagnosis and management of IBS. Nat Rev Gastroenterol Hepatol 2010;7(10):565–81.
11. Morcos A, Dinan T, Quigley EM. Irritable bowel syndrome: role of food in pathogenesis and management. J Dig Dis 2009;10(4):237–46.
12. Drossman DA, Camilleri M, Mayer EA, et al. AGA technical review on irritable bowel syndrome. Gastroenterology 2002;123(6):2108–31.
13. Spiller R. Role of motility in chronic diarrhoea. Neurogastroenterol Motil 2006; 18(12):1045–55.
14. Gareau MG, Silva MA, Perdue MH. Pathophysiological mechanisms of stress-induced intestinal damage. Curr Mol Med 2008;8(4):274–81.
15. Santos J, Alonso C, Vicario M, et al. Neuropharmacology of stress-induced mucosal inflammation: implications for inflammatory bowel disease and irritable bowel syndrome. Curr Mol Med 2008;8(4):258–73.
16. Ohman L, Simren M. Pathogenesis of IBS: role of inflammation, immunity and neuroimmune interactions. Nat Rev Gastroenterol Hepatol 2010;7(3):163–73.
17. Sarna SK. Colonic motor activity. Surg Clin North Am 1993;73(6):1201–23.
18. Sethi AK, Sarna SK. Colonic motor activity in acute colitis in conscious dogs. Gastroenterology 1991;100(4):954–63.
19. Jadcherla SR. Inflammation inhibits muscarinic signaling in in vivo canine colonic circular smooth muscle cells. Pediatr Res 2002;52(5):756–62.
20. Tams TR. Irritable bowel syndrome. In: Kirk RW, Bonagura JD, editors. Kirk's current veterinary therapy. Small animal practice. 11th edition. Philadelphia: W.B. Saunders; 1992.

21. Henroteaux M. [Results of an endoscopical study of canine colonic diseases. Predominance of idopathic colitis]. Ann Vet Med 1990;134:389–92 [in French].
22. Leib MS. Chronic colitis in dogs. In: Bonagura JD, editor. Kirk's current veterinary therapy, volume XIII. Philadelphia: W.B. Saunders Company; 2000. p. 643–8.
23. Mège C, Beaumont-Graff E, Béata C, et al. Annexe: Grilles d'évaluation. Pathologie Comportementale du Chien [Annex: evaluation grids. Behavioral pathology in dogs]. Paris: Masson-AFVAC; 2003 [in French].
24. Simpson JW. Diet and large intestinal disease in dogs and cats. J Nutr 1998; 128(Suppl 12):2717S–22S.
25. Zoran DL. Nutritional management of gastrointestinal conditions. In: Ettinger SJ, Feldman EC, editors. Textbook of veterinary internal medicine, vol. 1. St Louis (MO): Saunders Elsevier; 2010. p. 676–81.

Correlating Clinical Activity and Histopathologic Assessment of Gastrointestinal Lesion Severity: Current Challenges

Michael Willard, DVM, MS[a],*, Joanne Mansell, DVM, MS[b]

KEYWORDS

• Gastrointestinal • Histopathology • Clinical • Grading

Inflammatory bowel disease (IBD) was first reported in dogs and cats approximately 20 years ago. Since that time, it has become a fashionable and trendy diagnosis, and simultaneously there has been an ever-increasing tendency to rely upon histopathology of the intestine for diagnosis and therapy for patients with chronic disorders. This tendency is especially true for dogs with diarrhea and cats with either vomiting or diarrhea.

Historically, veterinarians used to biopsy the gastrointestinal tract infrequently because it generally required exploratory laparotomy to obtain the tissue samples, and biopsy was usually not seriously considered until patients were critically ill and had failed most therapeutic trials. However, with the advent of endoscopy and its widespread availability, intestinal biopsies suddenly became available and clients became more willing to allow the veterinarian to biopsy their pets. Initially there was what can almost be described as euphoria as veterinarians discovered that IBD could cause so many different clinical signs (diarrhea, mucoid stools, hematochezia, vomiting, anorexia, weight loss, abdominal pain, flatulence, borborygmus, lethargy).

This work was self funded.

The authors have nothing to disclose.

[a] Department of Small Animal Clinical Sciences, College of Veterinary Medicine, TAMU-4474, Texas A&M University, College Station, TX 77843-4474, USA

[b] Department of Pathobiology, College of Veterinary Medicine, 4467, Texas A&M University, College Station, TX 77843-4467, USA

* Corresponding author.

E-mail address: mwillard@cvm.tamu.edu

Vet Clin Small Anim 41 (2011) 457–463

doi:10.1016/j.cvsm.2011.01.005

0195-5616/11/$ – see front matter © 2011 Elsevier Inc. All rights reserved.

However, for some clinicians, this euphoria slowly turned into suspicion as they became increasingly concerned that essentially every patient that was biopsied received a histopathologic diagnosis of lymphoplasmacytic or eosinophilic enteritis. A few veterinarians noted that the word *normal* almost never appeared on intestinal histopathology reports, even when patients that were expected to have normal intestinal tissue (ie, patients with esophageal or foreign bodies) were biopsied. Thus, seeds of skepticism were sown in at least a few minds. To compound this problem, the observation that most patients were treated with the same drugs almost regardless of the histologic findings fueled the suspicion that intestinal biopsies were not as useful as initially thought.

Perhaps the first solid evidence that a problem existed in correlating histopathologic findings with clinical disease was the finding that the same histopathology slide of an intestinal biopsy could be interpreted differently by multiple pathologists.[1] Although histopathology is not an exact science and some variability is expected, the degree of disagreement between pathologists on some slides was substantial enough to cause concern among internists. Although some took this to be an indictment of pathologists, it was noted that the quality of the intestinal samples submitted to different laboratories, and by implication from veterinarians with different levels of training, also varied substantially.[2] A substantial number of biopsies from some laboratories were described as being so inadequate as to make it difficult at best, and impossible at worst, for a pathologist to be able to interpret the histopathologic lesions and render an accurate diagnosis (**Fig. 1**). Hence, the blame for the problems of

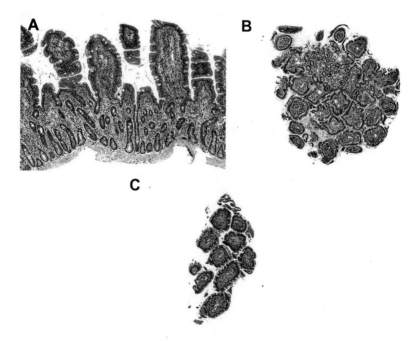

Fig. 1. (*A*) An adequate biopsy from canine duodenum. Full-thickness villus and lamina propria. (*B*) A marginal biopsy from canine duodenum. Villus tips and partial thickness of lamina propria. (*C*) An inadequate biopsy from canine duodenum. Only villus tips are present.

diagnosis needed to be shared between clinicians and pathologists because there appeared to be responsibility on both sides.

Another problem was that numerous systems or grading schemes for interpretation of intestinal histopathology were being reported (Jergens,[3–6] Hart,[7] Yamasaki,[8] Stonehewer,[9] Baez,[10] German,[11,12] Kull,[13] Zentek,[14] Waly,[15] Peters,[16] Wiinberg,[17] Garcia-Sancho,[18] Allenspach[19]). These grading schemes were generally not based upon outcome or prognosis, but an attempt to standardize grading. Unfortunately, no particular grading scheme gained widespread acceptance, adding to the difficulty when trying to compare results between different laboratories.

In view of the lack of consistency between pathologists when describing the histopathologic changes on a slide, the lack of agreement on a grading scheme for histologic evaluation of intestinal tissue, and the questionable quality of many tissue samples presented to the pathologist, it is not surprising that there was difficulty in correlating histopathologic findings with clinical findings.

Several studies from different institutions attempted to correlate histopathologic changes with clinical severity, clinical signs, or response to therapy. Studies by Allenspach,[19] Craven,[20] Garcia-Sancho,[18] McCann,[21] and Schreiner[22] totaled more than 150 dogs, and in no case was there a significant association between intestinal histopathology findings and clinical signs, serum biomarkers, or response to treatment. Jergens and coworkers[6] developed a canine inflammatory bowel disease activity index and found an association between histopathology and severity (as detected by the index), but other investigators could not repeat this finding, although they did find an association between the histopathologic score and the subjective assessment of the severity of the clinical illness.[23] One study found that clinically ill dogs had more histologic lesions than clinically normal control dogs,[14] but another group could not correlate clinical severity with numbers of plasma cells.[9] One study of cats showed that clinically ill cats with severe mucosal histologic changes were more likely to have worse clinical signs.[24]

In addition to the lack of undisputed or clear correlation between histopathologic diagnosis and clinical signs, investigators were unable to find improvement in the histopathology of intestinal samples when pretreatment samples were compared with post-treatment samples. In one study of nonhypoproteinemic dogs that responded clinically to treatment, no detectable difference was found between pretreatment and post-treatment histopathologic findings.[18] In addition, Allenspach and coworkers[19] did not find a difference in the numbers of intestinal mucosal plasma cells in dogs that were responding to treatment with cyclosporine. One possible interpretation of these findings is that histology does not reflect clinical signs; whereas, another possibility is that the current state of the art of evaluation of intestinal biopsies is deficient and therefore responsible.

If the latter is the reason, then it may be caused by (1) the quality of the tissue samples being submitted to the laboratory, either because the endoscopist is sampling the wrong area or the samples are from the correct area but are poor quality; (2) the quality of sample processing by the laboratory; or (3) the ability of the pathologist to interpret/describe the histopathologic lesions.

In an attempt to rectify some of these problems, the World Small Animal Veterinary Association sponsored a gastrointestinal standardization group that produced a pictorial/written template of histologic changes in the canine and feline stomach, duodenum, and colon.[25] It was hoped that an international effort would be more likely to engender widespread acceptance and use. The question then became whether use of such a template can solve some of the problems, especially the lack of consistency between pathologists. Willard and coworkers[26] found that simply using the template was not a panacea for the problems previously described. There was still a major lack of agreement between pathologists looking at the same histologic slide. This finding is similar to findings by another group of investigators looking at gastric samples.[17] Therefore, it appears that simply producing a template will not necessarily resolve problems of consistency, which is not to say that such a standard is not useful. It may be that there are additional factors that confuse the issue.

It is now known that the quality of the tissue samples submitted to the laboratory significantly impacts the ability to find specific lesions. Willard and coworkers[27] have shown that as the quality of the tissue samples improve (ie, going from inadequate samples containing just villus fragments to adequate samples including the entire thickness of the intestinal mucosa), the number of samples required to find lesions (ie, villus atrophy, lymphangiectasia, crypt abscesses, cellular infiltrates) significantly decreases. So many tissue samples are required to reliably find these lesions when the quality is inadequate that it is highly unlikely that an endoscopist would take a sufficient number of samples to find them. Not finding lesions because of poor quality of tissue samples would seriously impact the ability to correlate histology and clinical signs/outcome.

Recently, it was determined that tissue processing at the histopathology laboratory can significantly affect the ability to find changes, specifically eosinophilic and neutrophilic infiltrates.[26] Although it would seem that identification of eosinophils and neutrophils (which is fundamental in the training of pathologists) would be easy, variability in the application of hematoxylin and eosin staining by different laboratories was found to obscure their identification. It seems intuitively obvious that incorrectly identifying these cells could prevent finding some associations that might exist.

Despite these problems, some progress is occurring. A recent study was able to correlate the histologic finding of lymphangiectasia with hypoalbuminemia by 3 out of 4 pathologists.[26] Lymphangiectasia is expected to be correlated with hypoalbuminemia clinically, and being able to find this association is encouraging. Whether or not others will be able to confirm these findings remains to be seen.

Additional evidence of progress is the recent interest in ileal biopsies. Until recently, duodenal biopsies were the primary tissue sample taken from patients with suspected small bowel disease. Casamian-Sorrosal and others[28] compared the histology of duodenal and ileal biopsies and found that ileal biopsies often revealed lesions not found in duodenal samples. Before that, Evans and coworkers[29] found that lymphoma was much more likely to be found in the feline ileum than the feline duodenum. Failure to biopsy the right area of the intestines might play a role in why histopathology historically has not correlated with clinical signs.

One remaining question is whether rectifying the previously mentioned problems will allow correlation between clinical signs and histopathology. However, there is perhaps an even more important question, namely when should the gastrointestinal tract be biopsied?[30] Anecdotally, therapeutic trials (eg, dietary trials, antibiotic trials, anthelminthic trials, probiotic trials) are becoming more accepted by specialists. If patients that respond to these therapeutic trials are removed from the pool of animals that are biopsied, then it may be that we will be left with a group of patients in which histopathology is more appropriate, more helpful, and more predictive. Furthermore, it is important that clinicians have a realistic expectation of what information can be expected from gastrointestinal biopsies. Currently, we are not at the stage of reliably being able to correlate clinical activity and histopathologic diagnosis, especially in the diagnosis of IBD. At this time, it seems reasonable to expect to be able to use histopathology to differentiate certain gastrointestinal diseases (ie, mycotic enteritis from lymphoma or IBD, moderate IBD from lymphoma, eosinophilic enteritis from lymphoma). However, currently it does not appear realistic to expect to be able to accurately assess the severity of IBD or what therapies patients with IBD will respond best to based on histopathology. It should be understood by clinicians that differentiating between severe IBD and small cell lymphoma in cats may be difficult and of questionable usefulness.

Reaching a final diagnosis by gastrointestinal biopsy requires cooperation between clinician, pathologist, and laboratory. The studies cited earlier show that pathologists may only be able to accurately interpret gastrointestinal biopsies if they are of good quality and if the laboratory is accustomed to handling and staining these biopsies. What is clear is that (1) it is not appropriate to routinely biopsy all dogs and cats with chronic gastrointestinal disease, (2) adequate numbers of high-quality tissue samples appear to be necessary in order for the clinician to have confidence in the histopathology results, (3) processing at the laboratory may influence diagnosis, and (4) interpretation of gastrointestinal samples may require specialized training of the pathologist. The bottom line is that casually submitting tissues to the histopathology laboratory is not a panacea for diagnosing or prognosing patients with gastrointestinal disease.

REFERENCES

1. Willard MD, Jergens AE, Duncan RB, et al. Interobserver variation among histopathologic evaluations of intestinal tissues from dogs and cats. J Am Vet Med Assoc 2002;220:1177–82.
2. Willard MD, Lovering SL, Cohen ND, et al. Quality of tissue specimens obtained endoscopically from the duodenum of dogs and cats. J Am Vet Med Assoc 2001; 219:474–9.
3. Jergens AE, Moore FM, Haynes JS, et al. Idiopathic inflammatory bowel disease in dogs and cats: 84 cases (1987–1990). J Am Vet Med Assoc 1992;201(10): 1603–8.
4. Jergens AE, Moore FM, Kaiser MS, et al. Morphometric evaluation of Immunoglobulin A containing and Immunoglobulin G containing cells and T cells in duodenal mucosa from healthy dogs and from dogs with inflammatory bowel disease or nonspecific gastroenteritis. Am J Vet Res 1996;57(5):697–704.
5. Jergens AE, Gamet Y, Moore FM, et al. Colonic lymphocyte and plasma cell populations in dogs with lymphocytic-plasmocytic colitis. Am J Vet Res 1999;60: 515–20.
6. Jergens AE, Schreiner CA, Frank DE, et al. A scoring index for disease activity in canine inflammatory bowel disease. J Vet Intern Med 2003;17:291–7.
7. Hart JR, Shaker E, Patnaik AK, et al. Lymphocytic-plasmacytic enterocolitis in cats: 60 cases (1988–1990). J Am Anim Hosp Assoc 1994;30:505–14.
8. Yamasaki K, Suematsu H, Takahashi T. Comparison of gastric and duodenal lesions in dogs and cats with and without lymphocytic plasmacytic enteritis. J Am Vet Med Assoc 1996;209(1):95–7.
9. Stonehewer J, Simpson JW, Else RW, et al. Evaluation of B and T lymphocytes and plasma cells in colonic mucosa from healthy dogs and from dogs with inflammatory bowel disease. Res Vet Sci 1998;65:59–63.
10. Baez JL, Hendrick MJ, Walker LM, et al. Radiographic, ultrasonographic, and endoscopic findings in cats with inflammatory bowel disease of the stomach and small intestine: 33 cases (1990–1997). J Am Vet Med Assoc 1999;215: 349–54.

11. German AJ, Helps CR, Hall EJ, et al. Cytokine mRNA expression in mucosal biopsies from German Shepherd dogs with small intestinal enteropathies. Dig Dis Sci 2000;45:7–17.

12. German AJ, Hall EJ, Day MJ. Immune cell populations within the duodenal mucosa of dogs with enteropathies. J Vet Intern Med 2001;15:14–25.

13. Kull PA, Hess RS, Craig LE, et al. Clinical, clinicopathologic, radiographic, and ultrasonographic characteristics of intestinal lymphangiectasia in dogs: 17 cases (1996-1998). J Am Vet Med Assoc 2001;219:197–202.

14. Zentek J, Hall E, German A, et al. Morphology and Immunopathology of the small and large intestine in dogs with nonspecific dietary sensitivity. J Nutr 2002;132: 1652S–4S.

15. Waly NE, Stokes CR, Gruffydd-Jones TJ, et al. Immune cell populations in the duodenal mucosa of cats with inflammatory bowel disease. J Vet Intern Med 2004;18:816–25.

16. Peters I, Helps C, Calvert E, et al. Measurement of messenger RNA encoding the alpha-chain, polymeric immunoglobulin receptor, and J-chain in duodenal mucosa from dogs with and without chronic diarrhea by use of quantitative real-time reverse transcription-polymerase chain reaction assays. Am J Vet Res 2005;66:11–6.

17. Wiinberg B, Spohr A, Dietz H, et al. Quantitative analysis of inflammatory and immune responses in dogs with gastritis and their relationship to Helicobacter spp. infection. J Vet Intern Med 2005;19:4–14.

18. Garcia-Sancho M, Rodriguez-Franco F, Sainz A, et al. Evaluation of clinical, macroscopic, and histopathologic response to treatment in nonhypoproteinemic dogs with lymphocytic-plasmacytic enteritis. J Vet Intern Med 2007;21:11–7.

19. Allenspach K, Wieland B, Grone A, et al. Chronic enteropathies in dogs: evaluation of risk factors for negative outcome. J Vet Intern Med 2007;21:700–8.

20. Craven M, Simpson J, Ridyard A, et al. Canine inflammatory bowel disease: retrospective analysis of diagnosis and outcome in 80 cases (1995-2002). J Small Anim Pract 2004;45:336–42.

21. McCann T, Ridyard A, Else R, et al. Evaluation of disease activity markers in dogs with idiopathic inflammatory bowel disease. J Small Anim Pract 2007;48:620–5.

22. Schreiner N, Gaschen F, Grone A, et al. Clinical signs, histology and CD-3 positive cells before and after treatment of dogs with chronic enteropathies. J Vet Intern Med 2008;22:1079–83.

23. Münster M, Hörauf A, Bilzer T. Bestimmung des Krankheitsschweregrades und des Ergebnisses diatetischer, antibiotischer und immunsuppressiver Interventionen durch anwendung des caninen IBD Aktivitatsindex bei 21 Hunden mit chronisch entzundlicher Darmkrankheit [Assessment of disease severity and outcome of dietary, antibiotic, and immunosuppressive interventions by use of the canine IBD activity index in 21 dogs with chronic inflammatory bowel disease]. Berl Munch Tierarztl Wochenschr 2006;119:493–505 [in German].

24. Janeczko S, Atwater D, Bogel E, et al. The relationship of mucosal bacteria to duodenal histopathology cytokine mRNA and clinical disease activity in cats with inflammatory bowel disease. Vet Microbiol 2008;128:178–93.

25. Day M, Bilzer T, Mansell J, et al. Histopathologic standards for the diagnosis of gastrointestinal inflammation in endoscopic biopsy samples from the dog and cat: a report from the world small animal veterinary association. J Comp Pathol 2008;138:S1–43.

26. Willard M, Moore G, Denton B, et al. Effect of tissue processing on assessment of endoscopic intestinal biopsies in dogs and cats. J Vet Intern Med 2010;24:84–9.

27. Willard M, Mansell J, Fosgate G, et al. Effect of sample quality on the sensitivity of endoscopic biopsy for detecting gastric and duodenal lesions in dogs and cats. J Vet Intern Med 2008;22:1084–9.
28. Casamian-Sorrosal D, Willard M, Murray J, et al. Comparison of histopathologic findings in biopsies from the duodenum and ileum of dogs with enteropathy. J Vet Intern Med 2010;24:80–3.
29. Evans S, Bonczynski J, Broussard J, et al. Comparison of endoscopic and full-thickness biopsy specimens for diagnosis of inflammatory bowel disease and alimentary tract lymphoma in cats. J Am Vet Med Assoc 2006;229:1447–50.
30. Washabau R, Day M, Willard M, et al. 2009 Consensus statement: endoscopic, biopsy and histopathologic guidelines for the evaluation of gastrointestinal inflammation in companion animals. J Vet Intern Med 2010;24:10–26.

Index

Note: Page numbers of article titles are in **boldface** type.

A

Abscess(es), crypt, in dogs, treatment of, 394–395
Adherent and invasive *Escherichia coli* (AIEC), in Crohn disease, in Boxer dogs, 437–438
Adverse food reactions (AFRs)
    cutaneous, in dogs and cats, 366–368
    defined, 361
    in dogs and cats, **361–379**
        clinical signs of, 366–369
        described, 361–362
        diagnostic approach to, 370–373
            cutaneous form, 370
            GI form, 371–373
        differential diagnosis of, 369
        epidemiology of, 365–366
        pathogenesis of, 362–365
            allergens in, 363–365
            GI mucosal barrier in, 362–363
            gluten-sensitive enteropathy in, 364–365
            oral tolerance in, 363
        prognosis of, 376
        treatment of, 373–376
            client education and compliance in, 375
            dietary elimination trial in, 373–374
            dietary provocation test in, 375–376
            hydrolyzed diets in, 374–375
            novel protein diets in, 374
            oral medications in, 375
AFRs. See *Adverse food reactions (AFRs)*.
AIEC. See *Adherent and invasive Escherichia coli (AIEC)*.
Alimentary lymphoma
    in cats, **419–432**
        causes of, 419
        described, 419
        diagnosis of, 421–425
        pathogenesis of, 419
        patient history in, 420–421
        physical examination of, 420–421
        prognosis of, 425–429
        signalment of, 420–421
        treatment of, 425–429
    in dogs, **430**
Allergen(s), in pathogenesis of AFRs in dogs and cats, 363–365

Vet Clin Small Anim 41 (2011) 465–475
doi:10.1016/S0195-5616(11)00050-7
0195-5616/11/$ – see front matter © 2011 Elsevier Inc. All rights reserved.

vetsmall.theclinics.com

Moving?

Make sure your subscription moves with you!

To notify us of your new address, find your **Clinics Account Number** (located on your mailing label above your name), and contact customer service at:

Email: **journalscustomerservice-usa@elsevier.com**

800-654-2452 (subscribers in the U.S. & Canada)
314-447-8871 (subscribers outside of the U.S. & Canada)

Fax number: **314-447-8029**

Elsevier Health Sciences Division
Subscription Customer Service
3251 Riverport Lane
Maryland Heights, MO 63043

*To ensure uninterrupted delivery of your subscription, please notify us at least 4 weeks in advance of move.

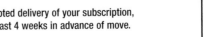